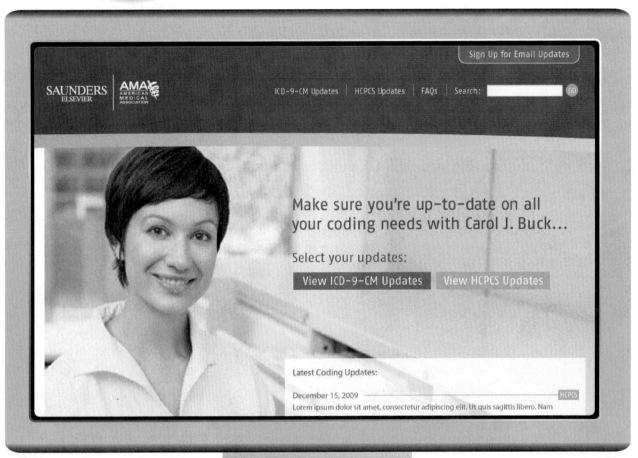

Standard Edition

2013
HCPCS Level II

Standard Edition

2013
HCPCS Level II

Carol J. Buck
MS, CPC, CPC-H, CCS-P

Former Program Director, Medical Secretary Programs
Northwest Technical College, East Grand Forks, Minnesota

AMERICAN MEDICAL
ASSOCIATION

3251 Riverport Lane
St. Louis, Missouri 63043

2013 HCPCS LEVEL II, STANDARD EDITION

ISBN: 978-1-4557-4528-9
ISSN: 2211-9485

Notices

Knowledge and best practice in this field are constantly changing. As new research and experience broaden our understanding, changes in research methods, professional practices, or medical treatment may become necessary.

Practitioners and researchers must always rely on their own experience and knowledge in evaluating and using any information, methods, compounds, or experiments described herein. In using such information or methods they should be mindful of their own safety and the safety of others, including parties for whom they have a professional responsibility.

With respect to any drug or pharmaceutical products identified, readers are advised to check the most current information provided (i) on procedures featured or (ii) by the manufacturer of each product to be administered, to verify the recommended dose or formula, the method and duration of administration, and contraindications. It is the responsibility of practitioners, relying on their own experience and knowledge of their patients, to make diagnoses, to determine dosages and the best treatment for each individual patient, and to take all appropriate safety precautions.

To the fullest extent of the law, neither the Publisher nor the authors, contributors, or editors, assume any liability for any injury and/or damage to persons or property as a matter of products liability, negligence or otherwise, or from any use or operation of any methods, products, instructions, or ideas contained in the material herein.

ISBN: 978-1-4557-4528-9

Content Strategy Director: Jeanne Olson
Senior Content Development Specialist: Jenna Price
Publishing Services Manager: Pat Joiner-Myers
Senior Designer: Amy Buxton

Printed in the United States of America

Last digit is the print number: 9   8   7   6   5   4   3   2   1

Working together to grow
libraries in developing countries

www.elsevier.com | www.bookaid.org | www.sabre.org

ELSEVIER   BOOK AID International   Sabre Foundation

TECHNICAL COLLABORATORS

Heidi Aguilar
Lead EHR Technical Collaborator
Grand Forks, North Dakota

Sheri Poe Bernard, CPC, CPC-H, CPC-I
Coding Education Specialist
Salt Lake City, Utah

Jacqueline Klitz Grass, MA, CPC
Coding Specialist
Grand Forks, North Dakota

Nancy Maguire, ACS, CRT, PCS, FCS, HCS-D, APC, AFC
Physician Consultant for Auditing and Education
Winchester, Virginia

CONTENTS

Updates will be posted on http://codingupdates.com when available.

Check the Centers for Medicare and Medicaid Services (http://www.cms.gov/Manuals/IOM/list.asp) website and http://codingupdates.com for IOMs.

Medical coding has long been a part of the health care profession. Through the years medical coding systems have become more complex and extensive. Today, medical coding is an intricate and immense process that is present in every health care setting. The increased use of electronic submissions for health care services only increases the need for coders who understand the coding process.

2013 HCPCS Level II was developed to help meet the needs of today's coder.

All material adheres to the latest government versions available at the time of printing.

Annotated

Throughout this text, revisions and additions are indicated by the following symbols:

◀ **New:** Additions to the previous edition are indicated by the color triangle.

← **Revised:** Revisions within the line or code from the previous edition are indicated by the color arrow.

✔ **Reinstated** indicates a code that was previously deleted and has now been reactivated.

✖ ~~deleted~~ words have been removed from this year's edition.

HCPCS Symbols

☼ **Special coverage instructions** apply to these codes. Usually these special coverage instructions are included in the Internet Only Manuals (IOM) select references at http:codingupdates.com.

◆ **Not covered or valid by Medicare** is indicated by the diamond. Usually the reason for the exclusion is included in the Internet Only Manuals (IOM) select references at http:codingupdates.com.

✳ **Carrier discretion** is an indication that you must contact the individual third-party payers to find out the coverage available for codes identified by this symbol.

NDC Drugs approved for Medicare Part B are listed as NDC (National Drug Code). All other FDA-approved drugs are listed as Other.

Color and/or *italic* typeface within the Table of Drugs and tabular section is added by the publisher and does not appear in the official code set. Information supplementing the official HCPCS Index produced by CMS is *italicized*.

SYMBOLS AND CONVENTIONS

HCPCS Symbols

Special coverage instructions apply to these codes. Usually these instructions are included in the Internet Only Manuals (IOM) select references located at http:codingupdates.com.

⊛ **L3540** Miscellaneous shoe additions, sole, full

IOM: 100-2, 15, 290

The Internet Only Manuals (IOM) give instructions regarding use of the code. IOM select references are located at http:codingupdates.com.

Not covered or valid by Medicare is indicated by the diamond. Usually the reason for the exclusion is included in the IOM references located at http:codingupdates.com.

◆ **A6533** Gradient compression stocking, thigh length, 18–30 mm Hg, each

IOM: 100-02, 15, 130; 100-03, 4, 280.1

Carrier discretion is an indication that you must contact the individual third-party payers for the coverage for these codes.

✳ **A6154** Wound pouch, each

Codes shown are for illustration purposes only and may not be current codes.

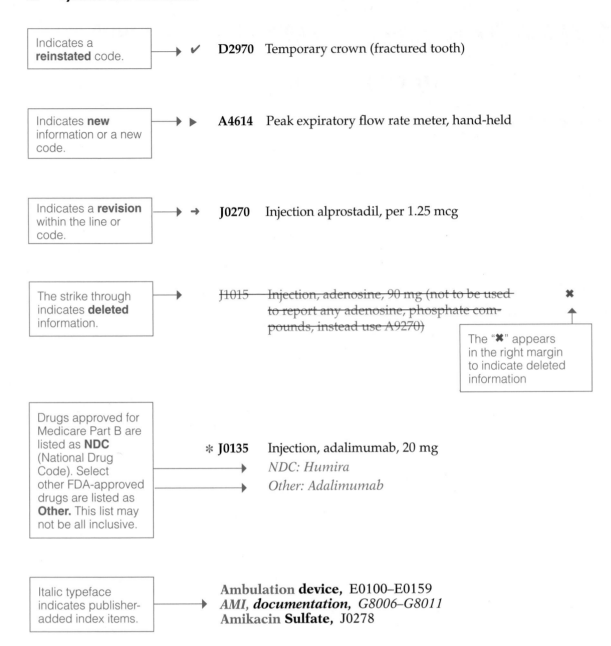

Indicates a **reinstated** code.

✔ **D2970** Temporary crown (fractured tooth)

Indicates **new** information or a new code.

▶ **A4614** Peak expiratory flow rate meter, hand-held

Indicates a **revision** within the line or code.

→ **J0270** Injection alprostadil, per 1.25 mcg

The strike through indicates **deleted** information.

▶ ~~J1015~~ ~~Injection, adenosine, 90 mg (not to be used to report any adenosine, phosphate compounds, instead use A9270)~~ ✖

The "✖" appears in the right margin to indicate deleted information

Drugs approved for Medicare Part B are listed as **NDC** (National Drug Code). Select other FDA-approved drugs are listed as **Other.** This list may not be all inclusive.

✳ **J0135** Injection, adalimumab, 20 mg
NDC: Humira
Other: Adalimumab

Italic typeface indicates publisher-added index items.

Ambulation device, E0100–E0159
AMI, documentation, G8006–G8011
Amikacin Sulfate, J0278

Codes shown are for illustration purposes only and may not be current codes.

2013 HCPCS UPDATES

2013 HCPCS New/Revised/Deleted Codes and Modifiers

HCPCS quarterly updates are posted on the companion website (http://www.codingupdates.com) when available.

NEW CODES/MODIFIERS

CH	C9600	G0457	G8922	G8939	G8956	G8973	G8990	G9157	G9173	J9002	S0354
CI	C9601	G0458	G8923	G8940	G8957	G8974	G8991	G9158	G9174	J9019	S0596
CJ	C9602	G8907	G8924	G8941	G8958	G8975	G8992	G9159	G9175	J9042	S1090
CK	C9603	G8908	G8925	G8942	G8959	G8976	G8993	G9160	G9176	L5859	S3721
CL	C9604	G8909	G8926	G8943	G8960	G8977	G8994	G9161	G9186	L7902	S8930
CM	C9605	G8910	G8927	G8944	G8961	G8978	G8995	G9162	J0178	L8605	S9110
CN	C9606	G8911	G8928	G8945	G8962	G8979	G8996	G9163	J0485	Q2034	V5281
LM	C9607	G8912	G8929	G8946	G8963	G8980	G8997	G9164	J0716	Q2049	V5282
RI	C9608	G8913	G8930	G8947	G8964	G8981	G8998	G9165	J0890	Q4131	V5283
A4435	C9733	G8914	G8931	G8948	G8965	G8982	G8999	G9166	J1050	Q4132	V5284
A9586	E0670	G8915	G8932	G8949	G8966	G8983	G9148	G9167	J1741	Q4133	V5285
C9290	E2378	G8916	G8933	G8950	G8967	G8984	G9149	G9168	J1744	Q4134	V5286
C9292	G0452	G8917	G8934	G8951	G8968	G8985	G9150	G9169	J2212	Q4135	V5287
C9293	G0453	G8918	G8935	G8952	G8969	G8986	G9151	G9170	J7178	Q4136	V5288
C9294	G0454	G8919	G8936	G8953	G8970	G8987	G9152	G9171	J7315	Q9969	V5289
C9295	G0455	G8920	G8937	G8954	G8971	G8988	G9153	G9172	J7527	S0353	V5290
C9296	G0456	G8921	G8938	G8955	G8972	G8989					

REVISED CODES/MODIFIERS

Change in Description	G8475	G8610	G8735	G8844	L8002	Q0486
CS	G8478	G8613	G8740	G8849	Q4119	Q0487
GS	G8483	G8616	G8751	G8850	Q4126	Q0488
A6021	G8484	G8619	G8756	G8854	Q4128	Q0489
A6022	G8485	G8622	G8757	G8855	V5267	Q0490
A6023	G8490	G8625	G8758	G8858		Q0491
C9724	G8494	G8632	G8759	G8863	Change in	Q0492
E0300	G8495	G8635	G8763	G8867	Administration	Q0493
E1020	G8499	G8650	G8769	G8873	SC	Q0494
E2368	G8509	G8654	G8773	G8876	A4619	Q0495
E2369	G8510	G8658	G8776	G8877	G0433	Q0496
E2370	G8511	G8662	G8779	G8880	G0434	Q0497
G0416	G8532	G8666	G8782	G8887	G9143	Q0498
G0446	G8536	G8670	G8783	G8889	L8680	Q0499
G0909	G8539	G8674	G8784	G8894	L8682	Q0500
G0921	G8541	G8682	G8785	G8895	L8683	Q0501
G0922	G8542	G8683	G8796	G8896	L8684	Q0502
G8400	G8543	G8685	G8801	G8897	L8685	Q0503
G8417	G8553	G8697	G8807	G8898	L8686	Q0504
G8418	G8558	G8698	G8808	G8899	L8687	Q0505
G8419	G8563	G8707	G8810	G8900	L8688	Q0506
G8427	G8568	G8714	G8811	G8904	Q0478	
G8428	G8577	G8717	G8812	J1561	Q0479	Change in Short Description
G8430	G8578	G8720	G8815	J1569	Q0480	J9208
G8431	G8592	G8722	G8817	J9020	Q0481	
G8432	G8594	G8724	G8833	J9280	Q0482	Miscellaneous Change
G8433	G8599	G8726	G8838	L5972	Q0483	J7665
G8450	G8602	G8728	G8841	L8000	Q0484	
G8452	G8604	G8732	G8843	L8001	Q0485	
	G8607	G8733				

DELETED CODES/MODIFIERS

DA	G0290	G8471	G8716	G8803	G8828	G8901	J9001	S3822	S3843
V8	G0291	G8472	G8727	G8805	G8829	G9141	K0741	S3823	S3847
V9	G0911	G8524	G8750	G8819	G8830	G9142	K0742	S3828	S3848
C9279	G0912	G8525	G8760	G8820	G8831	J1051	S3711	S3829	S3851
C9286	G8447	G8526	G8786	G8821	G8832	J1055	S3713	S3830	S3860
C9287	G8448	G8546	G8787	G8822	G8836	J1056	S3818	S3831	S3862
C9366	G8468	G8550	G8788	G8823	G8837	J1680	S3819	S3835	S8049
C9716	G8469	G8695	G8789	G8824	G8847	J8561	S3820	S3837	S9109
C9732	G8470	G8715	G8802						

ADDED AND DELETED DURING 2012

C9288	C9289	C9291	C9368	C9369	Q2045	Q2046	Q2047	Q2048

HCPCS 2013 INDEX

A

Abatacept, J0129
Abciximab, J0130
Abdomen
    dressing holder/binder, A4462
    pad, low profile, L1270
Abduction control, each, L2624
Abduction restrainer, A4566
Abduction rotation bar, foot, L3140–L3170
AbobotulinumtypeA, J0586
Absorption dressing, A6251–A6256
Access, site, occlusive, device, G0269
Access system, A4301
Accessories
    ambulation devices, E0153–E0159
    artificial kidney and machine (*see also* ESRD),
        E1510–E1699
    beds, E0271–E0280, E0300–E0326
    wheelchairs, E0950–E1030, E1050–E1298,
        E2201–E2295, E2300–E2399, K0001–K0109
ACE/ARB therapy, G8463–G8475
Acetaminophen, J0131
Acetazolamide sodium, J1120
Acetylcysteine
    inhalation solution, J7604, J7608
    injection, J0132
Activity, therapy, G0176
Acyclovir, J0133
Adalimumab, J0135
Adenosine, J0150, J0152
Adhesive, A4364
    bandage, A6413
    disc or foam pad, A5126
    remover, A4455, A4456
    support, breast prosthesis, A4280
    wound, closure, G0168
Administration, Part D
    supply, tositumomab, G3001
    vaccine, hepatitis B, G0010
    vaccine, influenza, G0008
    vaccine, pneumococcal, G0009
Admission, observation, G0379
Administrative, Miscellaneous and Investiga-
    tional, A9000–A9999
Adrenalin, J0171
*Advanced life support, A0390, A0426, A0427,
    A0433*
Aerosol
    compressor, E0572
    compressor filter, K0178–K0179
    mask, K0180
Aflibercept, J0178◄
AFO, E1815, E1830, L1900–L1990, L4392, L4396
Agalsidase beta, J0180
Aggrastat, J3245
A-hydroCort, J1710

Aide, home, health, G0156, S9122, T1021
    bath/toilet, E0160–E0162, E0235, E0240–E0249
    services, G0151–G0156, G0179–G0181, S5180,
        S5181, S9122, T1021, T1022
Air bubble detector, dialysis, E1530
Air fluidized bed, E0194
Air pressure pad/mattress, E0186, E0197
Air travel and nonemergency transportation,
    A0140
Alarm
    not otherwise classified, A9280
    pressure, dialysis, E1540
Alatrofloxacin mesylate, J0200
Albumin, human, P9041, P9042
Albuterol
    all formulations, inhalation solution, concen-
        trated, J7610, J7611
    all formulations, inhalation solution, unit
        dose, J7609, J7613
    all formulations, inhalation solution, J7620
Alcohol/substance, assessment, G0396, G0397,
    H0001, H0003, H0049
Alcohol, A4244
Alcohol wipes, A4245
Aldesleukin (IL2), J9015
Alefacept, J0215
Alemtuzumab, J9010
Alert device, A9280
Alginate dressing, A6196–A6199
Alglucerase, J0205
Alglucosidase, J0220
Alglucosidase alfa, J0221
Alphanate, J7186
Alpha-1-proteinase inhibitor, human, J0256, J0257
Alprostadil
    injection, J0270
    urethral supposity, J0275
ALS mileage, A0390
Alteplase recombinant, J2997
Alternating pressure mattress/pad, A4640, E0180,
    E0181, E0277
Ambulance, A0021–A0999
    air, A0430, A0431, A0435, A0436
    disposable supplies, A0382–A0398
    oxygen, A0422
Ambulation device, E0100–E0159
Amikacin Sulfate, J0278
Aminolevulinate, J7309
Aminolevulinic acid HCl, J7308
Aminophylline, J0280
Amiodarone HCl, J0282
Amitriptyline HCl, J1320
Ammonia N-13, A9526
Ammonia test paper, A4774
Amniotic membrane, V2790
Amobarbital, J0300
Amphotericin B, J0285
    Lipid Complex, J0287–J0289

◄ New   ← Revised   ✔ Reinstated   ~~deleted~~ Deleted

Ampicillin
  sodium, J0290
  sodium/sulbactam sodium, J0295
Amputee
  adapter, wheelchair, E0959
  prosthesis, L5000–L7510, L7520, L7900,
    L8400–L8465
  stump sock, L8470–L8485
  wheelchair, E1170–E1190, E1200, K0100
Amygdalin, J3570
Anadulafungin, J0348
Analysis
  semen, G0027
*Angiography, **iliac, artery,** G0278*
  non-ophthalmic fluorescent vascular, C9733
  reconstruction, G0288
  renal, artery, G0275
Anistreplase, J0350
Ankle **splint, recumbent,** K0126–K0130
Ankle-foot **orthosis (AFO),** L1900–L1990,
    L2106–L2116, L4361, L4392, L4396
Anterior-posterior-lateral **orthosis,** L0700, L0710
Antibiotic, G8708–G8712
*Antidepressant, **documentation,** G8126–G8128*
Anti-emetic, **oral,** Q0163–Q0181, J8498, J8597
Anti-hemophilic **factor (Factor VIII),** J7190–J7192
Anti-inhibitors, **per I.U.,** J7198
*Antimicrobial, **prophylaxis, documentation,** G8201*
Anti-neoplastic **drug, NOC,** J9999
Antithrombin **III,** J7197
Antithrombin **recombinant,** J7196
Apomorphine, J0364
Appliance
  cleaner, A5131
  pneumatic, E0655–E0673
*Application, **heat, cold,** E0200–E0239*
Aprotinin, J0365
Aqueous
  shunt, L8612
  sterile, J7051
*ARB/ACE **therapy,** G8468–G8475*
Arbutamine **HCl,** J0395
Arch **support,** L3040–L3100
  Intralesional, J3302
Arformoterol, J7605
Aripiprazole, J0400
Arm, **wheelchair,** E0973
Arsenic **trioxide,** J9017
Artificial
  Cornea, L8609
  kidney machines and accessories (*see also* Dialysis),
    E1510–E1699
  larynx, L8500
  saliva, A9155
*Arthrography, **injection, sacroiliac, joint,** G0259,*
    G0260
*Arthroscopy, **knee, surgical,** G0289, S2112, S2300*
Asparaginase, J9019–J9020◄

*Aspiration, **bone marrow,** G0364*
*Aspirator, **VABRA,** A4480*
Assessment
  alcohol/substance, G0396, G0397, H0001, H0003,
    H0049
  audiologic, V5008–V5020
  cardiac output, M0302
  speech, V5362–V5364
Assistive listening devices and accessories,
    V5281–V5290◄
Astramorph, J2275
Atherectomy, PTCA C9602, C9603
Atropine
  inhalation solution, concentrated, J7635
  inhalation solution, unit dose, J7636
Atropine **sulfate,** J0461
*Attachment, **walker,** E0154–E0159*
Audiologic **assessment,** V5008–V5020
Auditory **osseointegrated device, L8690–L8693**
Aurothioglucose, J2910
Azacitidine, J9025
Azathioprine, J7500, J7501
Azithromycin **injection,** J0456

B

Back **supports,** L0621–L0861, L0960
Baclofen, J0475, J0476
Bacterial **sensitivity study,** P7001
Bag
  drainage, A4357
  enema, A4458
  irrigation supply, A4398
  urinary, A4358, A5112
Basiliximab, J0480
*Bath, **aid,** E0160–E0162, E0235, E0240–E0249*
Bathtub
  chair, E0240
  stool or bench, E0245, E0247–E0248
  transfer rail, E0246
  wall rail, E0241, E0242
Battery, **L7360, L7364–L7368**
  charger, E1066, L7362, L7366
  replacement for blood glucose monitor,
    A4233–A4234
  replacement for cochlear implant device,
    L8623–L8624
  replacement for TENS, A4630
  ventilator, A4611–A4613
BCG **live, intravesical,** J9031
Beclomethasone **inhalation solution,** J7622
Bed
  accessories, E0271–E0280, E0300–E0326
  air fluidized, E0194
  cradle, any type, E0280
  drainage bag, bottle, A4357, A5102
  hospital, E0250–E0270, E0300–E0329

◄ New   ← Revised   ✔ Reinstated   ~~deleted~~ Deleted

Bed *(Continued)*
  pan, E0275, E0276
  rail, E0305, E0310
  safety enclosure frame/canopy, E0316
Behavioral, **health, treatment services, H0002–H2037**
Belatacept, J0485 ◀
Belimumab, J0490
Belt
  extremity, E0945
  ostomy, A4367
  pelvic, E0944
  safety, K0031
  wheelchair, E0978, E0979
Bench, bathtub *(see also* **Bathtub),** E0245
Bendamustine HCl, J9033
Benesch boot, L3212–L3214
Benztropine, J0515
Betadine, A4246, A4247
Betameth, *J0702*
Betamethasone
  acetate and betamethasone sodium phosphate, J0702
  inhalation solution, J7624
Bethanechol chloride, J0520
Bevacizumab, J9035, Q2024
Bifocal, glass or plastic, V2200–V2299
Bilirubin (phototherapy) light, E0202
Binder, A4465
Biofeedback device, E0746
Bioimpedance, electrical, cardiac output, M0302
Biperiden lactate, J0190
Bitolterol mesylate, inhalation solution
  concentrated, J7628
  unit dose, J7629
Bivalirudin, J0583
Bladder calculi irrigation solution, Q2004
Bleomycin sulfate, J9040
Blood
  count, G0306, G0307, S3630
  fresh frozen plasma, P9017
  glucose monitor, E0607, E2100, E2101, *S1030, S1031*
  glucose test, A4253
  granulocytes, pheresis, P9050
  ketone test, A4252
  leak detector, dialysis, E1560
  leukocyte poor, P9016
  mucoprotein, P2038
  platelets, P9019
  platelets, irradiated, P9032
  platelets, leukocytes reduced, P9031
  platelets, leukocytes reduced, irradiated, P9033
  platelets, pheresis, P9034
  platelets, pheresis, irradiated, P9036
  platelets, pheresis, leukocytes reduced, P9035
  platelets, pheresis, leukocytes reduced, irradiated, P9037
  pressure monitor, A4660, A4663, A4670
  pump, dialysis, E1620
  red blood cells, deglycerolized, P9039

Blood *(Continued)*
  red blood cells, irradiated, P9038
  red blood cells, leukocytes reduced, P9016
  red blood cells, leukocytes reduced, irradiated, P9040
  red blood cells, washed, P9022
  strips, A4253
  supply, P9010 P9022
  testing supplies, A4770
  tubing, A4750, A4755
Blood collection devices accessory, A4257, E0620
BMI, G8417–G8422
Body jacket
  scoliosis, L1300, L1310
Body sock, L0984
Body, mass, index, G8417–G8422
Bond or adhesive, ostomy skin, A4364
Bone
  density, study, G0130
  marrow, aspiration, G0364
Boot
  pelvic, E0944
  surgical, ambulatory, L3260
Bortezomib, J9041
Brachytherapy radioelements, Q3001
  brachytherapy, LDR, prostate, G0458
Breast prosthesis, L8000–L8035, L8600
  adhesive skin support, A4280
Breast pump
  accessories, A4281–A4286
  electric, any type, E0603
  heavy duty, hospital grade, E0604
  manual, any type, E0602
Breathing circuit, A4618
Brentuximab Vedotin, J9042 ◀
Brompheniramine maleate, J0945
Budesonide inhalation solution, J7626, J7627, J7633, J7634
Bulking agent, L8604
Buprenorphine hydrochloride, J0592
Bus, nonemergency transportation, A0110
Busulfan, J0594, J8510
Butorphanol tartrate, J0595
Bypass, graft, coronary, artery
  documentation, G8160–G8163
  surgery, S2205–S2209

C

C-1 Esterase Inhibitor, J0597–J0598
Cabazitaxel, J9043
Cabergoline, oral, J8515
Caffeine citrate, J0706
CABG, documentation, G8160–G8163
Cabinet/System, ultraviolet, E0691–E0694
CAD documentation, G8160–G8163
Calcitriol, J0636
Calcitonin-salmon, J0630

◀ New   ← Revised   ✔ Reinstated   ~~deleted~~ Deleted

Calcitrol, S0169
Calcium
  disodium edetate, J0600
  gluconate, J0610
  glycerophosphate and calcium lactate, J0620
  lactate and calcium glycerophosphate, J0620
  leucovorin, J0640
Calibrator solution, A4256
Canakinumab, J0638
Cancer, screening
  cervical or vaginal, G0101
  colorectal, G0104–G0106, G0120–G0122, G0328,
    S3890
  prostate, G0102, G0103
Cane, E0100, E0105
  accessory, A4636, A4637
Canister
  disposable, used with suction pump, A7000
  non-disposable, used with suction pump, A7001
Cannula, nasal, A4615
Capecitabine, oral, J8520, J8521
Capsaicin patch, J7335
Carbon filter, A4680
Carboplatin, J9045
Cardia Event, recorder, implantable, E0616
Cardiokymography, Q0035
Cardiovascular services, M0300–M0301
Cardioverter-defibrillator, G0448
Carmustine, J9050
Care, coordinated, G9001–G9011, H1002
Case management, T1016, T1017
Care plan, G0162
Caspofungin acetate, J0637
Cast
  hand restoration, L6900–L6915
  materials, special, A4590
  supplies, A4580, A4590, Q4001–Q4051
  thermoplastic, L2106, L2126
Caster
  front, for power wheelchair, K0099
  wheelchair, E0997, E0998
Catheter, A4300–A4355
  anchoring device, A5200, A4333, A4334
  cap, disposable (dialysis), A4860
  external collection device, A4327–A4330, A4347
  implanted, A7042, A7043
  indwelling, A4338–A4346
  insertion tray, A4354
  intermittent with insertion supplies, A4353
  irrigation supplies, A4355
  male external, A4324, A4325, A4348
  oropharyngeal suction, A4628
  starter set, A4329
  trachea (suction), A4609, A4610, A4624
  transtracheal oxygen, A4608
  vascular, A4300, A4301
Catheterization, specimen collection, P9612, P9615
CBC, G0306, G0307

Cefazolin sodium, J0690
Cefepime HCl, J0692
Cefotaxime sodium, J0698
Ceftaroline fosamil, J0712
Ceftazidime, J0713
Ceftizoxime sodium, J0715
Ceftriaxone sodium, J0696
Cefuroxime sodium, J0697
CellCept, K0412
Cellular therapy, M0075
Cement, ostomy, A4364
Centrifuge, A4650
Centruroides Immune F(ab), J0716 ◀
Cephalin Floculation, blood, P2028
Cephalothin sodium, J1890
Cephapirin sodium, J0710
Certification, physician, home, health, G0179–G0182
Certolizumab pegol, J0718
Cerumen, removal, G0268
Cervical
  cancer, screening, G0101
  cytopathology, G0123, G0124, G0141–G0148
  halo, L0810–L0830
  head harness/halter, E0942
  orthosis, L0100–L0200
  traction, E0855, E0856
Cervical cap contraceptive, A4261
Cervical-thoracic-lumbar-sacral orthosis (CTLSO),
  L0700, L0710
Cetuximab, J9055
Chair
  adjustable, dialysis, E1570
  lift, E0627
  rollabout, E1031
  sitz bath, E0160–E0162
  transport, E1035–E1039
Chelation therapy, M0300
Chemical endarterectomy, M0300
Chemistry and toxicology tests, P2028–P3001
Chemotherapy
  administration, Q0083–Q0085 (hospital reporting
    only)
  drug, oral, not otherwise classified, J8999
  drugs (*see also* drug by name), J9000–J9999
Chest shell (cuirass), E0457
Chest Wall Oscillation System, E0483
  hose, replacement, A7026
  vest, replacement, A7025
Chest wrap, E0459
Chin cup, cervical, L0150
Chloramphenicol sodium succinate, J0720
Chlordiazepoxide HCl, J1990
Chloromycetin Sodium Succinate, J0720
Chloroprocaine HCl, J2400
Chloroquine HCl, J0390
Chlorothiazide sodium, J1205
Chlorpromazine HCl, J3230
Choroid, lesion, destruction, G0186

Chorionic **gonadotropin,** J0725

Chromic **phosphate P32 suspension,** A9564

Chromium **CR-51 sodium chromate,** A9553

Cidofovir, J0740

Cilastatin **sodium, imipenem,** J0743

Ciprofloxacin, **for intravenous infusion,** J0744

Cisplatin, J9060

Cladribine, J9065

Clamp

   dialysis, A4910, A4918, A4920

   external urethral, A4356

Cleanser, **wound,** A6260

Cleansing **agent, dialysis equipment,** A4790

Clofarabine, J9027

Clonidine, J0735

Closure, wound, adhesive, tissue, G0168

Clotting **time tube,** A4771

Clubfoot **wedge,** L3380

Cochlear **prosthetic implant,** L8614

   accessories, L8615–L8617

   batteries, L8621–L8624

   replacement, L8619, L8627–L8629

Codeine **phosphate,** J0745

Colchicine, J0760

Cold/Heat, application, E0200–E0240

Colistimethate **sodium,** J0770

Collagen

   meniscus implant procedure, G0428

   skin test, G0025

   urinary tract implant, L8603

   wound dressing, A6020–A6024

Collagenase, **Clostridium Histolyticum,** J0775

Collar, **cervical**

   multiple post, L0180–L0200

   nonadjust (foam), L0120

Colorectal, screening, cancer, G0104–G0106,

   G0120–G0122, G0328, S3890

Coly-Mycin **M,** J0770

Comfort **items,** A9190

Complete, blood, count, G0306, G0307

Commode, E0160–E0175

   chair, E0170–E0171

   lift, E0625, E0172

   pail, E0167

   seat, wheelchair, E0968

Composite **dressing,** A6203–A6205

Compressed **gas system,** E0424–E0480

Compressor

   aerosol, E0572, E0575

   air, E0565

   nebulizer, E0570–E0585

   pneumatic, E0650–E0676

Compression

   bandage, A4460

   burn garment, A6501–A6512

   stockings, A6530–A6549

Compressor, E0565, E0570, E0572, E0650–E0652

Conductive gel/paste, A4558

Conductivity **meter, bath, dialysis,** E1550

Conference, team, G0175, G9007, S0220, S0221

Congo **red, blood,** P2029

Contact **layer,** A6206–A6208

Contact **lens,** V2500–V2599

Continent **device,** A5081, A5082, A5083

Continuous **glucose monitoring system**

   receiver, A9278

   sensor, A9276

   transmitter, A9277

Continuous **passive motion exercise device,** E0936

Continuous **positive airway pressure (CPAP) device,** E0601

   compressor, K0269

Contraceptive

   cervical cap, A4261

   condoms, A4267, A4268

   diaphragm, A4266

   intratubal occlusion device, A4264

   intrauterine, copper, J7300

   intrauterine, levonorgestrel releasing, J7302

   levonorgestrel, implants and supplies, A4260

   patch, J7304

   spermicide, A4269

   supply, A4267–A4269

   vaginal ring, J7303

Contracts, **maintenance, ESRD,** A4890

Contrast **material**

   injection during MRI, A4643

   low osmolar, A4644–A4646

Coordinated, care, G9001–G9011

Corneal **tissue processing,** V2785

Corset, **spinal orthosis,** L0970–L0976

Corticorelin **ovine triflutate,** J0795

Corticotropin, J0800

Corvert, *see* **Ibutilide fumarate**

Cosyntropin, J0833, J0834

Cough **stimulating device,** A7020, E0482

Counseling

   alcohol misuse, G0443

   cardiovascular disease, G0448

   obesity, G0447

   sexually transmitted infection, G0445

   smoking and tobacco cessation, G0436, G0437

Count, blood, G0306, G0307, S3636

Counterpulsation, external, G0166

Cover, **wound**

   alginate dressing, A6196–A6198

   foam dressing, A6209–A6214

   hydrogel dressing, A6242–A6248

   non-contact wound warming cover, and accessory, A6000, E0231, E0232

   specialty absorptive dressing, A6251–A6256

CPAP **(continuous positive airway pressure) device,** E0601

   headgear, K0185

   humidifier, A7046

   intermittent assist, E0452

◄ New   ← Revised   ✔ Reinstated   ~~deleted~~ Deleted

Cradle, **bed,** E0280
Crib, E0300
Cromolyn **sodium, inhalation solution, unit dose,** J7631, J7632
Crotalidae **polyvalent immune fab,** J0840
Crutches, E0110–E0118
    accessories, A4635–A4637, K0102
Cryoprecipitate, **each unit,** P9012
CTLSO, L1000–L1120, L0700, L0710
Cuirass, E0457
Culture **sensitivity study,** P7001
Cushion, **wheelchair,** E0977
Cyanocobalamin **Cobalt C057,** A9559
Cycler **dialysis machine,** E1594
Cyclophosphamide, J9070
    oral, J8530
Cyclosporine, J7502, J7515, J7516
Cytarabine, J9100
    liposome, J9098
Cytomegalovirus **immune globulin (human),** J0850
*Cytopathology, **cervical or vaginal,** G0123, G0124, G0141–G0148*

D

Dacarbazine, J9130
Daclizumab, J7513
Dactinomycin, J9120
Dalalone, J1100
Dalteparin **sodium,** J1645
Daptomycin, J0878
Darbepoetin **Alfa,** J0881–J0882
Daunorubicin
    Citrate, J9151
    HCl, J9150
DaunoXome, *see* **Daunorubicin citrate**
Decitabine, J0894
Decubitus **care equipment,** E0180–E0199
Deferoxamine **mesylate,** J0895
Defibrillator, **external,** E0617, K0606
    battery, K0607
    electrode, K0609
    garment, K0608
Degarelix, J9155
Deionizer, **water purification system,** E1615
Delivery/set-up/dispensing, A9901
Denileukin **diftitox,** J9160
Denosumab, J0897
*Density, **bone, study,** G0130*
Depo-estradiol **cypionate,** J1000
*Dermal **filler injection,** G0429*
Desmopressin **acetate,** J2597
*Destruction, **lesion, choroid,** G0186*
Detector, **blood leak, dialysis,** E1560
*Developmental **testing,** G0451*

Dexamethasone
    acetate, J1094
    inhalation solution, concentrated, J7637
    inhalation solution, unit dose, J7638
    intravitreal implant, J7312
    oral, J8540
    sodium phosphate, J1100
Dextran, J7100
Dextrose
    saline (normal), J7042
    water, J7060, J7070
Dextrostick, A4772
Diabetes
    evaluation, G0245, G0246
    shoes, A5500–A5508
    training, outpatient, G0108, G0109
Diagnostic
    radiology services, R0070–R0076
Dialysate
    concentrate additives, A4765
    solution, A4728
    testing solution, A4760
Dialysis
    air bubble detector, E1530
    bath conductivity, meter, E1550
    chemicals/antiseptics solution, A4674
    disposable cycler set, A4671
    emergency, G0257
    equipment, E1510–E1702
    extension line, A4672–A4673
    filter, A4680
    fluid barrier, E1575
    forceps, A4910
    home, S9335, S9339
    kit, A4820
    pressure alarm, E1540
    shunt, A4740
    supplies, A4650–A4927
    thermometer, A4910
    tourniquet, A4910
    unipuncture control system, E1580
    unscheduled, G0257
    venous pressure clamp, A4918
Dialyzer, A4690
Diaper, T1500, T4521–T4540
    adult incontinence garment, A4520
Diazepam, J3360
Diazoxide, J1730
Dicyclomine **HCl,** J0500
Diethylstilbestrol **diphosphate,** J9165
Digoxin, J1160
Digoxin **immune fab (ovine),** J1162
Dihydroergotamine **mesylate,** J1110
Dimenhydrinate, J1240
Dimercaprol, J0470
Dimethyl **sulfoxide (DMSO),** J1212
Diphenhydramine **HCl,** J1200
Dipyridamole, J1245

◀ New   ← Revised   ✔ Reinstated   ~~deleted~~ Deleted

Disarticulation
  lower extremities, prosthesis, L5000–L5999
  upper extremities, prosthesis, L6000–L6692
Disease
  status, oncology, G9063–G9139
Disposable supplies, ambulance, A0382, A0384,
  A0392–A0398
*Dispensing, **fee, pharmacy,** G0333, Q0510–Q0514,*
  S9430
DME
  miscellaneous, A9900–A9999
DMSO, J1212
Dobutamine HCl, J1250
Docetaxel, J9171
Documentation
  antidepressant, G8126–G8128
  blood pressure, G8476–G8478
  bypass, graft, coronary, artery, documentation,
    G8160–G8163
  CABG, G8160–G8163
  dysphagia, G8232
  dysphagia, screening, G8232, V5364
  ECG, 12-lead, G8705, G8706
  eye, functions, G8315–G8333
  influenza, immunization, G8482–G8484
  osteoporosis, G8401
  pharmacologic therapy for osteoporosis, G8634, G8635
  physician for DME, G0454
  prophylactic antibiotic, G8702, G8703
  prophylaxis, DVT, G8218
  prophylactic parenteral antibiotic, G8629–G8632
  prophylaxis, thrombosis, deep, vein, G8218
  urinary, incontinence, G8063, G8267
Dolasetron mesylate, J1260
Dome and mouthpiece (for nebulizer), A7016
Dopamine HCl, J1265
Doripenem, J1267
**Dornase alpha, inhalation solution, unit dose
  form,** J7639
Doxercalciferol, J1270
~~Doxil, J9001~~✖
Doxorubicin HCl, J9000, J9002 ←
Drainage
  bag, A4357, A4358
  board, postural, E0606
  bottle, A5102
Dressing (*see also* Bandage), A6020–A6406
  alginate, A6196–A6199
  collagen, A6020–A6024
  composite, A6200–A6205
  contact layer, A6206–A6208
  foam, A6209–A6215
  gauze, A6216–A6230, A6402–A6406
  holder/binder, A4462
  hydrocolloid, A6234–A6241
  hydrogel, A6242–A6248
  specialty absorptive, A6251–A6256
  transparent film, A6257–A6259

Dressing *(Continued)*
  tubular, A6457
  wound, K0744–K0746
Droperidol, J1790
  and fentanyl citrate, J1810
Dropper, A4649
*Drug **screen,** G0434*
Drugs (*see also* Table of Drugs)
  administered through a metered dose inhaler, J3535
  antiemetic, J8489, J8597, Q0163–Q0181
  chemotherapy, J8500–J9999
  disposable delivery system, 5 ml or less per hour,
    A4306
  disposable delivery system, 50 ml or greater per
    hour, A4305
  immunosuppressive, J7500–J7599
  infusion supplies, A4230–A4232, A4221, A4222
  inhalation solutions, J7608–J7699
  non-prescription, A9150
  not otherwise classified, J3490, J7599, J7699, J7799,
    J8499, J8999, J9999
  oral, NOS, J8499
  prescription, oral, J8499, J8999
Dry pressure pad/mattress, E0179, E0184, E0199
Durable medical equipment (DME), E0100–E1830,
  K Codes
Duraclon, *see* **Clonidine**
Dyphylline, J1180
*Dysphagia, **screening, documentation,** G8232, V5364*
*Dystrophic, **nails, trimming,** G0127*

E

Ear mold, V5264
Ecallantide, J1290
**Echocardiography injectable contrast mate-
  rial,** A9700
  ECG, 12-lead, G8704
Eculizumab, J1300
*ED, **visit,** G0380–G0384*
Edetate
  calcium disodium, J0600
  disodium, J3520
Eggcrate dry pressure pad/mattress, E0184, E0199
Elastic garments, A4466
Elbow
  disarticulation, endoskeletal, L6450
  orthosis (EO), E1800, L3700–L3740, L3760
  protector, E0191
Electric hand, L7007–L7008
*Electric, **nerve, stimulator, transcutaneous,** A4595,*
  E0720–E0749
Electrical work, dialysis equipment, A4870
*Electromagnetic, **therapy,** G0295, G0329*
*Electronic **medication compliance,** T1505*
Electrodes, per pair, A4556
Elevating leg rest, K0195

◄ New   ← Revised   ✔ Reinstated   ~~deleted~~ Deleted

Elliotts **b solution,** J9175

Emergency department, visit, G0380–G0384

EMG, E0746

Eminase, J0350

Endarterectomy, **chemical,** M0300

Endoscope **sheath,** A4270

Endoskeletal **system, addition,** L5848, L5856–L5857, L5925, *L5961*

Enfuvirtide, J1324

Enoxaparin **sodium,** J1650

Enema, bag, A4458

Enteral

   feeding supply kit (syringe) (pump) (gravity), B4034–B4036

   formulae, B4149–B4156

   nutrition infusion pump (with alarm) (without), B9000, B9002

   therapy, supplies, B4000–B9999

Epinephrine, J0171

Epirubicin **HCl,** J9178

Epoetin **alpha,** J0885–J0886, Q4081

Epoprostenol, J1325

Equipment

   decubitus, E0181–E0199

   exercise, A9300, E0935, E0936

   orthopedic, E0910–E0948, E1800–E8002

   oxygen, E0424–E0486, E1353–E1406

   pump, E0781, E0784, E0791

   respiratory, E0424–E0601

   safety, E0700, E0705

   traction, E0830–E0900

   transfer, E0705

   trapeze, E0910–E0912, E0940

   whirlpool, E1300, E1310

Erection device, tension ring, L7902

Ergonovine **maleate,** J1330

Eribulin **mesylate,** J9179

Ertapenem **sodium,** J1335

Erythromycin **lactobionate,** J1364

ESRD **(End-Stage Renal Disease;** *see also* **Dialysis)**

   machines and accessories, E1500–E1699

   plumbing, A4870

   supplies, A4651–A4929

Estrogen **conjugated,** J1410

Estrone **(5, Aqueous),** J1435

Ethanolamine **oleate,** J1430

Etidronate **disodium,** J1436

Etonogestrel **implant system,** J7307

Etoposide, J9181

   oral, J8560

Euflexxa, J7323

~~Everolimus, J8561~~ ✖

Euflexxa, J7323

Evaluation

   conformity, V5020

   contact lens, S0592

   diabetic, G0245, G0246

Evaluation (Continued)

   footwear, G8410–G8416

   fundus, G8325–G8328

   hearing, S0618, V5008, V5010

   hospice, G0337

   multidisciplinary, H2000

   nursing, T1001

   ocularist, S9150

   performance measurement, S3005

   resident, T2011

   speech, S9152

   team, T1024

   treatment response, G0254

Everolimus, J7527←

Examination

   gynecological, S0610–S0613

   ophthalmological, S0620, S0621

   pinworm, Q0113

   ringworm, S0605

Exercise

   class, S9451

   equipment, A9300, E0935, E0936

External

   ambulatory infusion pump, E0781, E0784

   ambulatory insulin delivery system, A9274

   power, battery components, L7360–L7368

   power, elbow, L7160–L7191

   urinary supplies, A4356-A4359

Extremity

   belt/harness, E0945

   traction, E0870–E0880

Eye

   case, V2756

   functions, documentation, G8315–G8333

   lens (contact) (spectacle), V2100–V2615

   prosthetic, V2623, V2629

   service (miscellaneous), V2700–V2799

F

Faceplate, **ostomy,** A4361

Face **tent, oxygen,** A4619

Factor **VIIA coagulation factor, recombinant,** J7189

Factor **VIII, anti-hemophilic factor,** J7185, J7190–J7192

Factor **IX,** J7193, J7194, J7195

Factor **XIII, anti-hemophilic factor,** J7180

Family **Planning Education,** H1010

Fee

   coordinated care, G9001–G9011

   dispensing, pharmacy, G0333, Q0510–Q0514, S9430

Fentanyl **citrate,** J3010

   and droperidol, J1810

Fern **test,** Q0114

Ferumoxytol, Q0138, Q0139

Filgrastim **(G-CSF),** J1440, J1441

◀ New   ← Revised   ✔ Reinstated   ~~deleted~~ Deleted

Filler, wound
  alginate dressing, A6199
  foam dressing, A6215
  hydrocolloid dressing, A6240, A6241
  hydrogel dressing, A6248
  not elsewhere classified, A6261, A6262
Film, transparent (for dressing), A6257–A6259
Filter
  aerosol compressor, A7014
  dialysis carbon, A4680
  ostomy, A4368
  tracheostoma, A4481
  ultrasonic generator, A7014
Fistula cannulation set, A4730
Flebogamma, J1572
Florbetapir F18, A9586 ◄
Flowmeter, E0440, E0555, E0580
Floxuridine, J9200
Fluconazole, injection, J1450
Fludarabine phosphate, J8562, J9185
Fluid barrier, dialysis, E1575
Flunisolide inhalation solution, J7641
Fluocinolone, J7311
Fluorodeoxyglucose F-18 FDG, A9552
Fluorouracil, J9190
Fluphenazine decanoate, J2680
Foam
  dressing, A6209–A6215
  pad adhesive, A5126
Folding walker, E0135, E0143
Foley catheter, A4312–A4316, A4338–A4346
Fomepizole, J1451
Fomivirsen sodium intraocular, J1452
Fondaparinux sodium, J1652
Footdrop splint, L4398
Footplate, E0175, E0970, L3031
Footwear, orthopedic, L3201–L3265
Forearm crutches, E0110, E0111
Formoterol, J7640
  fumarate, J7606
Fosaprepitant, J1453
Foscarnet sodium, J1455
Fosphenytoin, Q2009
Fracture
  bedpan, E0276
  frame, E0920, E0930, E0946–E0948
  orthosis, L2106–L2136, L3980–L3986
  orthotic additions, L2180–L2192, L3995
Fragmin, *see* **Dalteparin sodium**
Frames (spectacles), V2020, V2025
Fulvestrant, J9395
Furosemide, J1940

G

Gadobutrol, A9585
Gadofosveset trisodium, A9583

Gadoxetate disodium, A9581
Gait trainer, E8000–E8002
Gallium Ga67, A9556
Gallium nitrate, J1457
Galsulfase, J1458
Gammagard liquid, J1569
Gamma globulin, J1460, J1560
Gammaplex, J1557
Gamunex, J1561
Ganciclovir
  implant, J7310
  sodium, J1570
Garamycin, J1580
Gas system
  compressed, E0424, E0425
  gaseous, E0430, E0431, E0441, E0443
  liquid, E0434–E0440, E0442, E0444
Gatifloxacin, J1590
Gauze (*see also*** Bandage)**
  impregnated, A6222–A6233, A6266
  non-impregnated, A6402–A6404
Gefitinib, J8565
Gel
  conductive, A4558
  pressure pad, E0185, E0196
Gemcitabine HCl, J9201
Gemtuzumab ozogamicin, J9300
Generator
  ultrasonic with nebulizer, E0574
Gentamicin (Sulfate), J1580
Glasses
  air conduction, V5070
  binaural, V5120–V5150
  bone conduction, V5080
  frames, V2020, V2025
  hearing aid, V5230
Glaucoma
  screening, G0117, G0118
Gloves, A4927
Glucagon HCl, J1610
Glucose
  monitor with integrated lancing/blood sample collection, E2101
  monitor with integrated voice synthesizer, E2100
  test strips, A4253, A4772
Gluteal pad, L2650
Glycopyrrolate, inhalation solution, concentrated, J7642
Glycopyrrolate, inhalation solution, unit dose, J7643
Gold
  sodium thiomalate, J1600
Gomco drain bottle, A4912
Gonadorelin HCl, J1620
Goserelin acetate implant (*see also*** Implant),** J9202
Grab bar, trapeze, E0910, E0940
Gradient, compression stockings, A6530–A6549
Grade-aid, wheelchair, E0974

◄ New   ← Revised   ✔ Reinstated   ~~deleted~~ Deleted

Granisetron **HCl**, J1626
Gravity **traction device**, E0941
Gravlee **jet washer**, A4470
Guaiac, stool, G0394
Guidelines, practice, oncology, G9056–G9062

H

Hair **analysis (excluding arsenic)**, P2031
Hallus-Valgus **dynamic splint**, L3100
Hallux **prosthetic implant**, L8642
Haloperidol, J1630
   decanoate, J1631
Halo **procedures**, L0810–L0860
Halter, **cervical head**, E0942
Hand **finger orthosis, prefabricated**, L3923
Hand **restoration**, L6900–L6915
   partial prosthesis, L6000–L6020
   orthosis (WHFO), E1805, E1825, L3800–L3805,
      L3900-L3954
   rims, wheelchair, E0967
Handgrip **(cane, crutch, walker)**, A4636
Harness, E0942, E0944, E0945
Headgear **(for positive airway pressure device)**,
   K0185
Hearing
   assessment, S0618, V5008, V5010
   devices, V5000–V5299, L8614
   services, V5000–V5999
Heat
   application, E0200–E0239
   lamp, E0200, E0205
   infrared heating pad system, A4639, E0221
   pad, A9273, E0210, E0215, E0237, E0249
Heater **(nebulizer)**, E1372
Heavy duty, wheelchair, E1280–E1298, K0006,
   K0007, K0801–K0886
Heel
   elevator, air, E0370
   protector, E0191
   shoe, L3430–L3485
   stabilizer, L3170
Helicopter, **ambulance (*see also* Ambulance)**
Helmet
   cervical, L0100, L0110
   head, A8000–A8004
Hemin, J1640
Hemi-wheelchair, E1083–E1086
Hemipelvectomy **prosthesis**, L5280
Hemodialysis **machine**, E1590
Hemodialyzer, **portable**, E1635
Hemofil **M**, J7190
   hemoglobin, level, G0908, G0910
Hemophilia **clotting factor**, J7190–J7198
   NOC, J7199
Hemostats, A4850
Hemostix, A4773

Hepagam B
   IM, J1571
   IV, J1573
Heparin
   infusion pump, dialysis, E1520
   lock flush, J1642
   sodium, J1644
*Hepatitis **B**, vaccine, administration, G0010*
Hep-Lock **(U/P)**, J1642
Hexalite, A4590
High **osmolar contrast material**, Q9958–Q9964
Hip
   disarticulation prosthesis, L5250, L5270
   orthosis (HO), L1600–L1690
Hip-knee-ankle-foot **orthosis (HKAFO)**, L2040–L2090
Histrelin
   acetate, J1675
   implant, J9225
HKAFO, L2040–L2090
Home
   glucose, monitor, E0607, E2100, E2101, S1030,
      S1031
   health, aide, G0156, S9122, T1021
   health, clinical, social worker, G0155
   health, nursing, skilled, G0154
   health, occupational, therapist, G0152
   health, physical therapist, G0151
   health, physician, certification, G0179–G0182
   health, respiratory therapy, S5180, S5181
   therapist, speech, S9128
Home **Health Agency Services**, T0221
*HOPPS, **C1000–C9999***
*Hospice **home care**, Q5010*
Hospital
   bed, E0250–E0304, E0328, E0329
   observation, G0378, G0379
*Hospital **Outpatient Payment System**,*
   C1000–C9999
Hot **water bottle**, A9273
Human **fibrinogen concentrate**, J7178←
Humidifier, A7046, E0550–E0563
Hyalgan, J7321
Hyalomatrix, Q4117
Hyaluronan, J7326
Hyaluronate, **sodium**, J7317
Hyaluronidase, J3470
   ovine, J3471–J3473
Hydralazine **HCl**, J0360
Hydraulic **patient lift**, E0630
Hydrocollator, E0225, E0239
Hydrocolloid **dressing**, A6234–A6241
Hydrocortisone
   acetate, J1700
   sodium phosphate, J1710
   sodium succinate, J1720
Hydrogel **dressing**, A6242–A6248, A6231–A6233
Hydromorphone, J1170
Hydroxyprogesterone **caproate**, J1725

◄ New   ← Revised   ✔ Reinstated   ~~deleted~~ Deleted

Hydroxyzine **HCl,** J3410
Hylan **G-F 20,** *J7325*
Hyoscyamine **Sulfate,** J1980
Hyperbaric **oxygen chamber, topical,** A4575

I

Ibandronate **sodium,** J1740
Ibuprofen, **J1741** ◀
Ibutilide **Fumarate,** J1742
Icatibant, **J1744** ◀
Ice
  cap, E0230
  collar, E0230
Idarubicin **HCl,** J9211
Idursulfase, J1743
Ifosfamide, J9208
Iliac, artery, angiography, G0278
Iloprost, Q4074
Imiglucerase, J1786
Immune **globulin**
  Flebogamma, J1572
  Gammagard liquid, J1569
  Gammaplex, J1557
  Gamunex, J1561
  HepaGam B, J1571
  Hizentra, J1559
  NOS, J1566
  Octagam, J1568
  Privigen, J1459
  Rho(D), J2788, J2790
  Rhophylac, J2791
  Subcutaneous, J1562
Immunosuppressive **drug, not otherwise classi-
  fied,** J7599
Implant
  access system, A4301
  aqueous shunt, L8612
  breast, L8600
  cochlear, L8614, L8619
  collagen, urinary tract, L8603
  dextranomer/hyaluronic acid copolymer, L8604
  ganciclovir, J7310
  hallux, L8642
  urinary tract, L8603, L8606
  infusion pump, programmable, E0783, E0786
  joint, L8630, L8641, L8658
  lacrimal duct, A4262, A4263
  metacarpophalangeal joint, L8630
  metatarsal joint, L8641
  neurostimulator pulse generator, L8681–L8688
  not otherwise specified, L8699
  ocular, L8610
  ossicular, L8613
  osteogenesis stimulator, E0749
  percutaneous access system, A4301
  replacement implantable intraspinal catheter, E0785

Implant *(Continued)*
  synthetic, urinary, L8606
  vascular graft, L8670
Implantable **radiation dosimeter,** A4650
Impregnated **gauze dressing,** A6222–A6230
Incobotulinumtoxin **a,** J0588
Incontinence
  appliances and supplies, A4310, A4360,
    A5071–A5075, A5102–A5114, K0280, K0281
  garment, A4520, T4521–T4543
  supply, A4335, A4356–A4358
  treatment system, E0740
  urinary, documentation, G8063, G8067
Indium **IN-111**
  carpromab pendetide, A9507
  ibritumomab tiuxetan, A9542
  labeled autologous white blood cells, A9570
  labeled autologous platelets, A9571
  oxyquinoline, A9547
  pentetate, A9548
  pentetreotide, A9572
  satumomab, A4642
Infliximab **injection,** J1745
Influenza
  immunization, documentation, G8482–G8484
  vaccine, administration, G0008
  virus vaccine, Q2035–Q2039
Infusion
  pump, ambulatory, with administrative equipment,
    E0781
  pump, heparin, dialysis, E1520
  pump, implantable, E0782, E0783
  pump, implantable, refill kit, A4220
  pump, insulin, E0784
  pump, mechanical, reusable, E0779, E0780
  pump, uninterrupted infusion of Epiprostenol,
    K0455
  saline, J7030–J7060
  supplies, A4219, A4221, A4222, A4230–A4232,
    E0776–E0791
  therapy, other than chemotherapeutic drugs, Q0081
Inhalation **solution (*see also* drug name),**
    J7608–J7699, Q4074
*Injection **device, needle-free,** A4210*
Injections (*see also* **drug name),** J0120–J7320
  arthrography, sacroiliac, joint, G0259, G0260
  supplies for self-administered, A4211
*INR, **monitoring,** G0248–G0250*
Insertion **tray,** A4310–A4316
Insulin, J1815, J1817, S5550–S5571
  ambulatory, external, system, A9274
  treatment, outpatient, G9147
*Integra **flowable wound matrix,** Q4114*
Interferon
  Alpha, J9212–J9215
  Beta-1 a, J1826, Q3025–Q3026
  Beta-1 b, J1830
  Gamma, J9216

◀ New   ← Revised   ✔ Reinstated   ~~deleted~~ Deleted

Intermittent
assist device with continuous positive airway pressure device, E0470–E0472
limb compression device, E0676
peritoneal dialysis system, E1592
positive pressure breathing (IPPB) machine, E0500

Interphalangeal joint, prosthetic implant, L8658, L8659

Interscapular thoracic prosthesis
endoskeletal, L6570
upper limb, L6350–L6370

Intervention, tobacco, G9016

Intraconazole, J1835

Intraocular
lenses, V2630–V2632

Intrapulmonary percussive ventilation system, E0481

Intrauterine copper contraceptive, J7300

Iodine Iobenguane sulfate I-131, A9508

Iodine I-123 iobenguane, A9582

Iodine I-123 ioflupane, A9584

Iodine I-123 sodium iodide, A9509, A9516

Iodine I-125 serum albumin, A9532
sodium iodide, A9527
sodium iothalamate, A9554

Iodine I-131 iodinated serum albumin, A9524
sodium iodide capsule, A9517, A9528
sodium iodide solution, A9529–A9531
tositumomab, A9544–A9545

Iodine swabs/wipes, A4247

IPD
system, E1592

Ipilimumab, J9228

IPPB machine, E0500

Ipratropium bromide, inhalation solution, unit dose, J7644, J7645

Irinotecan, J9206

Iron
Dextran, J1750
sucrose, J1756

Irrigation/evacuation system, bowel
control unit, E0350
disposable supplies for, E0352

Irrigation solution for bladder calculi, Q2004

Irrigation supplies, A4320–A4322, A4355, A4397–A4400

Islet, transplant, G0341–G0343, S2102

Isoetharine HCl, inhalation solution
concentrated, J7647, J7648
unit dose, J7649, J7650

Isolates, B4150, B4152

Isoproterenol HCl, inhalation solution
concentrated, J7657, J7658
unit dose, J7659, J7660

Isosulfan blue, Q9968

Item, non-covered, A9270

IUD, J7300, S4989

IV pole, each, E0776, K0105

Ixabepilone, J9207

J

Jacket
scoliosis, L1300, L1310

Jaw, motion, rehabilitation system, E1700–E1702

Jenamicin, J1580

K

Kanamycin sulfate, J1840, J1850

Kartop patient lift, toilet or bathroom (see also Lift), E0625

Ketorolac thomethamine, J1885

Kidney
ESRD supply, A4650–A4927
machine, accessories, E1500–E1699
machine, E1500–E1699
system, E1510
wearable artificial, E1632

Kits
enteral feeding supply (syringe) (pump) (gravity), B4034–B4036
fistula cannulation (set), A4730
parenteral nutrition, B4220–B4224
surgical dressing (tray), A4550
tracheostomy, A4625

Knee
arthroscopy, surgical, G0289, S2112, S2300
disarticulation, prosthesis, L5150, L5160
joint, miniature, L5826
orthosis (KO), E1810, L1800–L1885

Knee-ankle-foot orthosis (KAFO), L2000–L2039, L2126–L2136
addition, high strength, lightweight material, L2755

Kyphosis pad, L1020, L1025

L

Laboratory
services, P0000–P9999

Laboratory tests
chemistry, P2028–P2038
microbiology, P7001
miscellaneous, P9010–P9615, Q0111–Q0115
toxicology, P3000–P3001, Q0091

Lacrimal duct implant
permanent, A4263
temporary, A4262

Lactated Ringer's infusion, J7120

Laetrile, J3570

Lancet, A4258, A4259

Lanreotide, J1930

Laronidase, J1931

◄ New   ← Revised   ✔ Reinstated   ~~deleted~~ Deleted

Larynx, artificial, L8500
Laser blood collection device and accessory,
  E0620, A4257
Lead investigation, T1029
Lead wires, per pair, A4557
Leg
  bag, A4358, A5105, A5112
  extensions for walker, E0158
  rest, elevating, K0195
  rest, wheelchair, E0990
  strap, replacement, A5113–A5114
Legg Perthes orthosis, L1700–L1755
Lens
  aniseikonic, V2118, V2318
  contact, V2500–V2599
  eye, V2100–V2615, V2700–V2799
  intraocular, V2630–V2632, *C1840*
  low vision, V2600–V2615
  progressive, V2781
Lepirudin, J1945
Lesion, destruction, choroid, G0186
Leucovorin calcium, J0640
Leukocyte poor blood, each unit, P9016
Leuprolide acetate, J9217, J9218, J9219,
  J1950
Levalbuterol, all formulations, inhalation solution
  concentrated, J7607, J7612
  unit dose, J7614, J7615
Levetiracetam, J1953
Levocarnitine, J1955
Levofloxacin, J1956
Levoleucovorin, J0641
Levonorgestrel, (contraceptive), implants and supplies, J7306
Levorphanol tartrate, J1960
Lexidronam, A9604
Lidocaine HCl, J2001
Lift
  patient (includes seat lift), E0621–E0635
  shoe, L3300–L3334
Lightweight, wheelchair, E1087–E1090,
  E1240–E1270, E2618
Lincomycin HCl, J2010
Linezolid, J2020
Listening devices, assistive, V5281–V5290
Liquid barrier, ostomy, A4363
Lodging, recipient, escort nonemergency transport, A0180, A0200
LOPS, G0245–G0247
Lorazepam, J2060
Loss of protective sensation, G0245–G0247
Low osmolar contrast material, Q9965–Q9967
LSO, L0621–L0640
Lubricant, A4402, A4332
Lumbar flexion, L0540
Lumbar-sacral orthosis (LSO), L0621–L0640
LVRS, services, G0302–G0305
Lymphocyte immune globulin, J7504, J7511

M

Machine
  IPPB, E0500
  kidney, E1500–E1699
Magnesium sulphate, J3475
Maintenance contract, ESRD, A4890
Mammography, screening, G0202
Mannitol, J2150, J7665
Mapping, vessel, for hemodialysis access,
  G0365
Marker, tissue, A4648
Mask
  aerosol, K0180
  oxygen, A4620
Mastectomy
  bra, L8000
  form, L8020
  prosthesis, L8030, L8600
  sleeve, L8010
Matristem, Q4118–Q4120
Mattress
  air pressure, E0186
  alternating pressure, E0277
  dry pressure, E0184
  gel pressure, E0196
  hospital bed, E0271, E0272
  non-powered, pressure reducing, E0373
  overlay, E0371–E0372
  powered, pressure reducing, E0277
  water pressure, E0187
Measurement period
  left ventricular function testing, G8682
  not an eligible candidate for left ventricular function testing, G8683
  left ventricular function testing not performed, NOS, G8685
Mecasermin, J2170
Mechlorethamine HCl, J9230
Medicaid, codes, T1000–T9999
Medical and surgical supplies, A4206–A8999
Medical nutritional therapy, G0270, G0271
Medical services, other, M0000–M9999
Medroxyprogesterone acetate, J1050 ←
~~Medroxyprogesterone acetate/estradiol cypionate, J1056~~ ✖
Melphalan
  HCl, J9245
  oral, J8600
Mental, health, training services, G0177
Meperidine, J2175
  and promethazine, J2180
Mepivacaine HCl, J0670
Meropenem, J2185
Mesna, J9209
Metacarpophalangeal joint, prosthetic implant,
  L8630, L8631

◄ New   ← Revised   ✔ Reinstated   ~~deleted~~ Deleted

Metaproterenol sulfate, inhalation solution
   concentrated, J7667, J7668
   unit dose, J7669, J7670
Metaraminol bitartrate, J0380
Metatarsal joint, prosthetic implant, L8641
Meter, bath conductivity, dialysis, E1550
Methacholine chloride, J7674
Methadone HCl, J1230
Methergine, *J2210*
Methocarbamol, J2800
Methotrexate
   oral, J8610
   sodium, J9250, J9260
Methyldopate HCl, J0210
Methylene blue, Q9968
Methylnaltrexone, J2212 ◀
Methylprednisolone
   acetate, J1020–J1040
   oral, J7509
   sodium succinate, J2920, J2930
Metoclopramide HCl, J2765
Micafungin sodium, J2248
Microbiology test, P7001
Midazolam HCl, J2250
Mileage
   ALS, A0390
   ambulance, A0380, A0390
Milrinone lactate, J2260
Mini-bus, nonemergency transportation, A0120
Minocycline hydrochloride, J2265
Mitomycin, J7315, J9280 ←
Mitoxantrone HCl, J9293
MNT, G0270, G0271
Mobility device, physician, service, G0372
Modalities, with office visit, M0005–M0008
Moisture exchanger for use with invasive mechanical ventilation, A4483
Moisturizer, skin, A6250
Molecular pathology procedure, G0452
Monitor
   blood glucose, E0607
   blood pressure, A4670
   pacemaker, E0610, E0615
Monitoring feature/device, A9279
Monitoring, INR, G0248–G0250
Monoclonal antibodies, J7505
Morphine sulfate, J2270, J2271
   sterile, preservative-free, J2275
Motion, jaw, rehabilitation system, E1700–E1702
Mouthpiece (for respiratory equipment), A4617
Moxifloxacin, J2280
Mucoprotein, blood, P2038
Multiaxial ankle, L5986
Multidisciplinary services, H2000–H2001, T1023–T1028
Multiple post collar, cervical, L0180–L0200
Multi-Podus type AFO, L4396
Muromonab-CD3, J7505

Mycophenolate mofetil, J7517
Mycophenolic acid, J7518

N

Nabilone, J8650
Nails, trimming, dystrophic, G0127
Nalbuphine HCl, J2300
Naloxone HCl, J2310
Naltrexone, J2315
Nandrolone
   decanoate, J2320
Narrowing device, wheelchair, E0969
Nasal
   application device, K0183
   pillows/seals (for nasal application device), K0184
   vaccine inhalation, J3530
Nasogastric tubing, B4081, B4082
Natalizumab, J2323
Nebulizer, E0570–E0585
   aerosol mask, A7015
   corrugated tubing, disposable, A7010
   corrugated tubing, non-disposable, A7011
   filter, disposable, A7013
   filter, non-disposable, A7014
   heater, E1372
   large volume, disposable, prefilled, A7008
   large volume, disposable, unfilled, A7007
   not used with oxygen, durable, glass, A7017
   pneumatic, administration set, A7003, A7005, A7006
   pneumatic, nonfiltered, A7004
   portable, E0570
   small volume, A7003–A7005
   ultrasonic, E0575
   ultrasonic, dome and mouthpiece, A7016
   ultrasonic, reservoir bottle, non-disposable, A7009
   water collection device, large volume nebulizer, A7012
Needle, A4215
   bone marrow biopsy, C1830
   non-coring, A4212
   with syringe, A4206–A4209
Negative pressure wound therapy pump, E2402
   accessories, A6550
   therapy, G0456, G0457
Nelarabine, J9261
Neonatal transport, ambulance, base rate, A0225
Neostigmine methylsulfate, J2710
Nerve, conduction, sensory, test, G0255
Nerve stimulator with batteries, E0765
Nesiritide injection, J2324
Neurophysiology, intraoperative, monitoring, G0453
Neuromuscular stimulator, E0745
Neurostimulator
   battery recharging system, L8695
   pulse generator, L8681–L8688

◀ New   ← Revised   ✔ Reinstated   ~~deleted~~ Deleted

Nitrogen **N-13 ammonia,** A9526
NMES, E0720–E0749
Nonchemotherapy drug, oral, NOS, J8499
Noncovered services, A9270
Nonemergency transportation, A0080–A0210
Nonimpregnated gauze dressing, A6216–A6221,
    A6402–A6404
Nonprescription drug, A9150
Not otherwise classified drug, J3490, J7599, J7699,
    J7799, J8499, J8999, J9999, Q0181
NPH, J1820
NPWT, pump, E2402
NTIOL category 3, Q1003
NTIOL category 4, Q1004
NTIOL category 5, Q1005
Nursing care, T1030–T1031
Nursing service, direct, skilled, outpatient, G0128
Nursing, skilled, home, health, G0154
Nutrition
    enteral infusion pump, B9000, B9002
    parenteral infusion pump, B9004, B9006
    parenteral solution, B4164–B5200
    therapy, medical, G0270, G0271

O

Observation
    admission, G0379
    hospital, G0378
    LPN or RN, G0163
Occipital/mandibular support, cervical, L0160
Occult, blood, G0394
Occupational, therapy, G0129, S9129
Octafluoropropane, Q9956
Octagam, J1568
Octreotide acetate, J2353, J2354
Ocular prosthetic implant, L8610
Ofatumumab, J9302
Olanzapine, J2358
Omalizumab, J2357
OnabotulinumtoxinA, J0585
Oncology
    disease status, G9063–G9139
    practice guidelines, G9056–G9062
    visit, G9050–G9055
Ondansetron HCl, J2405
Ondansetron oral, Q0162
One arm, drive attachment, K0101
Oprelvekin, J2355
O & P supply/accessory/service, L9900
Oral device/appliance, E0485–E0486
Oral/nasal mask, A7027
    nasal pillows, A7029
    oral cushion, A7028
Oral, NOS, drug, J8499
Oropharyngeal suction catheter, A4628
Orphenadrine, J2360

Orthopedic shoes
    arch support, L3040–L3100
    footwear, L3201–L3265, *L3000–L3649*
    insert, L3000–L3030
    lift, L3300–L3334
    miscellaneous additions, L3500–L3595
    positioning device, L3140–L3170
    transfer, L3600–L3649
    wedge, L3340–L3420
Orthotic additions
    carbon graphite lamination, L2755
    fracture, L2180–L2192, L3995
    halo, L0860
    lower extremity, L2200–L2999, L4320
    ratchet lock, L2430
    scoliosis, L1010–L1120, L1210–L1290
    shoe, L3300–L3595, L3649
    spinal, L0970–L0984
    upper limb, L3810–L3890, *L3900, L3901,*
        L3970–L3974, L3995
Orthotic devices
    ankle-foot (AFO; *see also* Orthopedic shoes), E1815,
        E1816, E1830, L1900–L1990, L2102–L2116,
        L3160, L4361
    anterior-posterior-lateral, L0700, L0710
    cervical, L0100–L0200
    cervical-thoracic-lumbar-sacral (CTLSO), L0700,
        L0710
    elbow (EO), E1800, E1801, L3700–L3740
    fracture, L2102–L2136, L3980–L3986
    halo, L0810–L0830
    hand, finger, prefabricated, L3923
    hand, (WHFO), E1805, E1825, L3807,
        L3900–L3954
    hip (HO), L1600–L1690
    hip-knee-ankle-foot (HKAFO), L2040–L2090
    interface material, E1820
    knee (KO), E1810, E1811, L1800–L1885
    knee-ankle-foot (KAFO; *see also* Orthopedic shoes),
        L2000–L2038, L2126–L2136
    Legg Perthes, L1700–L1755
    lumbar, L0625–L0640
    multiple post collar, L0180–L0200
    not otherwise specified, L0999, L1499, L2999,
        L3999, L5999, L7499, L8039, L8239
    pneumatic splint, L4350–*L4379*
    pronation/supination, E1818
    repair or replacement, L4000–L4210
    replace soft interface material, L4390–L4394
    sacroiliac, L0600–L0620
    scoliosis, L1000–L1499
    shoe, *see* Orthopedic shoes
    shoulder (SO), L1840, L3650, L3674
    shoulder-elbow-wrist-hand (SEWHO), L3960–L3978
    side bar disconnect, L2768
    spinal, cervical, L0100–L0200
    spinal, DME, K0112–K0116
    thoracic, L0210

◀ New   ← Revised   ✓ Reinstated   ~~deleted~~ Deleted

Orthotic devices *(Continued)*
  toe, E1830
  wrist-hand-finger (WHFO), E1805, E1806, E1825,
    L3900–L3954
Orthovisc, J7324
Ossicula prosthetic implant, L8613
Osteogenesis stimulator, E0747–E0749, E0760
Osteoporosis
  documentation, G8401
Ostomy
  accessories, A5093
  belt, A4396
  pouches, A4416–A4435, *A5056, A5057*←
  skin barrier, A4401–A4449
  supplies, A4361–A4421, A5051–A5149
Otto Bock, prosthesis, L7007
Overdoor, traction, E0860
Oxacillin sodium, J2700
Oxaliplatin, J9263
Oxygen
  ambulance, A0422
  battery charger, E1357
  battery pack/cartridge, E1356
  catheter, transtracheal, A7018
  chamber, hyperbaric, topical, A4575
  concentrator, E1390–E1391
  DC power adapter, E1358
  delivery system, topical NOS, E0446
  equipment, E0424–E0486, E1353–E1406
  Liquid oxygen system, E0433
  mask, A4620
  medication supplies, A4611–A4627
  rack/stand, E1355
  regulator, E1353
  respiratory equipment/supplies, A4611–A4627,
    E0424–E0480
  supplies and equipment, E0425–E0444, E0455
  tent, E0455
  tubing, A4616
  water vapor enriching system, E1405, E1406
  wheeled cart, E1354
Oxymorphone HCl, J2410
Oxytetracycline HCl, J2460
Oxytocin, J2590

P

Pacemaker monitor, E0610, E0615
Paclitaxel, J9265
Paclitaxel protein-bound particles, J9264
Pad
  correction, CTLSO, L1020–L1060
  gel pressure, E0185, E0196
  heat, *A9273,* E0210, E0215, E0217, E0238, E0249
  orthotic device interface, E1820
  sheepskin, E0188, E0189
  water circulating cold with pump, E0218

Pad *(Continued)*
  water circulating heat with pump, E0217
  water circulating heat unit, E0249
Pail, for use with commode chair, E0167
Pain assessment, G8730, G8731
Palate, prosthetic implant, L8618
Palifermin, J2425
Paliperidone palmitate, J2426
Palonosetron HCl, J2469
Pamidronate disodium, J2430
Pan, for use with commode chair, E0167
Panitumumab, J9303
Papanicolaou (Pap) screening smear, P3000, P3001,
    Q0091
Papaverine HCl, J2440
Paraffin, A4265
  bath unit, E0235
Parenteral nutrition
  administration kit, B4224
  pump, B9004, B9006
  solution, B4164–B5200
  supply kit, B4220, B4222
Paricalcitol, J2501
Parking fee, nonemergency transport, A0170
Paste, conductive, A4558
Pathology and laboratory tests, miscellaneous,
    P9010–P9615
Patient support system, E0636
Patient transfer system, E1035–E1036
Payment adjustment, hardship exemption, G8642,
    G8643
Pediculosis (lice) treatment, A9180
PEFR, peak expiratory flow rate meter, A4614
Pegademase bovine, J2504
Pegaptanib, J2503
Pegaspargase, J9266
Pegfilgrastim, J2505
Peginesatide, J0890◄
Pegloticase, J2507
Pelvic
  belt/harness/boot, E0944
  traction, E0890, E0900, E0947
Pemetrexed, J9305
Penicillin
  G benzathine/G benzathine and penicillin G pro-
    caine, J0558, J0561
  G potassium, J2540
  G procaine, aqueous, J2510
Pentamidine isethionate, J2545, J7676
Pentastarch, 10% solution, J2513
Pentazocine HCl, J3070
Pentobarbital sodium, J2515
Pentostatin, J9268
Percussor, E0480
Percutaneous access system, A4301
Perflexane lipid microspheres, Q9955
Perflutren lipid microspheres, Q9957
Peroneal strap, L0980

◄ New   ← Revised   ✔ Reinstated   ~~deleted~~ Deleted

Peroxide, A4244

Perphenazine, J3310

Personal **care services,** T1019–T1021

Pessary, A4561, A4562

PET, G0219, G0235, G0252

*Pharmacologic **therapy,** G8633*

Phenobarbital **sodium,** J2560

Phentolamine **mesylate,** J2760

Phenylephrine **HCl,** J2370

Phenytoin **sodium,** J1165

Phisohex **solution,** A4246

Photofrin, *see* **Porfimer sodium**

Phototherapy **light,** E0202

Phytonadione, J3430

Pillow, **cervical,** E0943

Pinworm **examination,** Q0113

Placement

　transcatheter, stent, S2211

Plasma

　single donor, fresh frozen, P9017

　multiple donor, pooled, frozen, P9023

Plastazote, L3002, L3252, L3253, L3265,
　　L5654–L5658

Platelet

　concentrate, each unit, P9019

　rich plasma, each unit, P9020

Platform **attachment**

　forearm crutch, E0153

　walker, E0154

Plerixafor, J2562

Plicamycin, J9270

Plumbing, **for home ESRD equipment,** A4870

Pneumatic

　appliance, E0655–E0673, L4350–*L4379*

　compressor, E0650–E0652

　splint, L4350–*L4379*

　ventricular assist device, Q0480–Q0505

Pneumatic **nebulizer**

　administration set, small volume, filtered, A7006

　administration set, small volume, nonfiltered, A7003

　administration set, small volume, nonfiltered, non-
　　disposable, A7005

　small volume, disposable, A7004

Pneumococcal

　vaccine, administration, G0009

Porfimer, J9600

Portable

　equipment transfer, R0070–R0076

　~~gaseous oxygen, K0741, K0742~~✖

　hemodialyzer system, E1635

　liquid oxygen system, E0433

　x-ray equipment, Q0092

Positioning **seat,** T5001

Positive **airway pressure device, accessories,**
　　A7030–A7039, E0561–E0562

Positive **expiratory pressure device,** E0484

Post-coital **examination,** Q0115

Postural **drainage board,** E0606

Potassium

　chloride, J3480

　hydroxide (KOH) preparation, Q0112

Pouch

　fecal collection, A4330

　ostomy, A4375–A4378, A5051–A5054, A5061–A5065

　urinary, A4379–A4383, A5071–A5075

Pralatrexate, J9307

*Practice, **guidelines, oncology,** G9056–G9062*

Pralidoxime **chloride,** J2730

Prednisolone

　acetate, J2650

　oral, J7506, J7510

Prednisone, J7506

Preparation **kits, dialysis,** A4914

Preparatory **prosthesis,** L5510–L5595

　chemotherapy, J8999

　nonchemotherapy, J8499

*Prescribing **privilege, eligible,** G8644*

Pressure

　alarm, dialysis, E1540

　pad, A4640, E0180–E0199

Privigen, J1459

Procainamide **HCl,** J2690

Procedure

　HALO, L0810–L0861

　noncovered, G0293, G0294

　scoliosis, L1000–L1499

Prochlorperazine, J0780

Prolotherapy, M0076

Promazine **HCl,** J2950

Promethazine

　HCl, J2550

　and meperdine, J2180

Prophylaxis

　DVT, documentation, G8218

　thrombosis, deep, vein, documentation, G8218

Propranolol **HCl,** J1800

*Prostate, **cancer, screening,** G0102, G0103*

Prosthesis

　artificial larynx battery/accessory, L8505

　breast, L8000–L8035, L8600

　eye, L8610, L8611, V2623–V2629

　fitting, L5400–L5460, L6380–L6388

　foot/ankle one piece system, L5979

　hand, L6000–L6020, L6025

　implants, L8600–L8690

　larynx, L8500

　lower extremity, L5700–L5999, L8640–L8642

　mandible, L8617

　maxilla, L8616

　maxillofacial, provided by a non-physician, L8040–
　　L8048

　miscellaneous service, L8499

　ocular, V2623–V2629

　repair of, L7520, L8049

　socks (shrinker, sheath, stump sock), L8400–L8485

　taxes, orthotic/prosthetic/other, L9999

◄ New　　← Revised　　✔ Reinstated　　~~deleted~~ Deleted

Prosthesis (*Continued*)
  tracheo-esophageal, L8507–L8509
  upper extremity, L6000–L6999
  vacuum erection system, L7900
Prosthetic **additions**
  lower extremity, L5610–L5999
  upper extremity, L6600–L7405
Protamine **sulfate**, J2720
Protectant, **skin**, A6250
Protector, **heel or elbow**, E0191
Protein **C Concentrate**, J2724
Protirelin, J2725
Pulse **generator**, E2120
Pump
  alternating pressure pad, E0182
  ambulatory infusion, E0781
  ambulatory insulin, E0784
  blood, dialysis, E1620
  breast, E0602–E0604
  enteral infusion, B9000, B9002
  external infusion, E0779
  heparin infusion, E1520
  implantable infusion, E0782, E0783
  implantable infusion, refill kit, A4220
  infusion, supplies, A4230, A4232
  negative pressure wound therapy, E2402
  parenteral infusion, B9004, B9006
  suction, portable, E0600
  water circulating pad, E0236
  wound, negative, pressure, E2402
Purification **system**, E1610, E1615
Pyridoxine **HCl**, J3415

Q

Quad **cane**, E0105
Quinupristin/dalfopristin, J2770

R

Rack/stand, **oxygen**, E1355
Radiesse, Q2026
Radioelements **for brachytherapy**, Q3001
Radiology **service**, R0070–R0076
Radiological, supplies, A4641, A4642
Radiopharmaceutical **diagnostic and therapeutic**
    imaging agent, A4641, A4642, A9500–A9699←
*Radiopharmaceutical, **therapeutic**, A9600, A9605*
*Radiosurgery, **stereotactic**, G0173, G0251, G0339,*
    G0340
Rail
  bathtub, E0241, E0242, E0246
  bed, E0305, E0310
  toilet, E0243
Ranibizumab, J2778
Rasburicase, J2783
Reaching/grabbing **device**, A9281

Reagent **strip**, A4252
Reciprocating **peritoneal dialysis system, E1630**
Reclast, J3488
*Reclining, **wheelchair**, E1014, E1050–E1070, E1100–*
    E1110
*Reconstruction, **angiography**, G0288*
Red **blood cells**, P9021, P9022
Regadenoson, J2785
Regular **insulin**, J1820
Regulator, **oxygen**, E1353
Rehabilitation
  cardiac, S9472, S9473
  program, H2001
  psychosocial, H2017, H2018
  services, G8699–G8701
  system, jaw, motion, E1700–E1702
  vestibular, S9476
*Removal, **cerumen**, G0268*
*Renal, **artery, angiography**, G0275*
Repair
  contract, ESRD, A4890
  maxillofacial prosthesis, L8049
  orthosis, L4000–L4130
  prosthetic, L7510
Replacement
  battery, A4630
  pad (alternating pressure), A4640
  tanks, dialysis, A4880
  tip for cane, crutches, walker, A4637
  underarm pad for crutches, A4635
*Reporting, **asthma measures group**, G8645, G8646*
RespiGam, *see* **Respiratory syncytial virus immune**
    globulin
Respiratory
  DME, A7000–A7527
  equipment, E0424–E0601
  function, therapeutic, procedure, G0237–G0239,
    S5180, S5181
  supplies, A4604–A4629
Restraint, **any type**, E0710
Reteplase, J2993
Revascularization, C9603–C9608
Rho(D) **immune globulin, human**, J2788, J2790,
    J2791, J2792
Rib **belt, thoracic**, A4572, L0220
Rilanocept, J2793
RimabotulinumtoxinB, J0587
Ringers **lactate infusion**, J7120
Ring, **ostomy**, A4404
*Risk-adjusted **functional status***
  elbow, wrist or hand, G8667–G8670
  hip, G8651-G8654
  knee, G8647–G8650
  lower leg, foot or ankle, G8655–G8658
  lumbar spine, G8659–G8662
  neck, cranium, mandible, thoracic spine, ribs, or
    other, G8671–G8674
  shoulder, G8663–G8666

◄ New   ← Revised   ✔ Reinstated   ~~deleted~~ Deleted

Risperidone, J2794
Rituximab, J9310
Robin-Aids, L6000, L6010, L6020, L6855, L6860
Rocking **bed,** E0462
Rollabout **chair,** E1031
Romidepsin, J9315
Romiplostim, J2796
Ropivacaine **HCl,** J2795
Rubidium **Rb-82,** A9555

S

Sacral **nerve stimulation test lead,** A4290
Safety **equipment,** E0700
  vest, wheelchair, E0980
Saline
  infusion, J7030–J7060
  solution, J7030–J7050, A4216–A4218
Saliva
  analysis, A0418
  artificial, A9155
Sargramostim **(GM-CSF),** J2820
Scoliosis, L1000–L1499
  additions, L1010–L1120, L1210–L1290
Screening
  alcohol misuse, G0442
  cancer, cervical or vaginal, G0101
  colorectal, cancer, G0104–G0106, G0120–G0122,
    G0328, S3890
  cytopathology cervical or vaginal, G0123, G0124,
    G0141–G0148
  depression, G0444
  dysphagia, documentation, G8232, V5364
  enzyme immunoassay, G0432
  glaucoma, G0117, G0118
  infectious agent antibody detection, G0433, G0435
  language, V5363
  prostate, cancer, G0102, G0103
  speech, V5362
Sculptra, Q2027
Sealant
  skin, A6250
Seat
  attachment, walker, E0156
  insert, wheelchair, E0992
  lift (patient), E0621, E0627–E0629
  upholstery, wheelchair, E0975
Secretin, J2850
Semen **analysis,** G0027
*Semi-reclining, **wheelchair,** E1100, E1110*
Sensitivity **study,** P7001
*Sensory **nerve conduction test,** G0255*
Sermorelin **acetate,** Q0515
Serum **clotting time tube,** A4771
Service
  hearing, V5000–V5999
  laboratory, P0000–P9999

Service (Continued)
  mental, health, training, G0177
  non-covered, A9270
  physician, for mobility device, G0372
  pulmonary, for LVRS, G0302–G0305
  speech-language, V5336–V5364
  vision, V2020–V2799
SEWHO, L3960–L3974
SEXA, G0130
Sheepskin **pad,** E0188, E0189
Shoes
  arch support, L3040–L3100
  for diabetics, A5500–A5508
  insert, L3000–L3030
  lift, L3300–L3334
  miscellaneous additions, L3500–L3595
  orthopedic, L3201–L3265
  positioning device, L3140–L3170
  transfer, L3600–L3649
  wedge, L3340–L3485
Shoulder
  disarticulation, prosthetic, L6300–L6320,
    L6550
  orthosis (SO), L3650–L3674
  spinal, cervical, L0100–L0200
Shoulder-elbow-wrist-hand **orthosis (SEWHO),**
  L3960–L3967
Shoulder **sling,** A4566
Shunt **accessory for dialysis,** A4740
  aqueous, L8612
Sigmoidoscopy, **cancer screening,** G0104,
  G0106
Sincalide, J2805
Sipuleucel-T, Q2043
Sirolimus, J7520
Sitz **bath,** E0160–E0162
Skin
  barrier, ostomy, A4362, A4363, A4369–A4373,
    A4385, A5120
  bond or cement, ostomy, A4364
  sealant, protectant, moisturizer, A6250
  substitute, Q4100–Q4136 ←
Sling, A4565
  patient lift, E0621, E0630, E0635
*Smear, **Papanicolaou, screening,** P3000, P3001,*
  Q0091
SNCT, G0255
*Social **worker, clinical, home, health,** G0155*
Social **worker, nonemergency transport,** A0160
Sock
  body sock, L0984
  prosthetic sock, L8420–L8435, L8470, L8480,
    L8485
  stump sock, L8470–L8485
Sodium
  chloride injection, J2912
  ferric gluconate complex in sucrose, J2916
  fluoride F-18, A9580

◄ New   ← Revised   ✔ Reinstated   ~~deleted~~ Deleted

Sodium *(Continued)*
  hyaluronate
    Euflexxa, J7323
    Hyalgan, J7321
    Orthovisc, J7324
    Supartz, J7321
    Synvisc and Synvisc-One, J7325
  phosphatc P32, A9563
  succinate, J1720
Solution
  calibrator, A4256
  dialysatc, A4760
  elliotts b, J9175
  enteral formulae, B4149–B4156
  parenteral nutrition, B4164–B5200
*Solvent, **adhesive remover,** A4455*
Somatrem, J2940
Somatropin, J2941
Sorbent cartridge, ESRD, E1636
*Special size, **wheelchair,** E1220–E1239*
Specialty absorptive dressing,
  A6251–A6256
Spectinomycin HCl, J3320
Speech assessment, V5362–V5364
Speech generating device, E2500–E2599
*Speech-Language, **services,** V5336–V5364*
*Speech, **pathologist,** G0153*
Spinal orthosis
  cervical, L0100, L0200
  cervical-thoracic-lumbar-sacral (CTLSO), L0700,
    L0710
  DME, K0112–K0116
  halo, L0810–L0830
  multiple post collar, L0180–L0200
  scoliosis, L1000–L1499
  torso supports, L0960
Splint, A4570, L3100, L4350–*L4379*
  ankle, L4390–L4398
  dynamic, E1800, E1805, E1810, E1815, E1825,
    E1830, E1840
  footdrop, L4398
  supplies, miscellaneous, Q4051
*Standard, **wheelchair,** E1130, K0001*
Static progressive stretch, E1801, E1806, E1811,
  E1816, E1818, E1821
Status
  disease, oncology, G9063–G9139
*Stent, **transcatheter, placement,** C9600, C9601,*
  S2211
Sterile cefuroxime sodium, J0697
Sterile water, A4216–A4217
*Stereotactic, **radiosurgery,** G0173, G0251, G0339,*
  G0340
Stimulators
  neuromuscular, E0744, E0745
  osteogenesis, electrical, E0747–E0749
  ultrasound, E0760
  salivary reflex, E0755

Stimulators *(Continued)*
  stoma absorptive cover, A5083
  transcutaneous, electric, nerve, A4595, E0720–E0749
Stockings
  gradient, compression, A6530–A6549
  surgical, A4490–A4510
Stomach tube, B4083
*Stool, **guaiac,** G0394*
Streptokinase, J2995
Streptomycin, J3000
Streptozocin, J9320
Strip, blood glucose test, A4253, A4772
  urine reagent, A4250
*Strontium-89 **chloride, supply of,** A9600*
*Study, **bone density,** G0130*
Stump sock, L8470–L8485
Stylet, A4212
*Substance/Alcohol, **assessment,** G0396, G0397,*
  H0001, H0003, H0049
Succinylcholine chloride, J0330
Suction pump
  gastric, home model, E2000
  portable, E0600
  respiratory, home model, E0600
Sumatriptan succinate, J3030
Supartz, J7321
Supply/accessory/service, A9900
Supplies
  battery, A4233–A4236, A4601, A4611–A4613, A4638
  cast, A4580, A4590, Q4001–Q4051
  catheters, A4300–A4306
  contraceptive, A4267–A4269
  diabetic shoes, A5500–A5513
  dialysis, A4653–A4927
  DME, other, A4630–A4640
  dressings, A6000–A6513
  enteral, therapy, B4000–B9999
  incontinence, A4310–A4355, A5102–5200
  infusion, A4221, A4222, A4230–A4232, E0776–E0791
  ostomy, A4361–A4434, A5051–A5093, A5120–A5200
  parenteral, therapy, B4000–B9999
  radiological, A4641, A4642
  respiratory, A4604–A4629
  splint, Q4051
  surgical, miscellaneous, A4649
  syringe, A4206–A4209, A4213, A4232
  urinary, external, A4356–A4360
Support
  arch, L3040–L3090
  cervical, L0100–L0200
  spinal, L0960
  stockings, L8100–L8239
Surgical
  arthroscopy, knee, G0289, S2112, S2113
  boot, L3208–L3211
  brush, dialysis, A4910
  dressing, A6196–A6406
  procedure, noncovered, G0293, G0294

◄ New   ← Revised   ✔ Reinstated   ~~deleted~~ Deleted

Surgical *(Continued)*
  stocking, A4490–A4510
  supplies, A4649
  tray, A4550
Swabs, betadine or iodine, A4247
Syringe, A4213
  with needle, A4206–A4209
Synvisc and Synvisc-One, J7325
System
  external, ambulatory insulin, A9274
  rehabilitation, jaw, motion, E1700–E1702
  transport, E1035–E1039

T

Tables, bed, E0274, E0315
Tacrolimus
  oral, J7507
  parenteral, J7525
Tape, A4450–A4452
Taxi, non emergency transportation, A0100
Team, conference, G0175, G9007, S0220, S0221
Technetium TC 99M
  Arcitumomab, A9568
  Bicisate, A9557
  Depreotide, A9536
  Disofenin, A9510
  Exametazine, A9521
  Exametazine labeled autologous white blood cells, A9569
  Fanolesomab, A9566
  Glucepatate, A9550
  Labeled red blood cells, A9560
  Macroaggregated albumin, A9540
  Mebrofenin, A9537
  Mertiatide, A9562
  Oxidronate, A9561
  Pentetate, A9539, A9567
  Pertechnetate, A9512
  Pyrophosphate, A9538
  Sestamibi, A9500
  Succimer, A9551
  Sulfur colloid, A9541
  Teboroxime, A9501
  Tetrofosmin, A9502
TEEV, J0900
Telavancin, J3095
Telehealth, Q3014
Telehealth transmission, T1014
Temozolomide
  injection, J9328
  oral, J8700
Temporary codes, Q0000–Q9999, S0009–S9999
Temsirolimus, J9330
Tenecteplase, J3101
Teniposide, Q2017
TENS, A4595, E0720–E0749

Tent, oxygen, E0455
Terbutaline sulfate, J3105
  inhalation solution, concentrated, J7680
  inhalation solution, unit dose, J7681
Teriparatide, J3110
Terminal devices, L6700–L6895
Test
  occult, blood, G0394
  sensory, nerve, conduction, G0255
Testosterone
  aqueous, J3140
  cypionate and estradiol cypionate, J1060
  enanthate, J3120, J3130
  enanthate and estradiol valerate, J0900
  propionate, J3150
  suspension, J3140
Tetanus immune globulin, human, J1670
Tetracycline, J0120
Thallous Chloride TL 201, A9505
Theophylline, J2810
Therapeutic lightbox, A4634, E0203
Therapy
  ACE/ARB, G8463–G8475
  activity, G0176
  electromagnetic, G0295, G0329
  enteral, supplies, B4000–B9999
  medical, nutritional, G0270, G0271
  occupational, H5300, *G0129, S9129*
  occupational, health, G0152
  respiratory, function, procedure, G0237–G0239, S5180, S5181
  parenteral, supplies, B4000–B9999
  speech, home, G0153, S9128
  wound, negative, pressure, pump, E2402
Theraskin, Q4121
Thermometer, A4931–A4932
  dialysis, A4910
Thiamine HCl, J3411
Thiethylperazine maleate, J3280
Thiotepa, J9340
Thoracic-lumbar-sacral orthosis (TLSO)
  scoliosis, L1200–L1290
  spinal, L0430–L0492
Thoracic orthosis, L0210
Thymol turbidity, blood, P2033
Thyrotropin Alfa, J3240
Tigecycline, J3243
Tinzarparin sodium, J1655
Tip (cane, crutch, walker) replacement, A4637
Tire, wheelchair, E0999
Tirofiban, J3246
Tissue marker, A4648
TLSO, L0430–L0492, L1200–L1290
Tobacco
  intervention, G9016
Tobramycin
  inhalation solution, unit dose, J7682, J7685
  sulfate, J3260

◀ New   ← Revised   ✔ Reinstated   ~~deleted~~ Deleted

Tocilizumab, J2362

Toe device, E1831

Toilet **accessories,** E0167–E0179, E0243, E0244, E0625

Tolazoline **HCl,** J2670

Toll, **non emergency transport,** A0170

Topical **hyperbaric oxygen chamber,** A4575

Topotecan, J8705, J9351

Torsemide, J3265

Tositumomab, administration and supply, G3001

Tracheostoma **heat moisture exchange system,** A7501–A7509

Tracheostomy
   care kit, A4629
   filter, A4481
   speaking valve, L8501
   supplies, A4623, A4629, A7523–A7524
   tube, A7520–A7522

Tracheotomy **mask or collar,** A7525–A7526

Traction
   cervical, E0855, E0856
   extremity, E0870–E0880
   device, ambulatory, E0830
   equipment, E0840–E0948
   pelvic, E0890, E0900, E0947

Training
   diabetes, outpatient, G0108, G0109
   home health or hospice, G0164
   services, mental, health, G0177

Transcatheter, placement, stent, S2211

Transcutaneous **electrical nerve stimulator (TENS),** E0720–E0770

Transducer **protector, dialysis,** E1575

Transfer **(shoe orthosis),** L3600–L3640

Transfer **system with seat,** E1035

Transplant
   islet, G0341–G0343, S2102

Transparent **film (for dressing),** A6257–A6259

Transport
   chair, E1035–E1039
   system, E1035–E1039
   x-ray, R0070–R0076

Transportation
   ambulance, A0021–A0999, Q3019, Q3020
   corneal tissue, V2785
   EKG (portable), R0076
   handicapped, A0130
   non emergency, A0080–A0210, T2001–T2005
   service, including ambulance, A0021–A0999, T2006
   taxi, non emergency, A0100
   toll, non emergency, A0170
   volunteer, non emergency, A0080, A0090
   x-ray (portable), R0070, R0075

Transtracheal **oxygen catheter,** A7018

Trapeze **bar,** E0910–E0912, E0940

Trauma, response, team, G0390

Tray
   insertion, A4310–A4316
   irrigation, A4320
   surgical (*see also* kits), A4550
   wheelchair, E0950

Treatment
   pediculosis (lice), A9180
   services, behavioral health, H0002–H2037

Treprostinil, J3285

Triamcinolone, J3301–J3303
   acetonide, J3300, J3301
   diacetate, J3302
   hexacetonide, J3303
   inhalation solution, concentrated, J7683
   inhalation solution, unit dose, J7684

Triflupromazine **HCl,** J3400

Trifocal, **glass or plastic,** V2300–V2399

Trimethobenzamide **HCl,** J3250

Trimetrexate **glucuoronate,** J3305

Trimming, nails, dystrophic, G0127

Triptorelin **pamoate,** J3315

Truss, L8300–L8330

Tube/Tubing
   anchoring device, A5200
   blood, A4750, A4755
   drainage extension, A4331
   gastrostomy, B4087, B4088
   irrigation, A4355
   larynectomy, A4622
   nasogastric, B4081, B4082
   oxygen, A4616
   serum clotting time, A4771
   stomach, B4083
   suction pump, each, A7002
   tire, K0091, K0093, K0095, K0097
   tracheostomy, A4622
   urinary drainage, K0280

U

Ultrasonic **nebulizer,** E0575

Ultrasound, G0389, S8055, S9024

Ultraviolet, cabinet/system, E0691–E0694

Ultraviolet **light therapy system,** A4633, E0691–E0694

Unclassified **drug,** J3490

Underpads, disposable, A4554

Unipuncture **control system, dialysis,** E1580

Upper **extremity addition, locking elbow,** L6693

Upper **extremity fracture orthosis,** L3980–L3999

Upper **limb prosthesis,** L6000–L7499

Urea, J3350

Ureterostomy **supplies,** A4454–A4590

Urethral **suppository, Alprostadil,** J0275

Urinal, E0325, E0326

◀ New   ← Revised   ✔ Reinstated   ~~deleted~~ Deleted

Urinary
catheter, A4338–A4346, A4351–A4353
collection and retention (supplies), A4310–A4360
incontinence, documentation, G8063, G8067
supplies, external, A4335, A4356–A4358
tract implant, collagen, L8603
tract implant, synthetic, L8606
Urine
sensitivity study, P7001
tests, A4250
Urofollitropin, J3355
Urokinase, J3364, J3365
Ustekinumab, J3357
U-V lens, V2755

V

Vabra aspirator, A4480
Vaccination, administration
hepatitis B, G0010
influenza virus, G0008
pneumococcal, G0009
Vaccine
administration, influenza, G0008
administration, pneumococcal, G0009
hepatitis B, administration, G0010
Vaginal
cancer, screening, G0101
cytopathology, G0123, G0124,
G0141–G0148
Vancomycin HCl, J3370
Vaporizer, E0605
Vascular
catheter (appliances and supplies), A4300–A4306
graft material, synthetic, L8670
Vasoxyl, J3390
Velaglucerase alfa, J3385
Venous pressure clamp, dialysis, A4918
Ventilator
battery, A4611–A4613
moisture exchanger, disposable, A4483
negative pressure, E0460
volume, stationary or portable, E0450, E0461–
E0464
Ventricular assist device, Q0478–Q0506
Verteporfin, J3396
Vest, safety, wheelchair, E0980
Vinblastine sulfate, J9360
Vincristine sulfate, J9370
Vinorelbine tartrate, J9390
Vision service, V2020–V2799
Visit, emergency department, G0380–G0384
Visual, function, postoperative cataract surgery,
G0915–G0918
Vitamin B-12 cyanocobalamin, J3420
Vitamin K, J3430

Voice
amplifier, L8510
prosthesis, L8511–L8514
Von Willebrand Factor Complex, human, J7183,
J7187
Voriconazole, J3465

W

Waiver, T2012–T2050
Walker, E0130–E0149
accessories, A4636, A4637
attachments, E0153–E0159
Walking splint, L4386
Washer, Gravlee jet, A4470
Water
dextrose, J7042, J7060, J7070
distilled (for nebulizer), A7018
pressure pad/mattress, E0187, E0198
purification system (ESRD), E1610, E1615
softening system (ESRD), E1625
sterile, A4714
WBC/CBC, G0306
Wedges, shoe, L3340–L3420
Wellness visit; annual, G0438, G0439
Wet mount, Q0111
Wheel attachment, rigid pickup walker, E0155
Wheelchair, E0950–E1298, K0001–K0108,
K0801–K0899
accessories, E0192, E0950–E1030, E1065–E1069,
E2211–E2230, E2300–E2399, *E2626–E2633*
amputee, E1170–E1200
back, fully reclining, manual, E1226
component or accessory, not otherwise specified,
K0108
cushions, E2601–E2625
heavy duty, E1280–E1298, K0006, K0007,
K0801–K0886
lightweight, E1087–E1090, E1240–E1270, E2618
narrowing device, E0969
power add-on, E0983–E0984
reclining, fully, E1014, E1050–E1070, E1100–E1110
semi-reclining, E1100, E1110
shock absorber, E1015–E1018
specially sized, E1220, E1230
standard, E1130, K0001
stump support system, K0551
tire, E0999
transfer board or device, E0705
tray, K0107
van, non-emergency, A0130
youth, E1091
WHFO with inflatable air chamber, L3807
WHO, wrist extension, L3914
Whirlpool equipment, E1300–E1310
Wig, A9282

◄ New   ← Revised   ✔ Reinstated   ~~deleted~~ Deleted

X

Y

Z

2013
TABLE OF DRUGS

IA	Intra-arterial administration
IV	Intravenous administration
IM	Intramuscular administration
IT	Intrathecal
SC	Subcutaneous administration
INH	Administration by inhaled solution
VAR	Various routes of administration
OTH	Other routes of administration
ORAL	Administered orally

Intravenous administration includes all methods, such as gravity infusion, injections, and timed pushes. The "VAR" posting denotes various routes of administration and is used for drugs that are commonly administered into joints, cavities, tissues, or topical applications, in addition to other parenteral administrations. Listings posted with "OTH" indicate other administration methods, such as suppositories or catheter injections.

Blue typeface terms are added by publisher.

DRUG NAME	DOSAGE	METHOD OF ADMINISTRATION	HCPCS CODE	
A				
Abatacept	10 mg	IV	**J0129**	←
Abbokinase	5,000 IU vial	IV	J3364	
	250,000 IU vial	IV	J3365	
Abbokinase, Open Cath	5,000 IU vial	IV	J3364	
Abciximab	10 mg	IV	**J0130**	
Abelcet	10 mg	IV	J0287	
Abilify	0.25 mg		J0400	
Ablavar	1 ml		A9583	
ABLC	50 mg	IV	J0285	
AbobotulinumtoxintypeA	5 units	IM	**J0586**	←
Abraxane	1 mg		J9264	
Accuneb	1 mg		J7613	
Acetadote	100 mg		J0132	
Acetaminophen	10 mg	IV	**J0131**	←
Acetazolamide sodium	up to 500 mg	IM, IV	**J1120**	
Acetylcysteine				
injection	100 mg	IV	**J0132**	←
unit dose form	per gram	INH	**J7604, J7608**	
Achromycin	up to 250 mg	IM, IV	J0120	
Actemra	1 mg		J3262	
ACTH	up to 40 units	IV, IM, SC	J0800	
Acthar	up to 40 units	IV, IM, SC	J0800	
Acthib			J3490	
Acthrel	1 mcg		J0795	
Actimmune	0.25 mg	SC	J1830	
	3 million units	SC	J9216	
Activase	1 mg	IV	J2997	
Acyclovir	5 mg		**J0133**	
			J8499	

◀ New   ← Revised   ✔ Reinstated   ~~deleted~~ Deleted

DRUG NAME	DOSAGE	METHOD OF ADMINISTRATION	HCPCS CODE	
Adagen	25 IU		J2504	
Adalimumab	20 mg	SC	**J0135**	←
Adcetis	1 mg	IV	J9042	◄
Adenocard	6 mg	IV	J0150	
	30 mg	IV	J0152	
Adenoscan	30 mg	IV	**J0152**	
Adenosine	6 mg	IV	**J0150**	
	30 mg	IV	**J0152**	
Adrenalin Chloride	up to 1 ml ampule	SC, IM	J0171	
Adrenalin, epinephrine	0.1 mg	SC, IM	**J0171**	
Adriamycin, PFS, RDF	10 mg	IV	J9000	
Adornaq-50	50 mg	IV	J3140	
Adrucil	500 mg	IV	J9190	
Advate	per IU		J7192	
Aflibercept	1 mg	OTH	**J0178**	◄
Agalsidase beta	1 mg	IV	**J0180**	
Aggrastat	0.25 mg	IM, IV	J3246	
Aglucosidase alfa	10 mg	IV	J0220	
A-hydroCort	up to 50 mg	IV, IM, SC	J1710	
	up to 100 m		J1720	
Akineton	per 5 mg	IM, IV	J0190	
Alatrofloxacin mesylate, injection	100 mg	IV	**J0200**	
Albumin			P9041, P9045 P9046, P9047	
Albuterol	0.5 mg	INH	**J7620**	
concentrated form	1 mg	INH	**J7610, J7611**	
unit dose form	1 mg	INH	**J7609, J7613**	
Aldesleukin	per single use vial	IM, IV	**J9015**	
Aldomet	up to 250 mg	IV	J0210	
Aldurazyme	0.1 mg		J1931	
Alefacept	0.5 mg	IM, IV	**J0215**	←
Alemtuzumab	10 mg	IV	**J9010**	←
Alferon N	250,000 IU	IM	J9215	
Alglucerase	per 10 units	IV	**J0205**	
Alglucosidase alfa	10 mg	IV	**J0220, J0221**	←
Alimta	10 mg		J9305	
Alkaban-AQ	1 mg	IV	J9360	
Alkeran	2 mg	ORAL	J8600	
	50 mg	IV	J9245	
Allopurinol Sodium			J9999	
Aloxi	25 mcg		J2469	
Alpha 1-proteinase inhibitor, human	10 mg	IV	**J0256 , J0257**	

◄ New   ← Revised   ✔ Reinstated   ~~deleted~~ Deleted

DRUG NAME	DOSAGE	METHOD OF ADMINISTRATION	HCPCS CODE
Alphanate			**J7186**
AlphaNine SD	per IU		J7193
Alprostadil			
injection	1.25 mcg	OTH injection	**J0270**
urethral suppository	EA	OTH	**J0275**
Alteplase recombinant	1 mg	IV	**J2997**
Alupent	per 10 mg	INH	**J7667, J7668**
noncompounded, unit dose	10 mg	INH	J7669
AmBisome	10 mg	IV	J0289
Amcort	per 5 mg	IM	J3302
A-methaPred	up to 40 mg	IM, IV	J2920
	up to 125 mg	IM, IV	J2930
Amevive	0.5 mg		J0215
Amgen	1 mcg	SC	J9212
Amifostine	500 mg	IV	**J0207**
Amikin	100 mg	IM, IV	J0278
Amikacin sulfate	100 mg	IM, IV	**J0278**
Aminocaproic Acid			J3490
Aminolevalinic acid HCl	unit dose (354 mg)	OTH	**J7308**
Aminolevulinate	1 g	OTH	**J7309**
Aminophylline	up to 250 mg	IV	**J0280**
Amiodarone HCl	30 mg	IV	**J0282**
Amitriptyline HCl	up to 20 mg	IM	**J1320**
Amobarbital	up to 125 mg	IM, IV	**J0300**
Amphadase	up to 150 units		J3470
Amphocin	50 mg	IV	J0285
Amphotec	10 mg	IV	J0288
Amphotericin B	50 mg	IV	**J0285**
Amphotericin B, lipid complex	10 mg	IV	**J0287–J0289**
Ampicillin			
sodium	up to 500 mg	IM, IV	**J0290**
sodium/sulbactam sodium	per 1.5 g	IM, IV	**J0295**
Amygdalin			J3570
Amytal	up to 125 mg	IM, IV	J0300
Anabolin LA 100	up to 50 mg	IM	J2320
Anadulafungin	1 mg	IV	**J0348** ←
Anascorp	up to 120 mg	IV	J0716 ◄
Ancef	500 mg	IV, IM	J0690
Andrest 90-4	up to 1 cc	IM	J0900
Andro-Cyp	up to 100 mg	IM	J1070
	1 cc, 200 mg	IM	J1080

◄ New   ← Revised   ✔ Reinstated   ~~deleted~~ Deleted

DRUG NAME	DOSAGE	METHOD OF ADMINISTRATION	HCPCS CODE
Andro-Cyp 200	up to 100 mg	IM	J1070
	1 cc, 200 mg	IM	J1080
Andro L.A. 200	up to 100 mg	IM	J3120
	up to 200 mg	IM	J3130
Andro-Estro 90-4	up to 1 cc	IM	J0900
Andro/Fem	up to 1 ml	IM	J1060
Androgyn L.A	up to 1 cc	IM	J0900
Androlone-50	up to 50 mg		J2320
Androlone-D 100	up to 50 mg	IM	J2320
Andronaq-50	up to 50 mg	IM	J3140
Andronaq-LA	up to 100 mg	IM	J1070
	1 cc, 200 mg	IM	J1080
Andronate-200	up to 100 mg	IM	J1070
	1 cc, 200 mg	IM	J1080
Andronate-100	up to 100 mg	IM	J1070
	1 cc, 200 mg	IM	J1080
Andropository 100	up to 100 mg	IM	J3120
	up to 200 mg	IM	J3130
Andryl 200	up to 100 mg	IM	J3120
	up to 200 mg	IM	J3130
Anectine	up to 20 mg	IM, IV	J0330
Anergan 25	up to 50 mg	IM, IV	J2550
	12.5 mg	ORAL	Q0169
	25 mg	ORAL	Q0170
Anergan 50	up to 50 mg	IM, IV	J2550
	12.5 mg	ORAL	Q0169
	25 mg	ORAL	Q0170
Angiomax	1 mg		J0583
Anidulafungin	1 mg	IV	J0348
Anistreplase	30 units	IV	**J0350**
Antiflex	up to 60 mg		J2360
Anti-Inhibitor	per IU	IV	**J7198**
Antispas	up to 20 mg	IM	J0500
Antithrombin III (human)	per IU	IV	**J7197**
Antithrombin recombinant	50 IU	IV	**J7196** ←
Antizol	15 mg		J1451
Anzemet	10 mg	IV	J1260
	50 mg	ORAL	S0174
	100 mg	ORAL	Q0180
A.P.L.	per 1,000 USP units	IM	J0725
Apokyn	1 mg		J0364
Apomorphine Hydrochloride	1 mg	SC	**J0364** ←

◀ New   ← Revised   ✔ Reinstated   deleted Deleted

DRUG NAME	DOSAGE	METHOD OF ADMINISTRATION	HCPCS CODE
Aprepitant	5 mg	ORAL	J8501
Apresoline	up to 20 mg	IV, IM	J0360
Aprotinin	10,000 kiu		**J0365**
AquaMEPHYTON	per 1 mg	IM, SC, IV	J3430
Aralast	10 mg	IV	J0256
Aralen	up to 250 mg	IM	J0390
Aramine	per 10 mg	IV, IM, SC	J0380
Aranesp			
ESRD use	1 mcg		J0882
Non-ESRD use	1 mcg		J0881
Arbutamine	1 mg	IV	**J0395**
Arcalyst	1 mg		J2793
Aredia	per 30 mg	IV	J2430
Arfonad, see Trimethaphan camsylate			
Arformoterol tartrate	15 mcg	INH	**J7605** ←
Aridol	25% in 50 ml	IV	J2150
	5 mg	INH	J7665
Arimidex			J8999
Aripiprazole	0.25 mg	IM	**J0400** ←
Aristocort Forte	per 5 mg	IM	J3302
Aristocort Intralesional	per 5 mg	IM	J3302
Aristopan	per 5 mg		J3303
Aristospan Intra-Articular	per 5 mg	VAR	J3303
Aristospan Intralesional	per 5 mg	VAR	J3303
Arixtra	per 0.5 m		J1652
Aromasin			J8999
Arranon	50 mg		J9261
Arrestin	up to 200 mg	IM	J3250
	250 mg	ORAL	Q0173
Arsenic trioxide	1 mg	IV	**J9017**
Arzerra	10 mg		J9302
Asparaginase	1,000 units	IV, IM	**J9019** ◄
	10,000 units	IV, IM	**J9020**
Astramorph PF	up to 10 mg	IM, IV, SC	J2270, J2275
	100 mg	IM, IV, SC	J2271
Atgam	250 mg	IV	J7504
Ativan	2 mg	IM, IV	J2060
Atropine			
concentrated form	per mg	INH	**J7635**
unit dose form	per mg	INH	**J7636**
sulfate	0.01 mg, per mg	IV, IM, SC	**J0461,** J7636
Atrovent	per mg	INH	J7644, J7645

◄ New   ← Revised   ✔ Reinstated   ~~deleted~~ Deleted

DRUG NAME	DOSAGE	METHOD OF ADMINISTRATION	HCPCS CODE	
Atryn	50 IU		J7196	
Aurothioglucose	up to 50 mg	IM	J2910	
Autologous cultured chondrocytes implant		OTH	J7330	←
Autoplex T	per IU	IV	J7198, J7199	
Avastin	10 mg		J9035	
Avelox	100 mg		J2280	
Avonex	11 mcg	IM	Q3025	
	11 mcg	SC	Q3026	
	33 mcg	IM	J1826	
Azacitidine	1 mg	SC	J9025	←
Azasan	50 mg		J7500	
Azathioprine	50 mg	ORAL	J7500	
Azathioprine				
parenteral	100 mg	IV	J7501	
dihydrate	1 gm	ORAL	Q0144	
injection	500 mg	IV	J0456	
Azithromycin	500 mg		J0456	
B				
Baci-RX			J3490	
Baciim			J3490	
Bacitracin			J3490	
Baclofen	10 mg	IT	J0475	
Baclofen for intrathecal trial	50 mcg	OTH	J0476	
Bacteriostatic	10 ml		A4216	
Bactocill	up to 250 mg	IM, IV	J2700	
BAL in oil	per 100 mg	IM	J0470	
Banflex	up to 60 mg	IV, IM	J2360	
Basiliximab	20 mg	IV	J0480	
Bayhep B			J3590	
BayRho-D	50 mcg		J2788	
BCG (Bacillus Calmette and Guérin), live	per vial	IV	J9031	
Bebulin VH	per IU		J7194	
Beclomethasone inhalation solution, unit dose form	per mg	INH	J7622, J7624	
Belatacept	1 mg	IV	J0485	◀
Belimumab	10 mg	IV	J0490	←
Bena-D 10	up to 50 mg	IV, IM	J1200	
Bena-D 50	up to 50 mg	IV, IM	J1200	
Benadryl	up to 50 mg	IV, IM	J1200	
Benahist 10	up to 50 mg	IV, IM	J1200	
Benahist 50	up to 50 mg	IV, IM	J1200	
Ben-Allergin-50	up to 50 mg	IV, IM	J1200	
	50 mg	ORAL	Q0163	

◀ New   ← Revised   ✔ Reinstated   ~~deleted~~ Deleted

DRUG NAME	DOSAGE	METHOD OF ADMINISTRATION	HCPCS CODE	
Bendamustine HCl	1 mg	IV	**J9033**	←
Benefix	per IU	IV	J7195	
Benlysta	10 mg		J0490	
Benoject-10	up to 50 mg	IV, IM	J1200	
Benoject-50	up to 50 mg	IV, IM	J1200	
Bentyl	up to 20 mg	IM	J0500	
Benzocaine			J3490	
Benztropine mesylate	per 1 mg	IM, IV	**J0515**	
Berinert, see C-1 esterase inhibitor				
Berubigen	up to 1,000 mcg	IM, SC	J3420	
Betalin 12	up to 1,000 mcg	IM, SC	J3420	
Betameth	per 3 mg	IM, IV	J0702	
Betamethasone acetate & betamethasone sodium phosphate	per 3 mg	IM	**J0702**	
Betamethasone inhalation solution, unit dose form	per mg	INH	**J7624**	
Betaseron	0.25 mg	SC	J1830	
Bethanechol chloride	up to 5 mg	SC	**J0520**	
Bevacizumab	10 mg	IV	**J9035**	←
Bicillin C-R	100,000 units		J0558	
Bicillin C-R 900/300	100,000 units	IM	J0558, J0561	
Bicillin L-A	100,000 units	IM	J0561	
BiCNU	100 mg	IV	J9050	
Biperiden lactate	per 5 mg	IM, IV	**J0190**	
Bitolterol mesylate				
concentrated form	per mg	INH	**J7628**	
unit dose form	per mg	INH	**J7629**	
Bivalirudin	1 mg	IV	**J0583**	←
Blenoxane	15 units	IM, IV, SC	J9040	
Bleomycin sulfate	15 units	IM, IV, SC	**J9040**	
Boniva	1 mg		J1740	
Bortezomib	0.1 mg	IV	**J9041**	←
Botox	1 unit		J0585	
Bravelle	75 IU		J3355	
Brentuximab Vedotin	1 mg	IV	**J9042**	◄
Brethine				
concentrated form	per 1 mg	INH	J7680	
unit dose	per 1 mg	INH	J7681	
	up to 1 mg	SC, IV	J3105	
Brevital Sodium			J3490	
Bricanyl Subcutaneous	up to 1 mg	SC, IV	J3105	
Brompheniramine maleate	per 10 mg	IM, SC, IV	**J0945**	
Broncho Saline	10 ml		A4216	
Bronkephrine, see Ethylnorepinephrine HCl				

◄ New   ← Revised   ✔ Reinstated   ~~deleted~~ Deleted

DRUG NAME	DOSAGE	METHOD OF ADMINISTRATION	HCPCS CODE	
Bronkosol				
concentrated form	per mg	INH	J7647, J7648	
unit dose form	per mg	INH	J7649, J7650	
Brovana			J7605, J7699	
Budesonide inhalation solution				
concentrated form	0.25 mg	INH	J7633, J7634	
unit dose form	0.5 mg	INH	J7626, J7627	
Bumetanide			J3490	
Bupivacaine			J3490	
Buprenorphine Hydrochloride	0.1 mg	IM	J0592	←
Busulfan	1 mg	IV	J0594	←
	2 mg	ORAL	J8510	
Butorphanol tartrate	1 mg		J0595	
C				
C1 Esterase Inhibitor	10 units	IV	J0597, J0598	←
Cabazitaxel	1 mg	IV	J9043	←
Cabergoline	0.25 mg	ORAL	J8515	
Cafcit	5 mg	IV	J0706	
Caffeine citrate	5 mg	IV	J0706	
Caine-1	10 mg	IV	J2001	
Caine-2	10 mg	IV	J2001	
Calcijex	0.1 mcg	IM	J0636	
Calcimar	up to 400 units	SC, IM	J0630	
Calcitonin-salmon	up to 400 units	SC, IM	J0630	
Calcitriol	0.1 mcg	IM	J0636	
Calcitriol in almond oil	0.1 mcg		J0636	
Calcium Disodium Versenate	up to 1,000 mg	IV, SC, IM	J0600	
Calcium folinate (Hungarian import)	per 50 mg		J0640	
Calcium gluconate	per 10 ml	IV	J0610	
Calcium glycerophosphate and calcium lactate	per 10 ml	IM, SC	J0620	
Caldolor	100 mg	IV	J1741	◄
Calphosan	per 10 ml	IM, SC	J0620	
Campath	10 mg		J9010	
Camptosar	20 mg	IV	J9206	
Canakinumab	1 mg	SC	J0638	←
Cancidas	5 mg		J0637	
Capecitabine	150 mg	ORAL	J8520	
	500 mg	ORAL	J8521	
Capsaicin patch	per 10 sq cm	OTH	J7335	
Carbocaine with Neo-Cobefrin	per 10 ml	VAR	J0670	
Carbocaine	per 10 ml	VAR	J0670	
Carboplatin	50 mg	IV	J9045	

◄ New   ← Revised   ✔ Reinstated   ~~deleted~~ Deleted

2013 TABLE OF DRUGS   B–C

DRUG NAME	DOSAGE	METHOD OF ADMINISTRATION	HCPCS CODE
Carimune	500 mg		J1566
Carmustine	100 mg	IV	J9050
Carnitor	per 1 g	IV	J1955
Carticel			J7330
Caspofungin acetate	5 mg	IV	J0637
Cathflo Activase	1 mg		J2997
Cayston, see Aztreonam			
Ceenu		ORAL	J8799, J8999
Cefadyl	up to 1 g	IV, IM	J0710
Cefazolin sodium	500 mg	IV, IM	J0690
Cefepime hydrochloride	500 mg	IV	J0692
Cefizox	per 500 mg	IM, IV	J0715
Cefotaxime sodium	per 1 g	IV, IM	J0698
Cefotetan			J3490
Cefoxitin sodium	1 g	IV, IM	J0694
Ceftazidime	per 500 mg	IM, IV	J0713
Cefteroline fosamil	1 mg		J0712
Ceftizoxime sodium	per 500 mg	IV, IM	J0715
Ceftriaxone sodium	per 250 mg	IV, IM	J0696
Cefuroxime sodium, sterile	per 750 mg	IM, IV	J0697
Celestone Soluspan	per 3 mg	IM	J0702
	per mg	ORAL	J7624
CellCept	250 mg	ORAL	J7517
Cel-U-Jec	per 4 mg	IM, IV	Q0511
Cenacort A-40	per 10 mg	IM	J3301
	per 5 mg		J3302
Cenacort Forte	per 5 mg	IM	J3302
Centruroides Immune F(ab)	up to 120 mg	IV	J0716 ◄
Cephalothin sodium	up to 1 g	IM, IV	J1890
Cephapirin sodium	up to 1 g	IV, IM	J0710
Ceprotin	10 IU		J2724
Cerebyx	50 mg		Q2009
Ceredase	per 10 units	IV	J0205
Cerezyme	10 units		J1786
Certolizumab pegol	1 mg	SC	J0718 ←
Cerubidine	10 mg	IV	J9150
Cetuximab	10 mg	IV	J9055 ←
Chealamide	per 150 mg	IV	J3520
Chirhostim	1 mcg	IV	J2850
Chloramphenicol sodium succinate	up to 1 g	IV	J0720
Chlordiazepoxide HCl	up to 100 mg	IM, IV	J1990
Chloromycetin Sodium Succinate	up to 1 g	IV	J0720

◄ New   ← Revised   ✔ Reinstated   deleted Deleted

DRUG NAME	DOSAGE	METHOD OF ADMINISTRATION	HCPCS CODE
Chloroprocaine HCl	per 30 ml	VAR	J2400
	10 mg	ORAL	Q0171
	25 mg	ORAL	Q0172
	up to 50 mg	IM, IV	J3230
Chloroquine HCl	up to 250 mg	IM	J0390
Chlorothiazide sodium	per 500 mg	IV	J1205
Chlorpromazine HCl	up to 50 mg	IM, IV	J3230
	10 mg	ORAL	Q0171
	25 mg	ORAL	Q0172
Cholografin Meglumine	per ml		Q9961
Chorex-5	per 1,000 USP units	IM	J0725
Chorex-10	per 1,000 USP units	IM	J0725
Chorignon	per 1,000 USP units	IM	J0725
Chorionic gonadotropin	per 1,000 USP units	IM	J0725
Choron 10	per 1,000 USP units	IM	J0725
Cidofovir	375 mg	IV	J0740
Cimzia	1 mg		J0718
Cinryze	10 units		J0598
Cilastatin sodium, imipenem	per 250 mg	IV, IM	J0743
Cimetidine HCl			J3490
Cipro IV	200 mg	IV	J0706
Ciprofloxacin	200 mg	IV	J0706
			J3490
Cisplatin, powder or solution	per 10 mg	IV	J9060
Cladribine	per mg	IV	J9065
Claforan	per 1 gm	IM, IV	J0698
Cleocin Phosphate			J3490
Clincacort	per 5 mg		J3302
Clofarabine	1 mg	IV	J9027 ←
Clolar	1 mg		J9027
Clonidine Hydrochloride	1 mg	epidural	J0735
Cobex	up to 1,000 mcg	IM, SC	J3420
Cobulin-M	up to 1,000 mcg		J3420
Codeine phosphate	per 30 mg	IM, IV, SC	J0745
Codimal-A	per 10 mg	IM, SC, IV	J0945
Cogentin	per 1 mg	IM, IV	J0515
Colchicine	per 1 mg	IV	J0760
Colistimethate sodium	up to 150 mg	IM, IV	J0770, S0142
Collagenase, Clostridium Histolyticum	0.01 mg	OTH	J0775 ←
Coly-Mycin M	up to 150 mg	IM, IV	J0770
Compa-Z	up to 10 mg	IM, IV	J0780

◀ New   ← Revised   ✔ Reinstated   ~~deleted~~ Deleted

DRUG NAME	DOSAGE	METHOD OF ADMINISTRATION	HCPCS CODE
Compazine	up to 10 mg	IM, IV	J0780, J8498
	5 mg	ORAL	Q0164
	10 mg	ORAL	Q0165
Compro			J8498
Comptosar	20 mg		J9206
Conray	per ml		Q9961
Conray 30	per ml		Q9958
Conray 43	per ml		Q9960
Copaxone	20 mg		J1595
Cophene-B	per 10 mg	IM, SC, IV	J0945
Copper contraceptive, intrauterine		OTH	J7300
Cordarone	30 mg	IV	J0282
Corgonject-5	per 1,000 USP units	IM	J0725
Corticorelin ovine triflutate	1 mcg		J0795
Corticotropin	up to 40 units	IV, IM, SC	J0800
Cortisone Acetate			J3490
Cortrosyn	per 0.25 mg	IM, IV	J0835
Corvert	1 mg		J1742
Cosmegen	0.5 mg	IV	J9120
Cosyntropin	per 0.25 mg	IM, IV	J0833, J0834
Cotolone	up to 1 ml		J2650
	per 5 mg		J7510
Cotranzine	up to 10 mg	IM, IV	J0780
Crofab	up to 1 gram		J0840
Cromolyn sodium, unit dose form	per 10 mg	INH	J7631, J7632
Crotalidae Polyvalent Immune Fab	up to 1 gram	IV	J0840
Crysticillin 300 A.S.	up to 600,000 units	IM, IV	J2510
Crysticillin 600 A.S.	up to 600,000 units	IM, IV	J2510
Cubicin	1 mg		J0878
Cyanocobalamin	up to 1,000 mcg		J3420
Cyclophosphamide	100 mg	IV	J9070
oral	25 mg	ORAL	J8530
Cyclosporine	25 mg	ORAL	J7515, J7516
	100 mg	ORAL	J7502
parenteral	250 mg	IV	J7516
Cymetra	1 cc		Q4112
Cyomin	up to 1,000 mcg		J3420
Cysto-Cornray LI	per ml		Q9958
Cystografin	per ml		Q9958
Cystografin-Dilute	per ml		Q9958
Cytarabine	100 mg	SC, IV	J9100
Cytarabine liposome	10 mg	IT	J9098

◄ New   ← Revised   ✔ Reinstated   ~~deleted~~ Deleted

DRUG NAME	DOSAGE	METHOD OF ADMINISTRATION	HCPCS CODE	
CytoGam	per vial		J0850	
Cytomegalovirus immune globulin intravenous (human)	per vial	IV	**J0850**	
Cytosar-U	100 mg	SC, IV	J9100	
Cytovene	500 mg	IV	J1570	
Cytoxan	100 mg	IV	J8530, J9070	
D				
D-5-W, infusion	1000 cc	IV	**J7070**	
Dacarbazine	100 mg	IV	**J9130**	
Daclizumab	25 mg	IV	**J7513**	
Dactinomycin	0.5 mg	IV	**J9120**	
Dalalone	1 mg	IM, IV, OTH	J1100	
Dalalone L.A	1 mg	IM	J1094	
Dalteparin sodium	per 2500 IU	SC	**J1645**	
Daptomycin	1 mg	IV	**J0878**	←
Darbepoetin Alfa	1 mcg	IV, SC	**J0881, J0882**	←
Daunorubicin citrate, liposomal formulation	10 mg	IV	**J9151**	
Daunorubicin HCl	10 mg	IV	**J9150**	
Daunoxome	10 mg	IV	J9151	
DDAVP	1 mcg	IV, SC	J2597	
Decadron Phosphate	1 mg	IM, IV, OTH	J1100	
Decadron	1 mg	IM, IV, OTH	J1100	
	0.25 mg		J8540	
Decadron-LA	1 mg	IM	J1094	
Deca-Durabolin	up to 50 mg	IM	J2320	
Decaject	1 mg	IM, IV, OTH	J1100	
Decaject-L.A.	1 mg	IM	J1094	
Decitabine	1 mg	IV	**J0894**	←
Decolone-50	up to 50 mg	IM	J2320	
Decolone-100	up to 50 mg	IM	J2320	
De-Comberol	up to 1 ml	IM	J1060	
Deferoxamine mesylate	500 mg	IM, SC, IV	**J0895**	
Definity	per ml		J3490, Q9957	
Degarelix	1 mg	SC	**J9155**	←
Dehist	per 10 mg	IM, SC, IV	J0945	
Deladumone OB	up to 1 cc	IM	J0900	
Deladumone	up to 1 cc	IM	J0900	
Delatest	up to 100 mg	IM	J0990, J3120	
	up to 200 mg	IM	J3130	
Delatestadiol	up to 1 cc	IM	J0900	
Delatestryl	up to 100 mg	IM	J3120	
	up to 200 mg	IM	J3130	
Delta-Cortef	5 mg	ORAL	J7510	

◀ New   ← Revised   ✔ Reinstated   ~~deleted~~ Deleted

DRUG NAME	DOSAGE	METHOD OF ADMINISTRATION	HCPCS CODE	
Delestrogen	up to 10 mg	IM	J1380	
Demadex	10 mg/ml	IV	J3265	
Demerol HCl	per 100 mg	IM, IV, SC	J2175	
Denileukin diftitox	300 mcg	IV	**J9160**	←
Denosumab	1 mg	SC	**J0897**	←
DepAndro 100	up to 100 mg	IM	J1070	
	1 cc, 200 mg	IM	J1080	
	up to 100 mg		J3150	
DepAndro 200	up to 100 mg	IM	J1070	
	1 cc, 200 mg	IM	J1080	
DepAndrogyn	up to 1 ml	IM	J1060	
DepGynogen	up to 5 mg	IM	J1000	
DepoCyt	10 mg		J9098	
DepMedalone 40	20 mg	IM	J1020	
	40 mg	IM	J1030	
	80 mg	IM	J1040	
DepMedalone 80	20 mg	IM	J1020	
	40 mg	IM	J1030	
	80 mg	IM	J1040	
Depo-estradiol cypionate	up to 5 mg	IM	**J1000**	
Depogen	up to 5 mg	IM	J1000	
Depoject	20 mg	IM	J1020	
	40 mg	IM	J1030	
	80 mg	IM	J1040	
Depo-Medrol	20 mg	IM	J1020	
	40 mg	IM	J1030	
	80 mg	IM	J1040	
Depopred-40	20 mg	IM	J1020	
	40 mg	IM	J1030	
	80 mg	IM	J1040	
Depopred-80	20 mg	IM	J1020	
	40 mg	IM	J1030	
	80 mg	IM	J1040	
Depotest	up to 100 mg	IM	J1070	
	1 cc, 200 mg	IM	J1080	
Depo-Testadiol	up to 1 ml	IM	J1060	
Depotestrogen	up to 1 ml	IM	J1060	
Depo-Testosterone	1 cc, 200 mg	IM	J1080	
	up to 100 mg	IM	J1070, J3120	
Dermagraft	per square centimeter		Q4106	
Desferal Mesylate	500 mg	IM, SC, IV	J0895	

◀ New   ← Revised   ✔ Reinstated   ~~deleted~~ Deleted

DRUG NAME	DOSAGE	METHOD OF ADMINISTRATION	HCPCS CODE
Desmopressin acetate	1 mcg	IV, SC	J2597
Dexacen LA-8	1 mg	IM	J1094
Dexacen-4	1 mg	IM, IV, OTH	J1100
Dexamethasone			
concentrated form	per mg	INH	J7637
intravitreal implant	0.1 mg	OTH	J7312
unit form	per mg	INH	J7638
oral	0.25 mg	ORAL	J8540
	1 mg		J1100
Dexamethasone acetate	1 mg	IM	J1094
Dexamethasone sodium phosphate	1 mg	IM, IV, OTH	J1100, J7638
Dexasone	1 mg	IM, IV, OTH	J1100
Dexasone L.A.	1 mg	IM	J1094
Dexferrum	50 mg		J1750
Dexone	0.25 mg	ORAL	J8540
	1 mg	IM, IV, OTH	J1100
Dexone LA	1 mg	IM	J1094
Dexpak	0.25 mg	ORAL	J8540
Dexrazoxane hydrochloride	250 mg	IV	J1190
Dextran 40	500 ml	IV	J7100
Dextran 70	500 ml		J7110
Dextran 75	500 ml	IV	J7110
Dextrose 5%/normal saline solution	500 ml = 1 unit	IV	J7042
Dextrose/water (5%)	500 ml = 1 unit	IV	J7060
D.H.E. 45	per 1 mg		J1110
Diamox	up to 500 mg	IM, IV	J1120
Diazepam	up to 5 mg	IM, IV	J3360
Diazoxide	up to 300 mg	IV	J1730
Dibent	up to 20 mg	IM	J0500
Dicyclocot	up to 20 mg		J0500
Dicyclomine HCl	up to 20 mg	IM	J0500
Didronel	per 300 mg	IV	J1436
Diethylstilbestrol diphosphate	250 mg	IV	J9165
Diflucan	200 mg	IV	J1450
Digibind	per vial		J1162
DigiFab	per vial		J1162
Digoxin	up to 0.5 mg	IM, IV	J1160
Digoxin immune fab (ovine)	per vial		J1162
Dihydrex	up to 50 mg	IV, IM	J1200
	50 mg	ORAL	Q0163
Dihydroergotamine mesylate	per 1 mg	IM, IV	J1110

◄ New   ← Revised   ✔ Reinstated   ~~deleted~~ Deleted

DRUG NAME	DOSAGE	METHOD OF ADMINISTRATION	HCPCS CODE
Dilantin	per 50 mg	IM, IV	J1165
Dilaudid	up to 4 mg	SC, IM, IV	J1170
	250 mg	OTH	S0092
Dilocaine	10 mg	IV	J2001
Dilomine	up to 20 mg	IM	J0500
Dilor	up to 500 mg	IM	J1180
Dimenhydrinate	up to 50 mg	IM, IV	J1240
Dimercaprol	per 100 mg	IM	J0470
Dimethyl sulfoxide	50%, 50 ml	OTH	J1212
Dinate	up to 50 mg	IM, IV	J1240
Dioval	up to 10 mg	IM	J1380
Dioval 40	up to 10 mg	IM	J1380
Dioval XX	up to 10 mg	IM	J1380
Diphenacen-50	up to 50 mg	IV, IM	J1200
	50 mg	ORAL	Q0163
Diphenhydramine HCl			
injection	up to 50 mg	IV, IM	J1200
oral	50 mg	ORAL	Q0163
Diprivan			J3490
Dipyridamole	per 10 mg	IV	J1245
Disotate	per 150 mg	IV	J3520
Di-Spaz	up to 20 mg	IM	J0500
Ditate-DS	up to 1 cc	IM	J0900
Diruril	per 500 mg	IV	J1205
Diuril Sodium	per 500 mg	IV	J1205
D-Med 80	20 mg	IM	J1020
	40 mg	IM	J1030
	80 mg	IM	J1040
DMSO, Dimethyl sulfoxide 50%	50 ml	OTH	J1212
Dobutamine HCl	per 250 mg	IV	J1250
Dobutrex	per 250 mg	IV	J1250
Docefrez	1 mg		J9171
Docetaxel	20 mg	IV	J9171
Dolasetron mesylate			
injection	10 mg	IV	J1260
tablets	100 mg	ORAL	Q0180
Dolophine HCl	up to 10 mg	IM, SC	J1230
Dommanate	up to 50 mg	IM, IV	J1240
Donbax	10 mg		J1267
Dopamine	40 mg		J1265
Dopamine HCl	40 mg		J1265

◄ New   ← Revised   ✔ Reinstated   ~~deleted~~ Deleted

DRUG NAME	DOSAGE	METHOD OF ADMINISTRATION	HCPCS CODE	
Doribax	10 mg		J1267	
Doripenem	10 mg	IV	**J1267**	←
Dornase alpha, unit dose form	per mg	INH	**J7639**	
Doxercalciferol	1 mcg	IV	**J1270**	
Doxil	10 mg	IV	Q2048	
Doxorubicin				
HCl	10 mg	IV	**J9000**	
HCl, all lipid	10 mg	IV	**J9002**	←
Dramamine	up to 50 mg	IM, IV	J1240	
Dramanate	up to 50 mg	IM, IV	J1240	
Dramilin	up to 50 mg	IM, IV	J1240	
Dramocen	up to 50 mg	IM, IV	J1240	
Dramoject	up to 50 mg	IM, IV	J1240	
Dronabinol	2.5 mg	ORAL	**Q0167**	
	5 mg	ORAL	**Q0168**	
Droperidol	up to 5 mg	IM, IV	**J1790**	
Droxia		ORAL	J8999	
Drug administered through a metered dose inhaler		INH	**J3535**	
Droperidol and fentanyl citrate	up to 2 ml ampule	IM, IV	**J1810**	
DTIC-Dome	100 mg	IV	J9130	
Dua-Gen L.A.	up to 1 cc		J0900	
DuoNeb	up to 2.5 mg		J7620	
	up to 0.5 mg		J7620	
Duoval P.A.	up to 1 cc	IM	J0900	
Durabolin	up to 50 mg	IM	J2320	
Duraclon	1 mg	epidural	J0735	
Dura-Estrin	up to 5 mg	IM	J1000	
Duracillin A.S.	up to 600,000 units	IM, IV	J2510	
Duragen-10	up to 10 mg	IM	J1380	
Duragen-20	up to 10 mg	IM	J1380	
Duragen-40	up to 10 mg	IM	J1380	
Duralone-40	20 mg	IM	J1020	
	40 mcg	IM	J1030	
	80 mg	IM	J1040	
Duralone-80	20 mg	IM	J1020	
	40 mg	IM	J1030	
	80 mg	IM	J1040	
Duralutin, see Hydroxyprogesterone Caproate				
Duramorph	10 mg	IM, IV, SC	J2275	
	up to 10 mg	IM, IV, SC	J2270	
	100 mg	OTH	J2271	

◀ New   ← Revised   ✔ Reinstated   d̶e̶l̶e̶t̶e̶d̶ Deleted

DRUG NAME	DOSAGE	METHOD OF ADMINISTRATION	HCPCS CODE	
Duratest-100	up to 100 mg	IM	J1070	
	1 cc, 200 mg	IM	J1080	
Duratest-200	up to 100 mg	IM	J1070	
	1 cc, 200 mg	IM	J1080	
Duratestrin	up to 1 ml	IM	J1060	
Durathate-200	up to 100 mg	IM	J3120	
	up to 200 mg	IM	J3130	
Dymenate	up to 50 mg	IM, IV	J1240	
Dyphylline	up to 500 mg	IM	**J1180**	
Dysport	5 units		J0586	
E				
Ecallantide	1 mg	SC	**J1290**	←
Eculizumab	10 mg	IV	**J1300**	←
Edetate calcium disodium	up to 1,000 mg	IV, SC, IM	**J0600**	
Edetate disodium	per 150 mg	IV	**J3520**	
Elaprase	1 mg		J1743	
Elavil	up to 20 mg	IM	J1320	
Eligard	7.5 mg		J9217	
Elitek	0.5 mg		J2783	
Ellence	2 mg		J9178	
Elliotts b solution	1 ml	OTH	**J9175**	
Eloxatin	0.5 mg		J9263	
Elspar	10,000 units	IV, IM	J9020	
Emend	1 mg		J1453	
Ememd	5 mg	ORAL	J8501	
Emete-Con, see Benzquinamide				
Eminase	30 units	IV	J0350	
Enbrel	25 mg	IM, IV	J1438	
Endrate ethylenediamine-tetra-acetic acid	per 150 mg	IV	J3520	
Enfuvirtide	1 mg	SC	**J1324**	←
Enovil	up to 20 mg	IM	J1320	
Enoxaparin sodium	10 mg	SC	**J1650**	
Eovist	1 ml		A9581	
Epinephrine, adrenalin	0.1 mg	SC, IM	**J0171**	
Epirubicin hydrochloride	2 mg		**J9178,** J7799	
Epoetin alfa	1,000 units	IV, SC	J0885, J0886, **Q4081**	←
Epogen	1,000 units		J0885	
			J0886	
			Q4081	
Epoprostenol	0.5 mg	IV	**J1325**	
Eptifibatide, injection	5 mg	IM, IV	**J1327**	

◀ New   ← Revised   ✔ Reinstated   ~~deleted~~ Deleted

DRUG NAME	DOSAGE	METHOD OF ADMINISTRATION	HCPCS CODE	
Eraxis	1 mg	IV	J0348	
Erbitux	10 mg		J9055	
Ergonovine maleate	up to 0.2 mg	IM, IV	**J1330**	
Eribulin mesylate	0.1 mg	IV	**J9179**	←
Ertapenem sodium	500 mg	IM, IV	**J1335**	←
Erwinase	1,000 units	IV, IM	J9019	◄
	10,000 units	IV, IM	J9020	◄
Erythromycin lactobionate	500 mg	IV	**J1364**	
Estra-D	up to 5 mg	IM	J1000	
Estra-L 20	up to 10 mg	IM	J1380	
	up to 40 mg	IM	J1370	
Estra-L 40	up to 10 mg	IM	J1380	
	up to 40 mg	IM	J1370	
Estra-Testrin	up to 1 cc	IM	J0900	
Estradiol Cypionate	up to 5 mg	IM	J1000, J1060	
Estradiol				
L.A.	up to 10 mg	IM	J1380	
	up to 40 mg	IM	J1370	
L.A. 20	up to 10 mg	IM	J1380	
	up to 40 mg	IM	J1370	
L.A. 40	up to 10 mg	IM	J1380	
	up to 40 mg	IM	J1370	
Estradiol valerate	up to 10 mg	IM	**J1380**	
Estragyn 5	per 1 mg		J1435	
Estro-Cyp	up to 5 mg	IM	J1000	
Estrogen, conjugated	per 25 mg	IV, IM	**J1410**	
Estroject L.A.	up to 5 mg	IM	J1000	
Estrone	per 1 mg	IM	**J1435**	
Estrone 5	per 1 mg	IM	J1435	
Estrone Aqueous	per 1 mg	IM	J1435	
Estronol	per 1 mg	IM	J1435	
Estronol-L.A.	up to 5 mg	IM	J1000	
Etanercept, injection	25 mg	IM, IV	**J1438**	
Ethamolin	100 mg		J1430	
Ethanolamine	100 mg		J1430, J3490	
Ethyol	500 mg	IV	J0207	
Etidronate disodium	per 300 mg	IV	**J1436**	
Etonogestrel implant			**J7307**	
Etopophos	10 mg	IV	J9181	
Etoposide	10 mg	IV	**J9181**	
oral	50 mg	ORAL	**J8560**	
Euflexxa	per dose	OTH	**J7323**	←

◄ New   ← Revised   ✔ Reinstated   ~~deleted~~ Deleted

DRUG NAME	DOSAGE	METHOD OF ADMINISTRATION	HCPCS CODE	
Everolimus	0.25 mg	ORAL	**J7527**	←
Everone	up to 100 mg	IM	J3120	
	up to 200 mg	IM	J3130	
Eylea			J0178	
Eylen	1 mg	OTH	J0178	◄
F				
Fabrazyme	1 mg	IV	J0180	
Factor VIIa (coagulation factor, recombinant)	1 mcg	IV	**J7189**	
Factor VIII (anti-hemophilic factor)				
human	per IU	IV	**J7190**	
porcine	per IU	IV	**J7191**	
recombinant	per IU	IV	**J7185, J7192**	
Factor IX				
anti-hemophilic factor, purified, non-recombinant	per IU	IV	**J7193**	
anti-hemophilic factor, recombinant	per IU	IV	**J7195**	
complex	per IU	IV	**J7194**	
Factors, other hemophilia clotting	per IU	IV	**J7196**	
Factrel	per 100 mcg	SC, IV	J1620	
Famotidine			J3490	
Faraheme	1 mg		Q0138, Q0139	
Faslodex	25 mg		J9395	
Feiba VH Immuno	per IU	IV	J7196	
Fentanyl citrate	0.1 mg	IM, IV	**J3010**	
Ferrlecit	12.5 mg		J2916	
Ferumoxytol	1 mg		**Q0138, Q0139**	
Filgrastim (G-CSF)	300 mcg	SC, IV	**J1440**	
	480 mcg	SC, IV	**J1441**	
Firazyr	1 mg	SC	J1744	◄
Firmagon	1 mg		J9155	
Flebogamma	500 mg	IV	**J1572**	
	1 cc		J1460	
Flexoject	up to 60 mg	IV, IM	J2360	
Flexon	up to 60 mg	IV, IM	J2360	
Flolan	0.5 mg	IV	J1325	
Floxuridine	500 mg	IV	**J9200**	
Fluconazole	200 mg	IV	**J1450**	
Fludara	1 mg	ORAL	J8562	
	50 mg	IV	J9185	
Fludarabine phosphate	50 mg	IV	**J9185**	
Flunisolide inhalation solution, unit dose form	per mg	INH	**J7641**	
Fluocinolone		OTH	**J7311**	←
Fluorouracil	500 mg	IV	**J9190**	

◄ **New**   ← **Revised**   ✔ **Reinstated**   ~~deleted~~ **Deleted**

DRUG NAME	DOSAGE	METHOD OF ADMINISTRATION	HCPCS CODE	
Fluphenazine decanoate	up to 25 mg		J2680	
Flutamide			J8999	
Folex	5 mg	IA, IM, IT, IV	J9250	
	50 mg	IA, IM, IT, IV	J9260	
Folex PFS	5 mg	IA, IM, IT, IV	J9250	
	50 mg	IA, IM, IT, IV	J9260	
Follutein	per 1,000 USP units	IM	J0725	
Folotyn	1 mg		J9307	
Fomepizole	15 mg		J1451	
Fomivirsen sodium	1.65 mg	Intraocular	J1452	
Fondaparinux sodium	0.5 mg	SC	J1652	←
Formoterol	12 mcg	INH	J7640	
Formoterol fumarate	20 mcg	INH	J7606	←
	12 mcg		J7640	
Fortaz	per 500 mg	IM, IV	J0713	
Forteo	10 mcg		J3110	
Fosaprepitant	1 mg	IV	J1453	←
Foscarnet sodium	per 1,000 mg	IV	J1455	
Foscavir	per 1,000 mg	IV	J1455	
Fosphenytoin	50 mg	IV	Q2009	←
Fragmin	per 2,500 IU		J1645	
FUDR	500 mg	IV	J9200	
Fulvestrant	25 mg	IM	J9395	←
Fungizone intravenous	50 mg	IV	J0285	
Furomide M.D.	up to 20 mg	IM, IV	J1940	
Furosemide	up to 20 mg	IM, IV	J1940	
Fuzeon	1 mg		J1324	
G				
Gablofen	10 mg		J0475	
	50 mcg		J0476	
Gadavist	0.1 ml		A9585	
Gadoxetate disodium	1 ml	IV	A9581	←
Gallium nitrate	1 mg	IV	J1457	←
Galsulfase	1 mg	IV	J1458	←
Gamastan	1 cc	IM	J1460	
	over 10 cc	IM	J1560	
Gammagard Liquid	500 mg	IV	J1569	←
Gammagard S/D			J1566	
Gamma globulin	1 cc	IM	J1460	
	over 10 cc	IM	J1560	
Gammaplex	500 mg	IV	J1557	←

◄ New   ← Revised   ✔ Reinstated   ~~deleted~~ Deleted

DRUG NAME	DOSAGE	METHOD OF ADMINISTRATION	HCPCS CODE	
GammaGraft	per square centimeter		Q4111	
Gammar	1 cc	IM	J1460	
	over 10 cc	IM	J1560	
Gammar-IV, see Immune globin intravenous (human)				
Gamulin RH				
immune globulin, human	100 IU		J2791	
	1 dose package, 300 mcg	IM	J2790	
immune globulin, human, solvent detergent	100 IU	IV	J2792	
Gamunex	500 mg	IV	J1561	←
Ganciclovir, implant	4.5 mg	OTH	J7310	
Ganciclovir sodium	500 mg	IV	J1570	
Ganirelix			J3490	
Ganite	1 mg		J1457	
Garamycin, gentamicin	up to 80 mg	IM, IV	J1580	
Gastrografin	per ml		Q9963	
Gastromark	per 100 ml		Q9954	
Gatifloxacin	10 mg	IV	J1590	
Gefitinib	250 mg	ORAL	J8565	←
Gel-One	per dose	OTH	J7326	←
Gemcitabine HCl	200 mg	IV	J9201	
Gemsar	200 mg	IV	J9201	
Gemtuzumab ozogamicin	5 mg	IV	J9300	
Gengraf	100 mg		J7502	
	25 mg	ORAL	J7515	
	250 mg		J7516	
Gentamicin Sulfate	up to 80 mg	IM, IV	J1580, J7699	
Gentran	500 ml	IV	J7100	
Gentran 75	500 ml	IV	J7110	
Gentropin	1 mg		J2941	
Geodon	10 mg		J3486	
Geref Diagnostic	1 mcg		Q0515	
Gesterol 50	per 50 mg		J2675	
Glassia	10 mg	IV	J0257	←
Glatiramer Acetate	20 mg	SC	J1595	←
GlucaGen	per 1 mg		J1610	
Glucagon HCl	per 1 mg	SC, IM, IV	J1610	
Glukor	per 1,000 USP units	IM	J0725	
Glycopyrrolate				
concentrated form	per 1 mg	INH	J7642	
unit dose form	per 1 mg	INH	J7643	

◄ New   ← Revised   ✔ Reinstated   ~~deleted~~ Deleted

DRUG NAME	DOSAGE	METHOD OF ADMINISTRATION	HCPCS CODE
Gold sodium thiomalate	up to 50 mg	IM	**J1600**
Gonadorelin HCl	per 100 mcg	SC, IV	**J1620**
Gonal-F			J3490
Gonic	per 1,000 USP units	IM	J0725
Goserelin acetate implant	per 3.6 mg	SC	**J9202**
Graftjacket	per square centimeter		Q4107
Graftjacket express	1 cc		Q4113
Granisetron HCl			
injection	100 mcg	IV	**J1626**
oral	1 mg	ORAL	**Q0166**
Gynogen L.A. A10	up to 10 mg	IM	J1380
Gynogen L.A. A20	up to 10 mg	IM	J1380
Gynogen L.A. A40	up to 10 mg	IM	J1380
H			
Halaven	0.1 mg		J9179
Haldol	up to 5 mg	IM, IV	J1630
Haloperidol	up to 5 mg	IM, IV	**J1630**
Haloperidol decanoate	per 50 mg	IM	**J1631**
Haloperidol Lactate	up to 5 mg		J1630
Heconia	per 1 mg	ORAL	J7505
Hectoral	1 mcg	IV	J1270
Helixate FS	per IU		J7192
Hemin	1 mg		**J1640**
Hemofil M	per IU	IV	J7190
Hemophilia clotting factors (e.g., anti-inhibitors)	per IU	IV	**J7198**
NOC	per IU	IV	**J7199**
Hepagam B	0.5 ml	IM	**J1571**
	0.5 ml	IV	**J1573**
Hep-Lock	10 units	IV	J1642
Hep-Lock U/P	10 units	IV	J1642
Heparin (Procine)	per 1,000 units		J1644
Heparin (Procine) Lock Flush	per 10 units		J1642
Heparin sodium	1,000 units	IV, SC	**J1644**
Heparin Sodium (Bovine)	per 1,000 units		J1644
Heparin Sodium Flush	per 10 units		J1642
Heparin sodium (heparin lock flush)	10 units	IV	**J1642**
Heparin Sodium (Procine)	per 1,000 units		J1644
Herceptin	10 mg	IV	J9355
Hexabrix 320	per ml		Q9967
Hexadrol Phosphate	1 mg	IM, IV, OTH	J1100
Histaject	per 10 mg	IM, SC, IV	J0945

◄ New   ← Revised   ✔ Reinstated   ~~deleted~~ Deleted

DRUG NAME	DOSAGE	METHOD OF ADMINISTRATION	HCPCS CODE	
Histerone 50	up to 50 mg	IM	J3140	
Histerone 100	up to 50 mg	IM	J3140	
Histrelin				
acetate	10 mcg		**J1675**	
implant	50 mg	OTH	**J9225**, J9226	←
Hizentra, see Immune globulin				
Humalog	per 5 units		J1815	
	per 50 units		J1817	
Human fibrinogen concentrate	100 mg	**IV**	**J7178**	←
Humate-P	per IU		J7187	
Humatrope	1 mg		J2941	
Humira	20 mg		J0135	
Humulin	per 5 units		J1815	
	per 50 units		J1817	
Hyalgan		OTH	**J7321**	←
Hyaluronic Acid			J3490	
Hyaluronidase	up to 150 units	SC, IV	**J3470**	
Hyaluronidase				
ovine	up to 999 units	VAR	**J3471**	←
ovine	per 1000 units	VAR	**J3472**	←
recombinant	1 usp	SC	**J3473**	←
Hyate:C	per IU	IV	J7191	
Hybolin Improved, see Nandrolone phenpropionate				
Hybolin Decanoate	up to 50 mg	IM	J2320	
Hycamtin	0.25 mg	ORAL	J8705	
	4 mg	IV	J9351	
Hydralazine HCl	up to 20 mg	IV, IM	**J0360**	
Hydrate	up to 50 mg	IM, IV	J1240	
Hydrea			J8999	
Hydrocortisone acetate	up to 25 mg	IV, IM, SC	**J1700**	
Hydrocortisone sodium phosphate	up to 50 mg	IV, IM, SC	**J1710**	
Hydrocortisone succinate sodium	up to 100 mg	IV, IM, SC	**J1720**	
Hydrocortone Acetate	up to 25 mg	IV, IM, SC	J1700	
Hydrocortone Phosphate	up to 50 mg	IM, IV, SC	J1710	
Hydromorphone HCl	up to 4 mg	SC, IM, IV	**J1170**	
Hydroxocobalamin	up to 1,000 mcg		J3420	
Hydroxyprogesterone Caproate	1 mg	IM	**J1725**	←
Hydroxyurea			J8999	
Hydroxyzine HCl	up to 25 mg	IM	**J3410**	
Hydroxyzine Pamoate	25 mg	ORAL	**Q0177**	
	50 mg	ORAL	**Q0178**	
Hylan G-F 20		OTH	J7325	←

◄ New   ← Revised   ✔ Reinstated   ~~deleted~~ Deleted

DRUG NAME	DOSAGE	METHOD OF ADMINISTRATION	HCPCS CODE	
Hyoscyamine sulfate	up to 0.25 mg	SC, IM, IV	J1980	
Hyperhep B			J3590	
Hyperrho S/D	300 mcg		J2790	
	100 IU		J2792	
Hyper-Sal	10 ml		A4216	
Hyperstat IV	up to 300 mg	IV	J1730	
Hyper-Tet	up to 250 units	IM	J1670	
HypRho-D	300 mcg	IM	J2790	
			J2791	
	50 mcg		J2788	
Hyrexin-50	up to 50 mg	IV, IM	J1200	
Hyzine-50	up to 25 mg	IM	J3410	
I				
Ibandronate sodium	1 mg	IV	J1740	←
Ibuprofen	100 mg	IV	J1741	◄
Ibutilide fumarate	1 mg	IV	J1742	
Icatibant	1 mg	SC	J1744	◄
Idamycin	5 mg	IV	J9211	
Idarubicin HCl	5 mg	IV	J9211	
Idursulfase	1 mg	IV	J1743	←
Ifex	1 g	IV	J9208	
Ifosfamide	1 g	IV	J9208	
Ilaris	1 mg		J0638	
Iloprost	20 mcg	INH	Q4074	←
Ilotycin, see Erythromycin gluceptate				
Imferon	50 mg		J1750, J1752	
Imiglucerase	10 units	IV	J1786	
Imitrex	6 mg	SC	J3030	
Immune globulin				
Flebogamma	500 mg	IV	J1572	
Gammagard Liquid	500 mg	IV	J1569	
Gammaplex	500 mg	IV	J1557	←
Gamunex	500 mg	IV	J1561	
HepaGam B	0.5 ml	IM	J1571	
	0.5 ml	IV	J1573	
Hizentra	100 mg	SC	J1559	←
NOS	500 mg	IV	J1566, J1599	
Octagam	500 mg	IV	J1568	
Privigen	500 mg	IV	J1459	
Rhophylac	100 IU	IM	J2791	
Subcutaneous	100 mg	SC	J1562	←
Immunosuppressive drug, not otherwise classified			J7599	

◄ New   ← Revised   ✔ Reinstated   ~~deleted~~ Deleted

DRUG NAME	DOSAGE	METHOD OF ADMINISTRATION	HCPCS CODE	
Imuran	50 mg	ORAL	J7500	
	100 mg		J7501	
Inapsine	up to 5 mg	IM, IV	J1790	
Incobotulinumtoxin type A	1 unit	IM	**J0588**	←
Increlex	1 mg		J2170	
Inderal	up to 1 mg	IV	J1800	
Infed	50 mg		J1750	
Infergen	1 mcg	SC	J9212	
Infliximab, injection	10 mg	IM, IV	**J1745**	
Innohep	1,000 IU	SC	J1655	
Innovar	up to 2 ml ampule	IM, IV	J1810	
Insulin	5 units	SC	**J1815**	
Insulin-Humalog	per 50 units		J1817	
Insulin lispro	50 units	SC	**J1817**	
Intal	per 10 mg	INH	J7631, J7632	
Integrilin	5 mg	IM, IV	J1327	
Integra				
Bilayer Matrix Wound Dressing (BMWD)	per square centimeter		Q4104	
Dermal Regeneration Template (DRT)	per square centimeter		Q4105	
Flowable Wound Matrix	1 cc		Q4114	
Matrix	per square centimeter		Q4108	
Interferon alphacon-1, recombinant	1 mcg	SC	**J9212**	
Interferon alfa-2a, recombinant	3 million units	SC, IM	**J9213**	
Interferon alfa-2b, recombinant	1 million units	SC, IM	**J9214**	
Interferon alfa-n3 (human leukocyte derived)	250,000 IU	IM	**J9215**	
Interferon beta-1a	30 mcg	IM	**J1826**	
	11 mcg	IM	**Q3025**	
	11 mcg	SC	**Q3026**	
Interferon beta-1b	0.25 mg	SC	**J1830**	
Interferon gamma-1b	3 million units	SC	**J9216**	
Intrauterine copper contraceptive		OTH	J7300	
Intron-A	1 million units		J9214	
Invanz	500 mg		J1335	
Invega Sustenna	1 mg		J2426	
Ipilimumab	1 mg	IV	**J9228**	←
Ipratropium bromide, unit dose form	per mg	INH	J7620, **J7644,** **J7645,** J3535	
Iressa	250 mg	ORAL	J8565	
Irinotecan	20 mg	IV	**J9206**	
Iron dextran	50 mg	IV, IM	**J1750**	←
Iron sucrose	1 mg	IV	J1756	
Irrigation solution for Tx of bladder calculi	per 50 ml	OTH	**Q2004**	

◄ New   ← Revised   ✔ Reinstated   ~~deleted~~ Deleted

DRUG NAME	DOSAGE	METHOD OF ADMINISTRATION	HCPCS CODE
Isocaine HCl	per 10 ml	VAR	J0670
Isoetharine HCl			
concentrated form	per mg	INH	**J7647, J7648**
unit dose form	per mg	INH	**J7649, J7650**
Isoproterenol HCl			
concentrated form	per mg	INH	**J7657, J7658**
unit dose form	per mg	INH	**J7659, J7660**
Isovue-200	per ml		Q9966, Q9967
Istodax	1 mg		J9315
Isuprel			
concentrated form	per mg	INH	J7657, J7658
unit dose form	per mg	INH	J7659, J7660
Itraconazole	50 mg	IV	**J1835**
Ixabepilone	1 mg	IV	**J9207**
Ixempra	1 mg		J9207
J			
Jenamicin	up to 80 mg	IM, IV	J1580
Jevtana	1 mg		J9043
K			
Kabikinase	per 250,000 IU	IV	J2995
Kalbitor	1 mg		J1290
Kaleinate	per 10 ml	IV	J0610
Kanamycin sulfate	up to 75 mg	IM, IV	**J1850**
	up to 500 mg	IM, IV	**J1840**
Kantrex	up to 75 mg	IM, IV	J1850
	up to 500 mg	IM, IV	J1840
Kay-Pred	up to 1 ml		J2650
Keflin	up to 1 g	IM, IV	J1890
Kefurox	per 750 mg		J0697
Kefzol	500 mg	IV, IM	J0690
Kenaject-40	per 10 mg	IM	J3301
	1 mg		J3300
Kenalog-10	per 10 mg	IM	J3301
	1 mg		J3300
Kenalog-40	per 10 mg	IM	J3301
	1 mg		J3300
Kepivance	50 mcg		J2425
Keppra	10 mg		J1953
Kestrone 5	per 1 mg	IM	J1435
Ketorolac tromethamine	per 15 mg	IM, IV	**J1885**
Key-Pred 25	up to 1 ml	IM	J2650
Key-Pred 50	up to 1 ml	IM	J2650

◄ New   ← Revised   ✔ Reinstated   ~~deleted~~ Deleted

DRUG NAME	DOSAGE	METHOD OF ADMINISTRATION	HCPCS CODE
Key-Pred-SP, see Prednisolone sodium phosphate			
K-Flex	up to 60 mg	IV, IM	J2360
Kineret			J3490
Kinlytic	250,000 IU		J3365
Klebcil	up to 75 mg	IM, IV	J1850
	up to 500 mg	IM, IV	J1840
Koate-HP (anti-hemophilic factor)			
human	per IU	IV	J7190
porcine	per IU	IV	J7191
recombinant	per IU	IV	J7192
Kogenate			
human	per IU	IV	J7190
porcine	per IU	IV	J7191
recombinant	per IU	IV	J7192
Konakion	per 1 mg	IM, SC, IV	J3430
Konyne-80	per IU	IV	J7194, J7195
Krystexxa	1 mg		J2507
Kytril	1 mg	ORAL	Q0166
	1 mg	IV	S0091
	100 mcg	IV	J1626
L			
Lactated Ringers	up to 1,000 cc		J7120
L.A.E. 20	up to 10 mg	IM	J1380
Laetrile, Amygdalin, vitamin B-17			**J3570**
Lanoxin	up to 0.5 mg	IM, IV	J1160
Lanreotide	1 mg	SC	**J1930** ←
Lantus	per 5 units		J1815
Largon, see Propiomazine HCl			
Laronidase	0.1 mg	IV	**J1931** ←
Lasix	up to 20 mg	IM, IV	J1940
L-Caine	10 mg	IV	J2001
L-Carnitine	per 1 gm		J1955
Lepirudin	50 mg		**J1945**
Leucovorin calcium	per 50 mg	IM, IV	**J0640**
Leukeran			J8999
Leukine	50 mcg	IV	J2820
Leuprolide acetate (for depot suspension)	per 3.75 mg	IM	**J1950**
	7.5 mg	IM	**J9217**
Leuprolide acetate	per 1 mg	IM	**J9218**
Leuprolide acetate implant	65 mg	OTH	**J9219** ←
Leustatin	per mg	IV	J9065

◄ New   ← Revised   ✔ Reinstated   ~~deleted~~ Deleted

DRUG NAME	DOSAGE	METHOD OF ADMINISTRATION	HCPCS CODE	
Levalbuterol HCl				
concentrated form	0.5 mg	INH	J7607, J7612	
unit dose form	0.5 mg	INH	J7614, J7615	
Levaquin I.U.	250 mg	IV	J1956	
Levetiracetam	10 mg	IV	J1953	←
Levocarnitine	per 1 gm	IV	J1955	
Levo-Dromoran	up to 2 mg	SC, IV	J1960	
Levofloxacin	250 mg	IV	J1956	
Levoleucovorin calcium	0.5 mg	IV	J0641	←
Levonorgestrel implant		OTH	J7306	←
Levonorgestrel-releasing intrauterine contraceptive system	52 mg	OTH	J7302	
Levorphanol tartrate	up to 2 mg	SC, IV	J1960	
Levsin	up to 0.25 mg	SC, IM, IV	J1980	
Levulan Kerastick	unit dose (354 mg)	OTH	J7308	
Lexiscan	0.1 mg		J2785	
Librium	up to 100 mg	IM, IV	J1990	
Lidocaine HCl	10 mg	IV	J2001	
Lidoject-1	10 mg	IV	J2001	
Lidoject-2	10 mg	IV	J2001	
Lincocin	up to 300 mg	IV	J2010	
Lincomycin HCl	up to 300 mg	IV	J2010	
Linezolid	200 mg	IV	J2020	
Lipodox			Q2049	
Liquaemin Sodium	1,000 units	IV, SC	J1644	
Lioresal	10 mg	IT	J0475	
			J0476	
LMD (10%)	500 ml	IV	J7100	
Lovenox	10 mg	SC	J1650	
Lorazepam	2 mg	IM, IV	J2060	
Lucentis	0.1 mg		J2778	
Lufyllin	up to 500 mg	IM	J1180	
Luminal Sodium	up to 120 mg	IM, IV	J2560	
Lumizyme	10 mg		J0220, J0221	
Lupon Depot	7.5 mg		J9217	
	3.75 mg		J1950	
Lupron	per 1 mg	IM	J9218	
	per 3.75 mg	IM	J1950	
	7.5 mg	IM	J9217	
Lymphocyte immune globulin				
anti-thymocyte globulin, equine	250 mg	IV	J7504	
anti-thymocyte globulin, rabbit	25 mg	IV	J7511	
Lyophilized			J1566	

◀ New   ← Revised   ✔ Reinstated   ~~deleted~~ Deleted

DRUG NAME	DOSAGE	METHOD OF ADMINISTRATION	HCPCS CODE	
M				
Macugen	0.3 mg		J2503	
Magnesium sulfate	500 mg		**J3475**	
Magnevist	per ml		A9579	
Makena	1 mg		J1725	
Malulane			J8999	
Mannitol	25% in 50 ml	IV	**J2150**	
	5 mg	INH	**J7665, J7799**	
Marcaine			J3490	
Marinol	2.5 mg	ORAL	Q0167	
	5 mg	ORAL	Q0168	
Marmine	up to 50 mg	IM, IV	J1240	
Maxipime	500 mg	IV	J0692	
MD-76R	per ml		Q9963	
MD Gastroview	per ml		Q9963	
Mecasermin	1 mg	SC	**J2170**	←
Mechlorethamine HCl (nitrogen mustard), HN2	10 mg	IV	**J9230**	
Medralone 40	20 mg	IM	J1020	
	40 mg	IM	J1030	
	80 mg	IM	J1040	
Medralone 80	20 mg	IM	J1020	
	40 mg	IM	J1030	
	80 mg	IM	J1040	
Medrol	per 4 mg	ORAL	J7509	
Medroxyprogesterone acetate	1 mg	IM	**J1050**	←
	~~150 mg~~	~~IM~~	~~J1055~~	✘
~~Medroxyprogesterone acetate/estradiol cypionate~~	~~5 mg/25 mg~~	~~IM~~	~~J1056~~	✘
Mefoxin	1 g	IV, IM	J0694	
Megace			J8999	
Megestrol Acetate			J8999	
Melphalan HCl	50 mg	IV	**J9245**	
Melphalan, oral	2 mg	ORAL	**J8600**	
Menoject LA	up to 1 ml	IM	J1060	
Mepergan Injection	up to 50 mg	IM, IV	J2180	
Meperidine HCl	per 100 mg	IM, IV, SC	**J2175**	
Meperidine and promethazine HCl	up to 50 mg	IM, IV	**J2180**	
Mepivacaine HCl	per 10 ml	VAR	**J0670**	
Mercaptopurine			J8999	
Meropenem	100 mg	IV	**J2185**	←
Merrem	100 mg		J2185	
Mesna	200 mg	IV	**J9209**	
Mesnex	200 mg	IV	J9209	

◄ New   ← Revised   ✔ Reinstated   ~~deleted~~ Deleted

DRUG NAME	DOSAGE	METHOD OF ADMINISTRATION	HCPCS CODE
Metaprel			
concentrated form	per 10 mg	INH	J7667, J7668
unit dose form	per 10 mg	INH	J7669, J7670
Metaproterenol sulfate			
concentrated form	per 10 mg	INH	J7667, J7668
unit dose form	per 10 mg	INH	J7669, J7670
Metaraminol bitartrate	per 10 mg	IV, IM, SC	J0380
Metastron	per millicurie		A9600
Methacholine chloride	1 mg	INH	J7674
Methadone HCl	up to 10 mg	IM, SC	J1230
Methergine	up to 0.2 mg		J2210
Methocarbamol	up to 10 ml	IV, IM	J2800
Methotrexate, oral	2.5 mg	ORAL	J8610
Methotrexate sodium	5 mg	IV, IM, IT, IA	J9250
	50 mg	IV, IM, IT, IA	J9260
Methotrexate LPF	5 mg	IV, IM, IT, IA	J9250
	50 mg	IV, IM, IT, IA	J9260
Methyldopate HCl	up to 250 mg	IV	J0210
Methylergonovine maleate	up to 0.2 mg		J2210
Methylnaltrexone	0.1 mg	SC	J2212
Methylpred	20 mg		J1020
Methylpred DP	per 4 mg		J7509
Methylprednisolone, oral	per 4 mg	ORAL	J7509
Methylprednisolone acetate	20 mg	IM	J1020
	40 mg	IM	J1030
	80 mg	IM	J1040
Methylprednisolone sodium succinate	up to 40 mg	IM, IV	J2920
	up to 125 mg	IM, IV	J2930
Metoclopramide HCl	up to 10 mg	IV	J2765
Metrodin	75 IU		J3355
Metronidazole			J3490
Metvixia	1 g	OTHO	J7309
Miacalcin	up to 400 units	SC, IM	J0630
Micafungin sodium	1 mg		J2248
MicRhoGAM	50 mcg		J2788
Midazolam HCl	per 1 mg	IM, IV	J2250
Millipred		ORAL	J8499
Milrinone lactate	5 mg	IV	J2260
Minocine	1 mg		J2265
Minocycline Hydrochloride	1 mg	IV	J2265
Mirena	52 mg	OTH	J7302
Mithracin	2,500 mcg	IV	J9270

◄ New   ← Revised   ✔ Reinstated   ~~deleted~~ Deleted

DRUG NAME	DOSAGE	METHOD OF ADMINISTRATION	HCPCS CODE	
Mitomycin	0.2 mg	Ophthalmic	**J7315**	←
	5 mg	IV	**J9280**	◄
Mitosol	0.2 mg	Ophthalmic	J7315	◄
	5 mg	IV	J9280	◄
Mitoxantrone HCl	per 5 mg	IV	**J9293**	
Monocid, see Cefonicic sodium				
Monoclate-P				
human	per IU	IV	J7190	
porcine	per IU	IV	J7191	
Monoclonal antibodies, parenteral	5 mg	IV	**J7505**	
Monoject Prefill Advanced	10 ml		A4216	
Mononine	per IU	IV	J7193	
Morphine sulfate	up to 10 mg	IM, IV, SC	**J2270**	
	100 mg	IM, IV, SC	**J2271**	
preservative-free	per 10 mg	SC, IM, IV	**J2275**	
Moxifloxacin	100 mg	IV	**J2280**	←
Mozobil	1 mg		J2562	
M-Prednisol-40	20 mg	IM	J1020	
	40 mg	IM	J1030	
	80 mg	IM	J1040	
M-Prednisol-80	20 mg	IM	J1020	
	40 mg	IM	J1030	
	80 mg	IM	J1040	
Mucomyst				
unit dose form	per gram	INH	J7604, J7608	
Mucosol				
injection	100 mg		J0132	
unit dose	per gram	INH	J7604, J7608	
MultiHance	per ml		A9577	
MultiHance Multipack	per ml		Aph78	
Muromonab-CD3	5 mg	IV	**J7505**	
Muse		OTH	J0275	
	1.25 mcg	OTH	J0270	
Mustargen	10 mg	IV	J9230	
Mutamycin	5 mg	IV	J9280	
Mycamine	1 mg		J2248	
Mycophenolic acid	180 mg	ORAL	**J7518**	←
Mycophenolate Mofetil	250 mg	ORAL	**J7517**	
Myfortic	180 mg		J7518	
Myleran	1 mg		J0594	
	2 mg	ORAL	J8510	
Mylotarg	5 mg	IV	J9300	

◄ **New**   ← **Revised**   ✔ **Reinstated**   ~~deleted~~ **Deleted**

DRUG NAME	DOSAGE	METHOD OF ADMINISTRATION	HCPCS CODE
Myobloc	per 100 units	IM	J0587
Myochrysine	up to 50 mg	IM	J1600
Myolin	up to 60 mg	IV, IM	J2360
Myozyme	10 mg		J0221
N			
Nabi-HB			J3590
Nabilone	1 mg	ORAL	**J8650**
N-acetyl-L-cysteine	per gram		J7604
Nafcillin			J3490
Naglazyme	1 mg		J1458
Nalbuphine HCl	per 10 mg	IM, IV, SC	**J2300**
Naloxone HCl	per 1 mg	IM, IV, SC	**J2310**, J3490
Naltrexone			J3490
Naltrexone, depot form	1 mg	IM	**J2315** ←
Nandrobolic L.A.	up to 50 mg	IM	J2320
Nandrolone decanoate	up to 50 mg	IM	**J2320**
Narcan	1 mg	IM, IV, SC	J2310
Naropin	1 mg		J2795
Nasahist B	per 10 mg	IM, SC, IV	J0945
Nasal vaccine inhalation		INH	**J3530**
Natalizumab	1 mg	IV	**J2323** ←
Natrecor	0.1 mg		J2325
Navane, see Thiothixene			
Navelbine	per 10 mg	IV	J9390
ND Stat	per 10 mg	IM, SC, IV	J0945
Nebcin	up to 80 mg	IM, IV	J3260
	per 300 mg		J7682
NebuPent	per 300 mg	INH	J2545, J7676
Nelarabine	50 mg	IV	**J9261**
Nembutal Sodium Solution	per 50 mg	IM, IV, OTH	J2515
Neocyten	up to 60 mg	IV, IM	J2360
Neo-Durabolic	up to 50 mg	IM	J2320
Neoral	100 mg		J7502
	25 mg		J7515
Neoquess	up to 20 mg	IM	J0500
Neosar	100 mg	IV	J9070
Neostigmine methylsulfate	up to 0.5 mg	IM, IV, SC	**J2710**
Neo-Synephrine	up to 1 ml	SC, IM, IV	J2370
Nervocaine 1%	10 mg	IV	J2001
Nervocaine 2%	10 mg	IV	J2001
Nesacaine	per 30 ml	VAR	J2400
Nesacaine-MPF	per 30 ml	VAR	J2400

◀ New   ← Revised   ✔ Reinstated   ~~deleted~~ Deleted

DRUG NAME	DOSAGE	METHOD OF ADMINISTRATION	HCPCS CODE	
Nesiritide	0.1 mg	IV	**J2325**	←
Neulasta	6 mg		J2505	
Neumega	5 mg	SC	J2355	
Neupogen	300 mcg	SC, IV	J1440	
	480 mcg	SC, IV	J1441	
Neuroforte-R	up to 1,000 mcg		J3420	
Neutrexin	per 25 mg	IV	J3305	
Nipent	per 10 mg	IV	J9268	
Nolvadex			J8999	
Nordryl	up to 50 mg	IV, IM	J1200	
	50 mg	ORAL	Q0163	
Norflex	up to 60 mg	IV, IM	J2360	
Norzine	up to 10 mg	IM	J3280	
Not otherwise classified drugs			**J3490**	
other than inhalation solution administered thru DME			**J7799**	
inhalation solution administered thru DME			**J7699**	
anti-neoplastic			**J9999**	
chemotherapeutic		ORAL	**J8999**	
immunosuppressive			**J7599**	
nonchemotherapeutic		ORAL	**J8499**	
Novantrone	per 5 mg	IV	J9293	
Novarel	per 1,000 USP Units		J0725	
Novolin	per 5 units		J1815	
	per 50 units		J1817	
Novolog	per 5 units		J1815	
	per 50 units		J1817	
Novo Seven	1 mcg	IV	J7189	
NPH	5 units	SC	J1815	
Nplate	100 units		J0587	
	10 mcg		J2796	
Nubain	per 10 mg	IM, IV, SC	J2300	
Nulecit	12.5 mg		J2916	
Nulicaine	10 mg	IV	J2001	
Nulojix	1 mg	IV	J0485	◄
Numorphan	up to 1 mg	IV, SC, IM	J2410	
Numorphan H.P.	up to 1 mg	IV, SC, IM	J2410	
Nutropin	1 mg		J2941	
O				
Oasis Burn Matrix	per square centimeter		Q4103	
Oasis Wound Matrix	per square centimeter		Q4102	
Octagam	500 mg	IV	**J1568**	←

◄ New   ← Revised   ✔ Reinstated   ~~deleted~~ Deleted

DRUG NAME	DOSAGE	METHOD OF ADMINISTRATION	HCPCS CODE
Octreotide Acetate, injection	1 mg	IM	J2353
	25 mcg	IV, SQ	J2354
Oculinum	per unit	IM	J0585
Ofatumumab	10 mg		J9302
Ofirmev	10 mg	IV	J0131	←
O-Flex	up to 60 mg	IV, IM	J2360
Oforta	10 mg		J8562
Olanzapine	1 mg	IM	J2358	←
Omalizumab	5 mg	SC	J2357	←
Omnipaque	per ml		Q9965, Q9966, Q9967
Omnipen-N	up to 500 mg	IM, IV	J0290
	per 1.5 gm	IM, IV	J0295
Omniscan	per ml		A9579
Omnitrope	1 mg		J2941
Omontys	0.1 mg	IV, SC	J0890	◄
OnabotulinumtoxinA	1 unit	IM	J0585	←
Oncaspar	per single dose vial	IM, IV	J9266
Oncovin	1 mg	IV	J9370
Ondansetron HCl	1 mg	IV	J2405
	1 mg	ORAL	Q0162
Ontak	300 mcg		J9160
Opana	up to 1 mg		J2410
Oprelvekin	5 mg	SC	J2355
Optimark	per ml		A9579
Optiray	per ml		Q9966, Q9967
Optison	per ml		Q9956
Oraminic II	per 10 mg	IM, SC, IV	J0945
Oraped	per 5 mg	ORAL	J7510
Orfro	up to 60 mg		J2360
Ormazine	10 mg	ORAL	Q0171
	25 mg	ORAL	Q0172
	up to 50 mg	IM, IV	J3230
Orphenadrine citrate	up to 60 mg	IV, IM	J2360
Orphenate	up to 60 mg	IV, IM	J2360
Orthoclone OKT3	5 mg		J7505
Orthovisc		OTH	J7324	←
Or-Tyl	up to 20 mg	IM	J0500
Osmitrol			J7799
Ovidrel			J3490
Oxacillin sodium	up to 250 mg	IM, IV	J2700
Oxaliplatin	0.5 mg	IV	J9263	←

◄ New   ← Revised   ✔ Reinstated   ~~deleted~~ Deleted

DRUG NAME	DOSAGE	METHOD OF ADMINISTRATION	HCPCS CODE	
Oxilan	per ml		Q9967	
Oxymorphone HCl	up to 1 mg	IV, SC, IM	J2410	
Oxytetracycline HCl	up to 50 mg	IM	J2460	
Oxytocin	up to 10 units	IV, IM	J2590	
Ozurdex	0.1 mg		J7312	
P				
Paclitaxel	30 mg	IV	J9265	
Paclitaxel protein-bound particles	1 mg	IV	J9264	←
Palifermin	50 mcg	IV	J2425	←
Paliperidone Palmitate	1 mg	IM	J2426	←
Palonosetron HCl	25 mcg	IV	J2469	←
Pamidronate disodium	per 30 mg	IV	J2430	
Panhematin	1 mg		J1640	
Panitumumab	10 mg	IV	J9303	←
Papaverine HCl	up to 60 mg	IV, IM	J2440	
Paragard T 380 A		OTH	J7300	
Paraplatin	50 mg	IV	J9045	
Paricalcitol, injection	1 mcg	IV, IM	J2501	
Pediapred	per 5 mg	ORAL	J7510	
Pegademase bovine	25 IU		J2504	
Pegaptinib	0.3 mg	OTH	J2503	←
Pegaspargase	per single dose vial	IM, IV	J9266	
Pegasys			J3490	
Pegfilgrastim	6 mg	SC	J2505	←
Peginesatide	0.1 mg	IV, SC	J0890	◄
Peg-Intron			J3490	
Pegloticase	1 mg	IV	J2507	←
Pemetrexed	10 mg	IV	J9305	←
Penicillin G benzathine	up to 100,000 units	IM	J0561	
Penicillin G benzathine and penicillin G procaine	100,000 units	IM	J0558	
Penicillin G potassium	up to 600,000 units	IM, IV	J2540	
Penicillin G procaine, aqueous	up to 600,000 units	IM, IV	J2510	
Penicillin G Sodium			J3490	
Pentam	per 300 mg		J7676	
Pentamidine isethionate	per 300 mg	INH, IM	J2545, J7676	
Pentastarch, 10%	100 ml		J2513	
Pentazocine HCl	30 mg	IM, SC, IV	J3070	
Pentobarbital sodium	per 50 mg	IM, IV, OTH	J2515	
Pentostatin	per 10 mg	IV	J9268	
Peforomist	20 mcg		J7606	
Permapen	up to 600,000	IM	J0561	

◄ New   ← Revised   ✔ Reinstated   ~~deleted~~ Deleted

DRUG NAME	DOSAGE	METHOD OF ADMINISTRATION	HCPCS CODE	
Perphenazine				
injection	up to 5 mg	IM, IV	**J3310**	
tablets	4 mg	ORAL	**Q0175**	
	8 mg	ORAL	**Q0176**	
Persantine IV	per 10 mg	IV	J1245	
Pfizerpen	up to 600,000 units	IM, IV	J2540	
Pfizerpen A.S.	up to 600,000 units	IM, IV	J2510	
Phenadoz			J8498	
Phenazine 25	up to 50 mg	IM, IV	J2550	
	12.5 mg	ORAL	Q0169	
	25 mg	ORAL	Q0170	
Phenazine 50	up to 50 mg	IM, IV	J2550	
	12.5 mg	ORAL	Q0169	
	25 mg	ORAL	Q0170	
Phenergan	12.5 mg	ORAL	Q0169	
	25 mg	ORAL	Q0170	
	up to 50 mg	IM, IV	J2550, J8498	
Phenobarbital sodium	up to 120 mg	IM, IV	**J2560**	
Phentolamine mesylate	up to 5 mg	IM, IV	**J2760**	
Phenylephrine HCl	up to 1 ml	SC, IM, IV	**J2370**, J7799	
Phenytoin sodium	per 50 mg	IM, IV	**J1165**	
Photofrin	75 mg	IV	J9600	
Phytonadione (Vitamin K)	per 1 mg	IM, SC, IV	**J3430**	
Piperacillin/Tazobactam Sodium, injection	1.125 g	IV	**J2543**, J3490	
Pitocin	up to 10 units	IV, IM	J2590	
Plantinol AQ	10 mg	IV	J9060	
Plas+SD	each unit	IV	P9023	
Plasma				
cryoprecipitate reduced	each unit	IV	**P9044**	←
pooled multiple donor, frozen	each unit	IV	**P9023**	
Platinol	10 mg	IV, IM	J9060	
Plerixafor	1 mg	SC	**J2562**	←
Plicamycin	2,500 mcg	IV	J9270	
Polocaine	per 10 ml	VAR	J0670	
Polycillin-N	up to 500 mg	IM, IV	J0290	
	per 1.5 gm	IM, IV	J0295	
Porfimer Sodium	75 mg	IV	**J9600**	
Potassium chloride	per 2 mEq	IV	**J3480**	
Pralatrexate	1 mg	IV	**J9307**	←
Pralidoxime chloride	up to 1 g	IV, IM, SC	**J2730**	
Predalone-50	up to 1 ml	IM	J2650	
Predcor-25	up to 1 ml	IM	J2650	

◀ New   ← Revised   ✔ Reinstated   ~~deleted~~ Deleted

2013 TABLE OF DRUGS P

DRUG NAME	DOSAGE	METHOD OF ADMINISTRATION	HCPCS CODE
Predcor-50	up to 1 ml	IM	J2650
Predicort-50	up to 1 ml	IM	J2650
Prelone	5 mg		J7510
Prednicot	5 mg		J7506, J7510
Prednisone	per 5 mg	ORAL	**J7506**
Prednisolone, oral	5 mg	ORAL	**J7510**
Prednisolone acetate	up to 1 ml	IM	**J2650**
Predoject-50	up to 1 ml	IM	J2650
Pregnyl	per 1,000 USP units	IM	J0725
Premarin Intravenous	per 25 mg	IV, IM	J1410
Prescription, chemotherapeutic, not otherwise specified		ORAL	**J8999**
Prescription, nonchemotherapeutic, not otherwise specified		ORAL	**J8499**
Prialt	1 mcg		J2278
Primacor	5 mg	IV	J2260
Primatrix	per square centimeter		Q4110
Primaxin	per 250 mg	IV, IM	J0743
Priscoline HCl	up to 25 mg	IV	J2670
Privigen	500 mg	IV	**J1459**	←
Pro-Depo, see Hydroxyprogesterone Caproate			
Procainamide HCl	up to 1 g	IM, IV	**J2690**
Prochlorperazine	up to 10 mg	IM, IV	**J0780**
			J8498
Prochlorperazine maleate	5 mg	ORAL	**Q0164**
	10 mg	ORAL	**Q0165**
			S0183
Procrit			J0885
			J0886
			Q4081
Prodrox			J3490
Profasi HP	per 1,000 USP units	IM	J0725
Profilnine Heat-Treated			
non-recombinant	per IU	IV	J7193
recombinant	per IU	IV	J7195
complex	per IU	IV	J7194
Profilnine-SD	per IU		J7193, J7194, J7195
Progestaject	per 50 mg		J2675
Progesterone	per 50 mg	IM	**J2675**	←
Prograf			
oral	per 1 mg	ORAL	J7507
parenteral	5 mg		J7525
Prohance Multipack	per ml		A9576

◀ New   ← Revised   ✔ Reinstated   ~~deleted~~ Deleted

DRUG NAME	DOSAGE	METHOD OF ADMINISTRATION	HCPCS CODE
Prokine	50 mcg	IV	J2820
Prolastin	10 mg	IV	J0256
Proleukin	per single use vial	IM, IV	J9015
Prolia	1 mg		J0897
Prolixin Decanoate	up to 25 mg		J2680
	25 mg	IM, SC	J2680
Promazine HCl	up to 25 mg	IM	J2950
Promethazine			J8498
Promethazine HCl			
injection	up to 50 mg	IM, IV	J2550
oral	12.5 mg	ORAL	Q0169
oral	25 mg	ORAL	Q0170
Promethegan			J8498
Pronestyl	up to 1 g	IM, IV	J2690
Proplex T			
non-recombinant	per IU	IV	J7193
recombinant	per IU	IV	J7195
complex	per IU	IV	J7194
Proplex SX-T			
non-recombinant	per IU	IV	J7193
recombinant	per IU	IV	J7195
complex	per IU	IV	J7194
Propofol			J3490
Propranolol HCl	up to 1 mg	IV	J1800
Prorex-25			
	up to 50 mg	IM, IV	J2550
	12.5 mg	ORAL	Q0169
	25 mg	ORAL	Q0170
Prorex-50			
	up to 50 mg	IM, IV	J2550
	12.5 mg	ORAL	Q0169
	25 mg	ORAL	Q0170
Prostaphlin	up to 1 g	IM, IV	J2690
Prostigmin	up to 0.5 mg	IM, IV, SC	J2710
Protamine sulfate	per 10 mg	IV	J2720
Protein C Concentrate	10 IU	IV	J2724
Protirelin	per 250 mcg	IV	J2725
Prothazine	up to 50 mg	IM, IV	J2550
	12.5 mg	ORAL	Q0169
	25 mg	ORAL	Q0170
Protonix			J3490
Protopam Chloride	up to 1 g	IV, IM, SC	J2730

◄ New   ← Revised   ✔ Reinstated   ~~deleted~~ Deleted

DRUG NAME	DOSAGE	METHOD OF ADMINISTRATION	HCPCS CODE	
Proventil				
concentrated form	1 mg	INH	J7610, J7611	
unit dose form	1 mg	INH	J7609, J7613	
Provocholine	per 1 mg		J7674	
Prozine-50	up to 25 mg	IM	J2950	
Pulmicort	0.25 mg	INH	J7633	
	up to 0.5 mg		J7626	
Pulmicort Respules	0.5 mg	INH	J7627, J7626	
	per 0.25 mg		J7633	
noncompounded, concentrated	up to 0.5 mg	INH	J7626	
Pulmozyme	per mg		J7639	
Purinethol	50 mg		J8999	
Pyridoxine HCl	100 mg		**J3415**	
Q				
Quelicin	up to 20 mg	IV, IM	J0330	
Quinupristin/dalfopristin	500 mg (150/350)	IV	**J2770**	
Qutenza	per 10 square cm		J7335	
R				
Ranibizumab	0.1 mg	OTH	**J2778**	←
Ranitidine HCl, injection	25 mg	IV, IM	**J2780**	
Rapamune	1 mg	ORAL	J7520	
Rasburicase	0.5 mg	IV	**J2783**	←
Rebif	11 mcg		Q3026	
Reclast	1 mg	IV	**J3488**	←
Recombinate (anti-hemophilic factor)				
human	per IU	IV	J7190	
porcine	per IU	IV	J7191	
recombinant	per IU	IV	J7192	
Recombivax			J3490	
Redisol	up to 1,000 mcg	IM, SC	J3420	
Regadenoson	0.1 mg	IV	**J2785**	←
Refacto	per IU		J7192	
Refludan	50 mg		J1945	
Regitine	up to 5 mg	IM, IV	J2760	
Reglan	up to 10 mg	IV	J2765	
Regular	5 units	SC	J1815	
Relefact TRH	per 250 mcg	IV	J2725	
Relistor	0.1 mg	SC	J2212	◄
Remicade	10 mg	IM, IV	J1745	
Remodulin	1 mg		J3285	
Reno-60	per ml		Q9961	

◄ New	← Revised	✔ Reinstated	~~deleted~~ Deleted

DRUG NAME	DOSAGE	METHOD OF ADMINISTRATION	HCPCS CODE	
Reno-Dip	per ml		Q9958	
ReoPro	10 mg	IV	J0130	
Rep-Pred 40	20 mg	IM	J1020	
	40 mg	IM	J1030	
	80 mg	IM	J1040	
Rep-Pred 80	20 mg	IM	J1020	
	40 mg	IM	J1030	
	80 mg	IM	J1040	
Resectisol			J7799	
Retavase	18.1 mg	IV	J2993	
Reteplase	18.1 mg	IV	J2993	
Retisert			J7311	
Retrovir	10 mg	IV	J3485	
Rheomacrodex	500 ml	IV	J7100	
Rhesonativ	1 dose package/ 300 mcg	IM	J2790	
	50 mg		J2788	
Rheumatrex Dose Pack	2.5 mg	ORAL	J8610	
Rho(D)				
immune globulin		IM, IV	J2791	←
immune globulin, human	1 dose package/ 300 mcg	IM	J2790	
	50 mg	IM	J2788	←
immune globulin, human, solvent detergent	100	IU, IV	J2792	
RhoGAM	1 dose package, 300 mcg	IM	J2790	
	50 mg		J2788	
Rhophylac	100 IU	IM, IV	J2791	←
Riastap	100 mg		J7178	
Rifadin			J3490	
Rifampin			J3490	
Rilonacept	1 mg	SC	J2793	←
RimabotulinumtoxinB	100 units	IM	J0587	←
Rimso-50	50 ml		J1212	
Ringers lactate infusion	up to 1,000 cc	IV	J7120	
Risperdal Costa	0.5 mg		J2794	
Risperidone	0.5 mg	IM	J2794	←
Rituxan	100 mg	IV	J9310	
Rituximab	100 mg	IV	J9310	
Robaxin	up to 10 ml	IV, IM	J2800	
Robinul	per mg		J7643	
Rocephin	per 250 mg	IV, IM	J0696	

◄ New   ← Revised   ✔ Reinstated   ~~deleted~~ Deleted

DRUG NAME	DOSAGE	METHOD OF ADMINISTRATION	HCPCS CODE	
Rodex	100 mg		J3415	
Roferon-A	3 million units	SC, IM	J9213	
Romidepsin	1 mg	IV	**J9315**	←
Romiplostim	10 mcg	SC	**J2796**	←
Ropivacaine Hydrochloride	1 mg	OTH	**J2795**	←
Rubex	10 mg	IV	J9000	
Rubramin PC	up to 1,000 mcg	IM, SC	J3420	
S				
Saizen	1 mg		J2941	
Saline solution	10 ml		A4216	
5% dextrose	500 ml	IV	**J7042**	
infusion	250 cc	IV	**J7050**	
	1,000 cc	IV	**J7030**	
sterile	500 ml = 1 unit	IV, OTH	**J7040**	
Sandimmune	25 mg	ORAL	J7515	
	100 mg	ORAL	J7502	
	250 mg	OTH	J7516	
Sandoglobulin, see Immune globin intravenous (human)				
Sandostatin, Lar Depot	25 mcg		J2354	
	1 mg	IM	J2353	
Sargramostim (GM-CSF)	50 mcg	IV	**J2820**	
Selestoject	per 4 mg	IM, IV	J0702	
Sensorcaine MPF			J3490	
Sermorelin acetate	1 mcg	SC	**Q0515**	←
Serostim	1 mg		J2941	
Simulect	20 mg		J0480	
Sincalide	5 mcg	IV	**J2805**	←
Sinografin	per ml		Q9963	
Sinusol-B	per 10 mg	IM, SC, IV	J0945	
Sirolimus	1 mg	ORAL	**J7520**	
Smz-TMP			J3490	
Sodium Chloride	1,000 cc		J7030	
	10 ml		A4216	
	500 ml = 1 unit		J7040	
	500 ml		A4217	
	250 cc		J7050	
inhalation solution			J7699	
Sodium Chloride Bacteriostatic	10 ml		A4216	
Sodium Chloride Concentrate			J7799	
Sodium ferricgluconate in sucrose	12.5 mg		**J2916**	

◀ New   ← Revised   ✔ Reinstated   ~~deleted~~ Deleted

DRUG NAME	DOSAGE	METHOD OF ADMINISTRATION	HCPCS CODE	
Sodium Hyaluronate			J3490	
Euflexxa			**J7323**	
Hyalgan			**J7321**	
Orthovisc			**J7324**	
Supartz			**J7321**	
Solganal	up to 50 mg	IM	J2910	
Soliris	10 mg		J1300	
Solu-Cortef	up to 50 mg	IV, IM, SC	J1710	
	100 mg		J1720	
Solu-Medrol	up to 40 mg	IM, IV	J2920	
	up to 125 mg	IM, IV	J2930	
Solurex	1 mg	IM, IV, OTH	J1100	
Solurex LA	1 mg	IM	J1094	
Somatrem	1 mg	SC	**J2940**	←
Somatropin	1 mg	SC	**J2941**	←
Somatulin Depot	1 mg		J1930	
Sparine	up to 25 mg	IM	J2950	
Spasmoject	up to 20 mg	IM	J0500	
Spectinomycin HCl	up to 2 g	IM	**J3320**	
Sporanox	50 mg	IV	J1835	
Stadol	1 mg		J0595	
Staphcillin, see Methicillin sodium				
Stelara	1 mg		J3357	
Stilphostrol	250 mg	IV	J9165	
Streptase	250,000 IU	IV	J2995	
Streptokinase	per 250,000	IU, IV	**J2995**	
Streptomycin Sulfate	up to 1 g	IM	**J3000**	
Streptomycin	up to 1 g	IM	**J3000**	
Streptozocin	1 gm	IV	**J9320**	
Strontium-89 chloride	per millicurie		**A9600**	
Sublimaze	0.1 mg	IM, IV	J3010	
Succinylcholine chloride	up to 20 mg	IV, IM	**J0330**	
Sufenta			J3490	
Sufentanil Citrate			J3490	
Sumarel Dosepro	6 mg		J3030	
Sumatriptan succinate	6 mg	SC	**J3030**	
Supartz		OTH	**J7321**	←
SurgiMend			C9358	
Surostrin	up to 20 mg	IV, IM	**J0330**	
Sus-Phrine	up to 1 ml ampule	SC, IM	J0171	

◀ New   ← Revised   ✔ Reinstated   ~~deleted~~ Deleted

DRUG NAME	DOSAGE	METHOD OF ADMINISTRATION	HCPCS CODE	
Synercid	500 mg (150/350)	IV	J2770	
Synkavite	per 1 mg	IM, SC, IV	J3430	
Syntocinon	up to 10 units	IV, IM	J2590	
Synvisc and Synvisc-One	1 mg	OTH	**J7325**	←
Syrex	10 ml		A4216	
Sytobex	1,000 mcg	IM, SC	J3420	
T				
Tacrolimus				
oral	per 1 mg	ORAL	**J7507**	
parenteral	5 mg	IV	**J7525**	←
Talwin	30 mg	IM, SC, IV	J3070	
Tamoxifen Citrate			J8999	
Taractan, see Chlorprothixene				
Taxol	30 mg	IV	J9265	
Taxotere	20 mg	IV	J9171	
Tazicef	per 500 mg		J0713	
Tazidime, see Ceftazidime Technetium TC Sestambi	per dose		**A9500**	
			J0713	
TEEV	up to 1 cc	IM	J0900	
Teflaro	1 mg		J0712	
Telavancin	10 mg	IV	**J3095**	←
Temodar	5 mg	ORAL	J8700, J9328	
Temozolomide	1 mg	IV	**J9328**	←
	5 mg	ORAL	**J8700**	
Temsirolimus	1 mg	IV	**J9330**	←
Tenecteplase	1 mg	IV	**J3101**	←
Teniposide	50 mg		**Q2017**	
Tequin	10 mg	IV	J1590	
Terbutaline sulfate	up to 1 mg	SC, IV	**J3105**	
concentrated form	per 1 mg	INH	**J7680**	
unit dose form	per 1 mg	INH	**J7681**	
Teriparatide	10 mcg	SC	**J3110**	←
Terramycin IM	up to 50 mg	IM	J2460	
Testa-C	up to 100 mg	IM	J1070	
	1 cc, 200 mg	IM	J1080	
Testadiate	up to 1 cc	IM	J0900	
Testadiate-Depo	up to 100 mg	IM	J1070	
	1 cc, 200 mg	IM	J1080	
Testaject-LA	up to 100 mg	IM	J1070	
	1 cc, 200 mg	IM	J1080	
Testaqua	up to 50 mg	IM	J3140	
Test-Estro Cypionates	up to 1 ml	IM	J1060	

◄ New   ← Revised   ✔ Reinstated   ~~deleted~~ Deleted

DRUG NAME	DOSAGE	METHOD OF ADMINISTRATION	HCPCS CODE
Test-Estro-C	up to 1 ml	IM	J1060
Testex	up to 100 mg	IM	J3150
Testo AQ	up to 50 mg		J3140
Testoject-50	up to 50 mg	IM	J3140
Testoject-LA	up to 100 mg	IM	J1070
	1 cc, 200 mg	IM	J1080
Testone			
LA 200	up to 100 mg	IM	J3120
	up to 200 mg	IM	J3130
LA 100	up to 100 mg	IM	J3120
	up to 200 mg	IM	J3130
Testosterone	up to 50 mg		J3140
Testosterone Aqueous	up to 50 mg	IM	J3140
Testosterone enanthate and estradiol valerate	up to 1 cc	IM	J0900
Testosterone enanthate	up to 100 mg	IM	J3120
	up to 200 mg	IM	J3130
Testosterone cypionate	up to 100 mg	IM	J1070
	1 cc, 200 mg	IM	J1080
Testosterone cypionate and estradiol cypionate	up to 1 ml	IM	J1060
Testosterone propionate	up to 100 mg	IM	J3150
Testosterone suspension	up to 50 mg	IM	J3140
Testradiol 90/4	up to 1 cc	IM	J0900
Testrin PA	up to 100 mg	IM	J3120
	up to 200 mg	IM	J3130
Testro AQ	up to 50 mg		J3140
Tetanus immune globulin, human	up to 250 units	IM	J1670
Tetracycline	up to 250 mg	IM, IV	J0120
Tev-Tropin	1 mg		J2941
Thallous Chloride TI–201	per MCI		A9505
Theelin Aqueous	per 1 mg	IM	J1435
Theophylline	per 40 mg	IV	J2810
TheraCys	per vial	IV	J9031
Thiamine HCl	100 mg		J3411
Thiethylenecthiophosphoramide/T	15 mg		J9340
Thiethylperazine maleate			
injection	up to 10 mg	IM	J3280
oral	10 mg	ORAL	Q0174
Thiotepa	15 mg	IV	J9340
Thorazine	10 mg	ORAL	Q0171
	25 mg	ORAL	Q0172
	up to 50 mg		J3230, J8498
Thrombate III	per IU		J7197

◄ New   ← Revised   ✔ Reinstated   ~~deleted~~ Deleted

DRUG NAME	DOSAGE	METHOD OF ADMINISTRATION	HCPCS CODE
Thymoglobulin, see Immune globin, anti-thymocyte			
	25 mg		J7511
Thypinone	per 250 mcg	IV	J2725
Thyrogen	0.9 mg	IM, SC	J3240
Thyrotropin Alfa, injection	0.9 mg	IM, SC	**J3240**
Tice BCG	per vial	IV	J9031
Ticon			
injection	up to 200 mg	IM	J3250
oral	250 mg	ORAL	Q0173
Tigan			
injection	up to 200 mg	IM	J3250
oral	250 mg	ORAL	Q0173
Tigecycline	1 mg	IV	**J3243** ←
Tiject-20	up to 200 mg	IM	J3250
	250 mg	ORAL	Q0173
Timentin			J3490
Tinzaparin	1,000 IU	SC	**J1655**
Tirofiban Hydrochloride, injection	0.25 mg	IM, IV	**J3246**
TNKase	1 mg		**J3101**
Tobi	300 mg	INH	J7682, J7685
Tobramycin, inhalation solution	300 mg	INH	**J7682, J7685**
Tobramycin sulfate	up to 80 mg	IM, IV	**J3260, J7685**
Tocilizumab	1 mg	IV	**J3262** ←
Tofranil, see Imipramine HCl			
Tolazoline HCl	up to 25 mg	IV	**J2670**
Topotecan	0.25 mg	ORAL	**J8705**
	0.1 mg	IV	**J9351**
Toradol	per 15 mg	IM, IV	J1885
Torecan	10 mg	ORAL	Q0174
	up to 10 mg	IM	J3280
Torisel	1 mg		**J9330**
Tornalate			
concentrated form	per mg	INH	J7628
unit dose	per mg	INH	J7629
Torsemide	10 mg/ml	IV	**J3265**
Totacillin-N	up to 500 mg	IM, IV	J0290
	per 1.5 gm	IM, IV	J0295
Trastuzumab	10 mg	IV	**J9355**
Trasylol	10,000 KIU		J0365
Treanda	1 mg		J9033
Trelstar Depot	3.75 mg		J3315
Trelstar LA	3.75 mg		J3315

◄ New   ← Revised   ✔ Reinstated   ~~deleted~~ Deleted

DRUG NAME	DOSAGE	METHOD OF ADMINISTRATION	HCPCS CODE
Treprostinil	1 mg		J3285, J7686
Trexall	2.5 mg	ORAL	J8610
Triethylenethosphoramide	15 mg		J9340
Tri-Kort	1 mg		J3300
	per 10 mg	IM	J3301
Triam-A	1 mg		J3300
	per 10 mg	IM	J3301
Triamcinolone			
concentrated form	per 1 mg	INH	J7683
unit dose	per 1 mg	INH	J7684
Triamcinolone acetonide	1 mg		J3300, J7684
	per 10 mg	IM	J3301
Triamcinolone diacetate	per 5 mg	IM	J3302
Triamcinolone hexacetonide	per 5 mg	VAR	J3303
Triamcot	per 5 mg		J3302
Triesence	1 mg		J3300
	per 10 mg	IM	J3301
Triflupromazine HCl	up to 20 mg	IM, IV	J3400
Trilafon	4 mg	ORAL	Q0175
	8 mg	ORAL	Q0176
	up to 5 mg	IM, IV	J3310
Trilog	1 mg		J3300
	per 10 mg	IM	J3301
Trilone	per 5 mg		J3302
Trimethobenzamide HCl			
injection	up to 200 mg	IM	J3250
oral	250 mg	ORAL	Q0173
Trimetrexate glucuronate	per 25 mg	IV	J3305
Triptorelin Pamoate	3.75 mg	SC	J3315
Trisenox	1 mg	IV	J9017
Trobicin	up to 2 g	IM	J3320
Trovan	100 mg	IV	J0200
Truxadryl	50 mg		J1200
Twinrix			J3490
Tysabri	1 mg		J2323
Tyvaso	1.74 mg		J7686
			J7699
U			
Ultravist 150	per ml		Q9965
Ultravist 240	per ml		Q9966
Ultravist 300	per ml		Q9966
Ultravist 370	per ml		Q9967

◄ New   ← Revised   ✔ Reinstated   ~~deleted~~ Deleted

DRUG NAME	DOSAGE	METHOD OF ADMINISTRATION	HCPCS CODE	
Ultrazine-10	up to 10 mg	IM, IV	J0780	
Unasyn	per 1.5 gm	IM, IV	J0295	
Unclassified drugs (see also Not elsewhere classified)			**J3490**	
Unspecified oral antiemetic			**Q0181**	
Urea	up to 40 g	IV	**J3350**	
Ureaphil	up to 40 g	IV	J3350	
Urecholine	up to 5 mg	SC	J0520	
Urofollitropin	75 IU		**J3355**	
Urokinase	5,000 IU vial	IV	**J3364**	
	250,000 IU vial	IV	**J3365**	
Ustekinumab	1 mg	SC	**J3357**	←
V				
V-Gan 25	up to 50 mg	IM, IV	J2550	
	12.5 mg	ORAL	Q0169	
	25 mg	ORAL	Q0170	
V-Gan 50	up to 50 mg	IM, IV	J2550	
	12.5 mg	ORAL	Q0169	
	25 mg	ORAL	Q0170	
Valcyte			J3490	
Valergen 10	10 mg	IM	J1380	
Valergen 20	10 mg	IM	J1380	
Valergen 40	up to 10 mg	IM	J1380	
Valertest No. 1	up to 1 cc	IM	J0900	
			J1060	
Valertest No. 2	up to 1 cc	IM	J0900	
Valium	up to 5 mg	IM, IV	J3360	
Valrubicin, intravesical	200 mg	OTH	**J9357**	
Valstar	200 mg	OTH	J9357	
Vancocin	500 mg	IV, IM	J3370	
Vancoled	500 mg	IV, IM	J3370	
Vancomycin HCl	500 mg	IV, IM	**J3370**	
Vantas	50 mg		J9226	
Vasceze	per 10 mg		J1642	
Vasceze Sodium Chloride	10 ml		A4216	
Vasoxyl, see Methoxamine HCl				
Vectibix	10 mg		J9303	
Velaglucerase alfa	100 units	IV	**J3385**	←
Velban	1 mg	IV	J9360	
Velcade	0.1 mg		J9041	
Velsar	1 mg	IV	J9360	
Venofer	1 mg	IV	J1756	
Ventavis	20 mcg		Q4074	

◄ New   ← Revised   ✔ Reinstated   ~~deleted~~ Deleted

DRUG NAME	DOSAGE	METHOD OF ADMINISTRATION	HCPCS CODE
Ventolin	0.5 mg	INH	J7620
concentrated form	1 mg	INH	J7610, J7611
unit dose form	1 mg	INH	J7609, J7613
VePesid			
	10 mg	IV	J9181
	50 mg	ORAL	J8560
Veritas Collagen Matrix			J3490
Versed	per 1 mg	IM, IV	J2250
Verteporfin	0.1 mg	IV	J3396
Vesprin	up to 20 mg	IM, IV	J3400
VFEND IV	10 mg		J3465
Viadur	65 mg		J9219
Vibativ	10 mg		J3095
Vidaza	1 mg		J9025
Vinblastine sulfate	1 mg	IV	J9360
Vincasar PFS	1 mg	IV	J9370
Vincristine sulfate	1 mg	IV	J9370
Vinorelbine tartrate	per 10 mg	IV	J9390
Vispaque	per ml		Q9966, Q9967
Vistacot	up to 25 mg		J3410
Vistaject-25	up to 25 mg	IM	J3410
Vistaril	up to 25 mg	IM	J3410
	25 mg	ORAL	Q0177
	50 mg	ORAL	Q0178
Vistide	375 mg	IV	J0740
Visudyne	0.1 mg	IV	J3396
Vita #12	up to 1,000 mcg		J3420
Vitamin K, phytonadione, menadione, menadiol sodium diphosphate	per 1 mg	IM, SC, IV	J3430
Vitamin B-12 cyanocobalamin	up to 1,000 mcg	IM, SC	J3420
Vitrase	up to 150 units		J3470
	per 1 USP unit		J3471
Vitrasert	4.5 mg		J7310
Vivaglobin	100 mg		J1562
Vivitrol	1 mg		J2315
Von Willebrand Factor Complex, human	per IU VWF:RCo	IV	J7187
	per IU VWF:RCo	IV	J7183 ←
Voriconazole	10 mg	IV	J3465 ←
Vpriv	100 units		J3385
Vumon	50 mg		Q2017
W			
Water for injection bacteriostatic	10 ml		A4216
Wehamine	up to 50 mg	IM, IV	J1240

◀ New   ← Revised   ✔ Reinstated   ~~deleted~~ Deleted

DRUG NAME	DOSAGE	METHOD OF ADMINISTRATION	HCPCS CODE
Wehdryl	up to 50 mg	IM, IV	J1200
	50 mg	ORAL	Q0163
Wellcovorin	per 50 mg	IM, IV	J0640
Wilate	per IU	IV	J7187
Win Rho SD	100 IU	IV	J2792
Wyamine Sulfate, see Mephentermine sulfate			
Wycillin	up to 600,000 units	IM, IV	J2510
Wydase	up to 150 units	SC, IV	J3470
X			
Xeloda	150 mg	ORAL	J8520
	500 mg	ORAL	J8521
Xeomin	1 unit		J0588
Xgera	1 mg		J0987
Xgeva	1 mg		J0897
Xiaflex	0.01 mg		J0775
Xolair	5 mg		J2357
Xopenex	0.5 mg	INH	J7620
concentrated form	1 mg	INH	J7610, J7611, J7612
unit dose form	1 mg	INH	J7609, J7613, J7614
Xylocaine HCl	10 mg	IV	J2001
Xyntha	per IU IV		J7185, J7192
Y			
Yervoy	1 mg		J9228
Z			
Zanosar	1 g	IV	J9320
Zantac	25 mg	IV, IM	J2780
Zemaira	10 mg	IV	J0256
Zemplar	1 mcg	IM, IV	J2501
Zenapax	25 mg	IV	J7513
Zetran	up to 5 mg	IM, IV	J3360
Ziconotide	1 mcg	OTH	**J2278**	←
Zidovudine	10 mg	IV	**J3485**
Zinacef	per 750 mg	IM, IV	J0697
Zinecard	per 250 mg		J1190
Ziprasidone Mesylate	10 mg	IM	**J3486**	←
Zithromax	500 mg	ORAL	J0456
I.V.	500 mg	IV	J0456
Zmax	1 g		Q0144
Zofran	1 mg	IV	J2405
	1 mg	ORAL	Q0162

◄ New ← Revised ✔ Reinstated ~~deleted~~ Deleted

DRUG NAME	DOSAGE	METHOD OF ADMINISTRATION	HCPCS CODE	
Zoladex	per 3.6 mg	SC	J9202	
Zoledronic Acid	1 mg	IV	J3488	←
Zolicef	500 mg	IV, IM	J0690	
Zometa	1 mg	IV	**J3487**	←
Zorbtive	1 mg		J2941	
Zortress	0.25 mg	ORAL	J7527	
Zosyn	1.125 g	IV	J2543	
Zovirax	5 mg		J8499	
Zyprexa Relprevv	1 mg		J2358	
Zyvox	200 mg	IV	J2020	

◀ New   ← Revised   ✔ Reinstated   ~~deleted~~ Deleted

HCPCS 2013: LEVEL II NATIONAL CODES

**2013 HCPCS quarterly updates available
on the companion website at:
http://www.codingupdates.com**

DISCLAIMER

Every effort has been made to make this text complete and accurate, but no guarantee, warranty, or representation is made for its accuracy or completeness. This text is based on the Centers for Medicare and Medicaid Services Healthcare Common Procedure Coding System (HCPCS).

INTRODUCTION

2013 HCPCS quarterly updates available on the companion website at: http:/evolve.elsevier.com/Buck/HCPCS/.

The Centers for Medicare and Medicaid Services (CMS) (formerly Health Care Financing Administration [HCFA]) Healthcare Common Procedure Coding System (HCPCS) is a collection of codes and descriptors that represent procedures, supplies, products, and services that may be provided to Medicare beneficiaries and to individuals enrolled in private health insurance programs. The codes are divided as follows:

Level I: Codes and descriptors copyrighted by the American Medical Association's (AMA's) Current Procedural Terminology, ed. 4 (CPT-4). These are 5 position numeric codes representing physician and nonphysician services.

Level II: Includes codes and descriptors copyrighted by the American Dental Association's current dental terminology, seventh edition (CDT-7/8). These are 5 position alpha-numeric codes comprising the D series. All other Level II codes and descriptors are approved and maintained jointly by the alpha-numeric editorial panel (consisting of CMS, the Health Insurance Association of America, and the Blue Cross and Blue Shield Association). These are 5 position alpha-numeric codes representing primarily items and nonphysician services that are not represented in the Level I codes.

Level III: The CMS eliminated Level III local codes. See Program Memorandum AB-02-113.

Headings are provided as a means of grouping similar or closely related items. The placement of a code under a heading does not indicate additional means of classification, nor does it relate to any health insurance coverage categories.

HCPCS also contains modifiers, which are two-position codes and descriptors used to indicate that a service or procedure that has been performed has been altered by some specific circumstance but not changed in its definition or code. Modifiers are grouped by the levels. Level I modifiers and descriptors are copyrighted by the AMA. Level II modifiers are HCPCS modifiers. Modifiers in the D series are copyrighted by the ADA.

HCPCS is designed to promote uniform reporting and statistical data collection of medical procedures, supplies, products, and services.

HCPCS Disclaimer

Inclusion or exclusion of a procedure, supply, product, or service does not imply any health insurance coverage or reimbursement policy.

HCPCS makes as much use as possible of generic descriptions, but the inclusion of brand names to describe devices or drugs is intended only for indexing purposes; it is not meant to convey endorsement of any particular product or drug.

Updating HCPCS

The primary updates are made annually. Quarterly updates are also issued by CMS.

Legend

CMS Updates:

▶   New
→   Revised
✔   Reinstated
✖   Deleted
✪   Special coverage instructions
◆   Not covered or valid by Medicare
✳   Carrier discretion

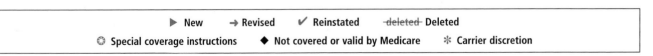

▶ New   → Revised   ✔ Reinstated   deleted Deleted
✪ Special coverage instructions   ◆ Not covered or valid by Medicare   ✳ Carrier discretion

LEVEL II NATIONAL MODIFIERS

✳ **A1** Dressing for one wound

✳ **A2** Dressing for two wounds

✳ **A3** Dressing for three wounds

✳ **A4** Dressing for four wounds

✳ **A5** Dressing for five wounds

✳ **A6** Dressing for six wounds

✳ **A7** Dressing for seven wounds

✳ **A8** Dressing for eight wounds

✳ **A9** Dressing for nine or more wounds

✺ **AA** Anesthesia services performed personally by anesthesiologist

IOM: 100-04, 12, 90.4

✺ **AD** Medical supervision by a physician: more than four concurrent anesthesia procedures

IOM: 100-04, 12, 90.4

✳ **AE** Registered dietician

✳ **AF** Specialty physician

✳ **AG** Primary physician

✺ **AH** Clinical psychologist

IOM: 100-04, 12, 170

✳ **AI** Principal physician of record

✺ **AJ** Clinical social worker

IOM: 100-04, 12, 170

IOM: 100-04, 12, 150

✳ **AK** Nonparticipating physician

✺ **AM** Physician, team member service

Not assigned for Medicare

✳ **AP** Determination of refractive state was not performed in the course of diagnostic ophthalmological examination

✳ **AQ** Physician providing a service in an unlisted health professional shortage area (HPSA)

✳ **AR** Physician provider services in a physician scarcity area

✳ **AS** Physician assistant, nurse practitioner, or clinical nurse specialist services for assistant at surgery

✳ **AT** Acute treatment (this modifier should be used when reporting service 98940, 98941, 98942)

✳ **AU** Item furnished in conjunction with a urological, ostomy, or tracheostomy supply

✳ **AV** Item furnished in conjunction with a prosthetic device, prosthetic or orthotic

✳ **AW** Item furnished in conjunction with a surgical dressing

✳ **AX** Item furnished in conjunction with dialysis services

✳ **AY** Item or service furnished to an ESRD patient that is not for the treatment of ESRD

◆ **AZ** Physician providing a service in a dental health professional shortage area for the purpose of an electronic health record incentive payment

✳ **BA** Item furnished in conjunction with parenteral enteral nutrition (PEN) services

✳ **BL** Special acquisition of blood and blood products

✳ **BO** Orally administered nutrition, not by feeding tube

✳ **BP** The beneficiary has been informed of the purchase and rental options and has elected to purchase the item

✳ **BR** The beneficiary has been informed of the purchase and rental options and has elected to rent the item

✳ **BU** The beneficiary has been informed of the purchase and rental options and after 30 days has not informed the supplier of his/her decision

✳ **CA** Procedure payable only in the inpatient setting when performed emergently on an outpatient who expires prior to admission

✳ **CB** Service ordered by a renal dialysis facility (RDF) physician as part of the ESRD beneficiary's dialysis benefit, is not part of the composite rate, and is separately reimbursable

✳ **CC** Procedure code change (Use CC when the procedure code submitted was changed either for administrative reasons or because an incorrect code was filed)

✺ **CD** AMCC test has been ordered by an ESRD facility or MCP physician that is part of the composite rate and is not separately billable

✺ **CE** AMCC test has been ordered by an ESRD facility or MCP physician that is a composite rate test but is beyond the normal frequency covered under the rate and is separately reimbursable based on medical necessity

---

▶ New → Revised ✔ Reinstated ~~deleted~~ Deleted

✺ Special coverage instructions ◆ Not covered or valid by Medicare ✳ Carrier discretion

○ **CF**   AMCC test has been ordered by an ESRD facility or MCP physician that is not part of the composite rate and is separately billable

＊ **CG**   Policy criteria applied

▶ ○ **CH**   0 percent impaired, limited or restricted

▶ ○ **CI**   At least 1 percent but less than 20 percent impaired, limited or restricted

▶ ○ **CJ**   At least 20 percent but less than 40 percent impaired, limited or restricted

▶ ○ **CK**   At least 40 percent but less than 60 percent impaired, limited or restricted

▶ ○ **CL**   At least 60 percent but less than 80 percent impaired, limited or restricted

▶ ○ **CM**   At least 80 percent but less than 100 percent impaired, limited or restricted

▶ ○ **CN**   100 percent impaired, limited or restricted

＊ **CR**   Catastrophe/Disaster related

→ ＊ **CS**   Item or service related, in whole or in part, to an illness, injury, or condition that was caused by or exacerbated by the effects, direct or indirect, of the 2010 oil spill in the Gulf of Mexico, including but not limited to subsequent clean-up activities

~~DA~~   ~~Oral health assessment by a licensed health professional other than a dentist~~ ✖

＊ **E1**   Upper left, eyelid

＊ **E2**   Lower left, eyelid

＊ **E3**   Upper right, eyelid

＊ **E4**   Lower right, eyelid

○ **EA**   Erythropoetic stimulating agent (ESA) administered to treat anemia due to anti-cancer chemotherapy

CMS requires claims for non-ESRD ESAs (J0881 and J0885) to include one of three modifiers: -EA, -EB, -EC.

○ **EB**   Erythropoetic stimulating agent (ESA) administered to treat anemia due to anti-cancer radiotherapy

CMS requires claims for non-ESRD ESAs (J0881 and J0885) to include one of three modifiers: -EA, -EB, -EC.

○ **EC**   Erythropoetic stimulating agent (ESA) administered to treat anemia not due to anti-cancer radiotherapy or anti-cancer chemotherapy

CMS requires claims for non-ESRD ESAs (J0881 and J0885) to include one of three modifiers: -EA, -EB, -EC.

○ **ED**   Hematocrit level has exceeded 39% (or hemoglobin level has exceeded 13.0 g/dl) for 3 or more consecutive billing cycles immediately prior to and including the current cycle

○ **EE**   Hematocrit level has not exceeded 39% (or hemoglobin level has not exceeded 13.0 g/dl) for 3 or more consecutive billing cycles immediately prior to and including the current cycle

○ **EJ**   Subsequent claims for a defined course of therapy, e.g., EPO, sodium hyaluronate, infliximab

○ **EM**   Emergency reserve supply (for ESRD benefit only)

＊ **EP**   Service provided as part of Medicaid early periodic screening diagnosis and treatment (EPSDT) program

＊ **ET**   Emergency services

＊ **EY**   No physician or other licensed health care provider order for this item or service

Items billed before a signed and dated order has been received by the supplier must be submitted with an -EY modifier added to each related HCPCS code.

＊ **F1**   Left hand, second digit

＊ **F2**   Left hand, third digit

＊ **F3**   Left hand, fourth digit

＊ **F4**   Left hand, fifth digit

＊ **F5**   Right hand, thumb

＊ **F6**   Right hand, second digit

＊ **F7**   Right hand, third digit

＊ **F8**   Right hand, fourth digit

＊ **F9**   Right hand, fifth digit

＊ **FA**   Left hand, thumb

◆ **FB**   Item provided without cost to provider, supplier or practitioner, or full credit received for replaced device (examples, but not limited to, covered under warranty, replaced due to defect, free samples)

○ **FC**   Partial credit received for replaced device

＊ **FP**   Service provided as part of family planning program

＊ **G1**   Most recent URR reading of less than 60

＊ **G2**   Most recent URR reading of 60 to 64.9

＊ **G3**   Most recent URR reading of 65 to 69.9

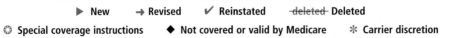

▶ **New**   → **Revised**   ✔ **Reinstated**   ~~deleted~~ **Deleted**
○ **Special coverage instructions**   ◆ **Not covered or valid by Medicare**   ＊ **Carrier discretion**

✳ **G4** Most recent URR reading of 70 to 74.9

✳ **G5** Most recent URR reading of 75 or greater

✳ **G6** ESRD patient for whom less than six dialysis sessions have been provided in a month

❂ **G7** Pregnancy resulted from rape or incest or pregnancy certified by physician as life threatening

IOM: 100-02, 15, 20.1; 100-03, 3, 170.3

✳ **G8** Monitored anesthesia care (MAC) for deep complex, complicated, or markedly invasive surgical procedure

✳ **G9** Monitored anesthesia care for patient who has history of severe cardiopulmonary condition

✳ **GA** Waiver of liability statement issued as required by payer policy, individual case

An item/service is expected to be denied as not reasonable and necessary and an ABN is on file. Modifier -GA can be used on either a specific or a miscellaneous HCPCS code. Modifiers -GA and -GY should never be reported together on the same line for the same HCPCS code.

✳ **GB** Claim being resubmitted for payment because it is no longer covered under a global payment demonstration

❂ **GC** This service has been performed in part by a resident under the direction of a teaching physician.

IOM: 100-04, 12, 90.4, 100

✳ **GD** Units of service exceeds medically unlikely edit value and represents reasonable and necessary services

❂ **GE** This service has been performed by a resident without the presence of a teaching physician under the primary care exception

✳ **GF** Non-physician (e.g., nurse practitioner (NP), certified registered nurse anesthetist (CRNA), certified registered nurse (CRN), clinical nurse specialist (CNS), physician assistant (PA)) services in a critical access hospital

✳ **GG** Performance and payment of a screening mammogram and diagnostic mammogram on the same patient, same day

✳ **GH** Diagnostic mammogram converted from screening mammogram on same day

✳ **GJ** "Opt out" physician or practitioner emergency or urgent service

✳ **GK** Reasonable and necessary item/service associated with a -GA or -GZ modifier

An upgrade is defined as an item that goes beyond what is medically necessary under Medicare's coverage requirements. An item can be considered an upgrade even if the physician has signed an order for it. When suppliers know that an item will not be paid in full because it does not meet the coverage criteria stated in the LCD, the supplier can still obtain partial payment at the time of initial determination if the claim is billed using one of the upgrade modifiers (GK or GL). (https://www.cms.gov/ manuals/downloads/clm104c01.pdf)

✳ **GL** Medically unnecessary upgrade provided instead of non-upgraded item, no charge, no Advance Beneficiary Notice (ABN)

✳ **GM** Multiple patients on one ambulance trip

✳ **GN** Services delivered under an outpatient speech language pathology plan of care

✳ **GO** Services delivered under an outpatient occupational therapy plan of care

✳ **GP** Services delivered under an outpatient physical therapy plan of care

✳ **GQ** Via asynchronous telecommunications system

✳ **GR** This service was performed in whole or in part by a resident in a department of Veterans Affairs medical center or clinic, supervised in accordance with VA policy

➜ ❂ **GS** Dosage of EPO or erythropoietin-stimulating agent has been reduced and maintained in response to hematocrit or hemoglobin level

❂ **GT** Via interactive audio and video telecommunication systems

✳ **GU** Waiver of liability statement issued as required by payer policy, routine notice

❂ **GV** Attending physician not employed or paid under arrangement by the patient's hospice provider

❂ **GW** Service not related to the hospice patient's terminal condition

---

▶ New   ➜ Revised   ✔ Reinstated   ~~deleted~~ Deleted
❂ Special coverage instructions   ◆ Not covered or valid by Medicare   ✳ Carrier discretion

✳ **GX**   Notice of liability issued, voluntary under payer policy

-GX modifier must be submitted with non-covered charges only. This modifier differentiates from the required uses in conjunction with ABN. (https://www .cms.gov/manuals/downloads/ clm104c01.pdf)

◆ **GY**   Item or service statutorily excluded, does not meet the definition of any Medicare benefit or, for non-Medicare insurers, is not a contract benefit

Examples of "statutorily excluded" include: Infusion drug not administered using a durable infusion pump, a wheelchair that is for use for mobility outside the home or hearing aids. -GA and -GY should never be coded together on the same line for the same HCPCS code. (https://www.cms.gov/ manuals/downloads/clm104c01.pdf)

◆ **GZ**   Item or service expected to be denied as not reasonable or necessary

Used when an ABN is not on file and can be used on either a specific or a miscellaneous HCPCS code. It would never be correct to place any combination of -GY, -GZ or -GA modifiers on the same claim line and will result in rejected or denied claim for invalid coding. (https://www.cms. gov/manuals/downloads/clm104c01.pdf)

◆ **H9**   Court-ordered

◆ **HA**   Child/adolescent program

◆ **HB**   Adult program, nongeriatric

◆ **HC**   Adult program, geriatric

◆ **HD**   Pregnant/parenting women's program

◆ **HE**   Mental health program

◆ **HF**   Substance abuse program

◆ **HG**   Opioid addiction treatment program

◆ **HH**   Integrated mental health/substance abuse program

◆ **HI**   Integrated mental health and mental retardation/developmental disabilities program

◆ **HJ**   Employee assistance program

◆ **HK**   Specialized mental health programs for high-risk populations

◆ **HL**   Intern

◆ **HM**   Less than bachelor degree level

◆ **HN**   Bachelors degree level

◆ **HO**   Masters degree level

◆ **HP**   Doctoral level

◆ **HQ**   Group setting

◆ **HR**   Family/couple with client present

◆ **HS**   Family/couple without client present

◆ **HT**   Multi-disciplinary team

◆ **HU**   Funded by child welfare agency

◆ **HV**   Funded by state addictions agency

◆ **HW**   Funded by state mental health agency

◆ **HX**   Funded by county/local agency

◆ **HY**   Funded by juvenile justice agency

◆ **HZ**   Funded by criminal justice agency

✳ **J1**   Competitive acquisition program no-pay submission for a prescription number

✳ **J2**   Competitive acquisition program, restocking of emergency drugs after emergency administration

✳ **J3**   Competitive acquisition program (CAP), drug not available through CAP as written, reimbursed under average sales price methodology

✳ **J4**   DMEPOS item subject to DMEPOS competitive bidding program that is furnished by a hospital upon discharge

✳ **JA**   Administered intravenously

This modifier is informational only (not a payment modifier) and may be submitted with all injection codes. According to Medicare, reporting this modifier is voluntary. (CMS Pub. 100-04, chapter 8, section 60.2.3.1 and Pub. 100-04, chapter 17, section 80.11)

✳ **JB**   Administered subcutaneously

✳ **JC**   Skin substitute used as a graft

✳ **JD**   Skin substitute not used as a graft

✳ **JW**   Drug amount discarded/not administered to any patient

Use -JW to identify unused drugs or biologicals from single use vial/package that are appropriately discarded. Bill on separate line for payment of discarded drug/biological.

✳ **K0**   Lower extremity prosthesis functional Level 0 - does not have the ability or potential to ambulate or transfer safely with or without assistance and a prosthesis does not enhance their quality of life or mobility.

✳ **K1**   Lower extremity prosthesis functional Level 1 - has the ability or potential to use a prosthesis for transfers or ambulation on level surfaces at fixed cadence. Typical of the limited and unlimited household ambulator.

▶ New   → Revised   ✔ Reinstated   ̶d̶e̶l̶e̶t̶e̶d̶ Deleted
☉ Special coverage instructions   ◆ Not covered or valid by Medicare   ✳ Carrier discretion

✳ **K2** Lower extremity prosthesis functional Level 2 - has the ability or potential for ambulation with the ability to traverse low level environmental barriers such as curbs, stairs or uneven surfaces. Typical of the limited community ambulator.

✳ **K3** Lower extremity prosthesis functional Level 3 - has the ability or potential for ambulation with variable cadence. Typical of the community ambulator who has the ability to traverse most environmental barriers and may have vocational, therapeutic, or exercise activity that demands prosthetic utilization beyond simple locomotion.

✳ **K4** Lower extremity prosthesis functional Level 4 - has the ability or potential for prosthetic ambulation that exceeds the basic ambulation skills, exhibiting high impact, stress, or energy levels, typical of the prosthetic demands of the child, active adult, or athlete.

✳ **KA** Add on option/accessory for wheelchair

✳ **KB** Beneficiary requested upgrade for ABN, more than 4 modifiers identified on claim

✳ **KC** Replacement of special power wheelchair interface

✳ **KD** Drug or biological infused through DME

✳ **KE** Bid under round one of the DMEPOS competitive bidding program for use with non-competitive bid base equipment

✳ **KF** Item designated by FDA as Class III device

✳ **KG** DMEPOS item subject to DMEPOS competitive bidding program number 1

✳ **KH** DMEPOS item, initial claim, purchase or first month rental

✳ **KI** DMEPOS item, second or third month rental

✳ **KJ** DMEPOS item, parenteral enteral nutrition (PEN) pump or capped rental, months four to fifteen

✳ **KK** DMEPOS item subject to DMEPOS competitive bidding program number 2

✳ **KL** DMEPOS item delivered via mail

✳ **KM** Replacement of facial prosthesis including new impression/moulage

✳ **KN** Replacement of facial prosthesis using previous master model

✳ **KO** Single drug unit dose formulation

✳ **KP** First drug of a multiple drug unit dose formulation

✳ **KQ** Second or subsequent drug of a multiple drug unit dose formulation

✳ **KR** Rental item, billing for partial month

☺ **KS** Glucose monitor supply for diabetic beneficiary not treated with insulin

✳ **KT** Beneficiary resides in a competitive bidding area and travels outside that competitive bidding area and receives a competitive bid item

✳ **KU** DMEPOS item subject to DMEPOS competitive bidding program number 3

✳ **KV** DMEPOS item subject to DMEPOS competitive bidding program that is furnished as part of a professional service

✳ **KW** DMEPOS item subject to DMEPOS competitive bidding program number 4

✳ **KX** Requirements specified in the medical policy have been met

✳ **KY** DMEPOS item subject to DMEPOS competitive bidding program number 5

✳ **KZ** New coverage not implemented by managed care

✳ **LC** Left circumflex coronary artery

✳ **LD** Left anterior descending coronary artery

✳ **LL** Lease/rental (use the LL modifier when DME equipment rental is to be applied against the purchase price)

▶ ✳ **LM** Left main coronary artery

✳ **LR** Laboratory round trip

☺ **LS** FDA-monitored intraocular lens implant

✳ **LT** Left side (used to identify procedures performed on the left side of the body)

✳ **M2** Medicare secondary payer (MSP)

✳ **MS** Six month maintenance and servicing fee for reasonable and necessary parts and labor which are not covered under any manufacturer or supplier warranty

✳ **NB** Nebulizer system, any type, FDA-cleared for use with specific drug

✳ **NR** New when rented (use the NR modifier when DME which was new at the time of rental is subsequently purchased)

✳ **NU** New equipment

✳ **P1** A normal healthy patient

✳ **P2** A patient with mild systemic disease

✳ **P3** A patient with severe systemic disease

▶ New　→ Revised　✔ Reinstated　~~deleted~~ Deleted

☺ Special coverage instructions　◆ Not covered or valid by Medicare　✳ Carrier discretion

✳ **P4**   A patient with severe systemic disease that is a constant threat to life

✳ **P5**   A moribund patient who is not expected to survive without the operation

✳ **P6**   A declared brain-dead patient whose organs are being removed for donor purposes

◆ **PA**   Surgical or other invasive procedure on wrong body part

◆ **PB**   Surgical or other invasive procedure on wrong patient

◆ **PC**   Wrong surgery or other invasive procedure on patient

✳ **PD**   Diagnostic or related non diagnostic item or service provided in a wholly owned or operated entity to a patient who is admitted as an inpatient within 3 days

✳ **PI**   Positron emission tomography (PET) or PET/computed tomography (CT) to inform the initial treatment strategy of tumors that are biopsy proven or strongly suspected of being cancerous based on other diagnostic testing

✳ **PL**   Progressive addition lenses

✳ **PS**   Positron emission tomography (PET) or PET/computed tomography (CT) to inform the subsequent treatment strategy of cancerous tumors when the beneficiary's treating physician determines that the PET study is needed to inform subsequent anti-tumor strategy

✳ **PT**   Colorectal cancer screening test; converted to diagnostic text or other procedure

   Assign this modifier with the appropriate CPT procedure code for colonoscopy, flexible sigmoidoscopy, or barium enema when the service is initiated as a colorectal cancer screening service but then becomes a diagnostic service. (MLN Matters article MM7012 (PDF, 75 KB)

☺ **Q0**   Investigational clinical service provided in a clinical research study that is in an approved clinical research study

☺ **Q1**   Routine clinical service provided in a clinical research study that is in an approved clinical research study

✳ **Q2**   HCFA/ORD demonstration project procedure/service

✳ **Q3**   Live kidney donor surgery and related services

✳ **Q4**   Service for ordering/referring physician qualifies as a service exemption

☺ **Q5**   Service furnished by a substitute physician under a reciprocal billing arrangement

   IOM: 100-04, 1, 30.2.10

☺ **Q6**   Service furnished by a locum tenens physician

   IOM: 100-04, 1, 30.2.11

✳ **Q7**   One Class A finding

✳ **Q8**   Two Class B findings

✳ **Q9**   One Class B and two Class C findings

✳ **QC**   Single channel monitoring

✳ **QD**   Recording and storage in solid state memory by a digital recorder

✳ **QE**   Prescribed amount of oxygen is less than 1 liter per minute (LPM)

✳ **QF**   Prescribed amount of oxygen exceeds 4 liters per minute (LPM) and portable oxygen is prescribed

✳ **QG**   Prescribed amount of oxygen is greater than 4 liters per minute (LPM)

✳ **QH**   Oxygen conserving device is being used with an oxygen delivery system

☺ **QJ**   Services/items provided to a prisoner or patient in state or local custody, however, the state or local government, as applicable, meets the requirements in 42 CFR 411.4 (B)

☺ **QK**   Medical direction of two, three, or four concurrent anesthesia procedures involving qualified individuals

   IOM: 100-04, 12, 50K, 90

✳ **QL**   Patient pronounced dead after ambulance called

✳ **QM**   Ambulance service provided under arrangement by a provider of services

✳ **QN**   Ambulance service furnished directly by a provider of services

☺ **QP**   Documentation is on file showing that the laboratory test(s) was ordered individually or ordered as a CPT-recognized panel other than automated profile codes 80002-80019, G0058, G0059, and G0060.

☺ **QS**   Monitored anesthesia care service

   IOM: 100-04, 12, 30.6, 501

✳ **QT**   Recording and storage on tape by an analog tape recorder

✳ **QW**   CLIA-waived test

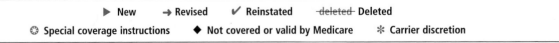

▶ New   → Revised   ✔ Reinstated   ~~deleted~~ Deleted
☺ Special coverage instructions   ◆ Not covered or valid by Medicare   ✳ Carrier discretion

✳ **QX** CRNA service: with medical direction by a physician

☺ **QY** Medical direction of one certified registered nurse anesthetist (CRNA) by an anesthesiologist

IOM: 100-04, 12, 50K, 90

✳ **QZ** CRNA service: without medical direction by a physician

✳ **RA** Replacement of a DME, orthotic or prosthetic item

Contractors will deny claims for replacement parts when furnished in conjunction with the repair of a capped rental item and billed with modifier -RB, including claims for parts submitted using code E1399, that are billed during the capped rental period (i.e., the last day of the 13th month of continuous use or before). Repair includes all maintenance, servicing, and repair of capped rental DME because it is included in the allowed rental payment amounts. (Pub 100-20 One-Time Notification Centers for Medicare & Medicaid Services, Transmittal: 901, May 13, 2011)

✳ **RB** Replacement of a part of a DME, orthotic or prosthetic item furnished as part of a repair

✳ **RC** Right coronary artery

✳ **RD** Drug provided to beneficiary, but not administered "incident-to"

✳ **RE** Furnished in full compliance with FDA-mandated risk evaluation and mitigation strategy (REMS)

▶ ✳ **RI** Ramus intermedius coronary artery

✳ **RR** Rental (use the 'RR' modifier when DME is to be rented)

✳ **RT** Right side (used to identify procedures performed on the right side of the body)

◆ **SA** Nurse practitioner rendering service in collaboration with a physician

◆ **SB** Nurse midwife

→ ✳ **SC** Medically necessary service or supply

◆ **SD** Services provided by registered nurse with specialized, highly technical home infusion training

◆ **SE** State and/or federally funded programs/services

✳ **SF** Second opinion ordered by a professional review organization (PRO) per Section 9401, P.L. 99-272 (100% reimbursement - no Medicare deductible or coinsurance)

✳ **SG** Ambulatory surgical center (ASC) facility service

◆ **SH** Second concurrently administered infusion therapy

◆ **SJ** Third or more concurrently administered infusion therapy

◆ **SK** Member of high risk population (use only with codes for immunization)

◆ **SL** State supplied vaccine

◆ **SM** Second surgical opinion

◆ **SN** Third surgical opinion

◆ **SQ** Item ordered by home health

◆ **SS** Home infusion services provided in the infusion suite of the IV therapy provider

◆ **ST** Related to trauma or injury

◆ **SU** Procedure performed in physician's office (to denote use of facility and equipment)

◆ **SV** Pharmaceuticals delivered to patient's home but not utilized

✳ **SW** Services provided by a certified diabetic educator

◆ **SY** Persons who are in close contact with member of high-risk population (use only with codes for immunization)

✳ **T1** Left foot, second digit

✳ **T2** Left foot, third digit

✳ **T3** Left foot, fourth digit

✳ **T4** Left foot, fifth digit

✳ **T5** Right foot, great toe

✳ **T6** Right foot, second digit

✳ **T7** Right foot, third digit

✳ **T8** Right foot, fourth digit

✳ **T9** Right foot, fifth digit

✳ **TA** Left foot, great toe

✳ **TC** Technical component; Under certain circumstances, a charge may be made for the technical component alone; under those circumstances the technical component charge is identified by adding modifier TC to the usual procedure number; technical component charges are institutional charges and not billed separately by physicians; however, portable x-ray suppliers only bill for technical component and should utilize modifier TC; the charge data from portable x-ray suppliers will then be used to build customary and prevailing profiles.

◆ **TD** RN

▶ New   → Revised   ✔ Reinstated   ~~deleted~~ Deleted

☺ Special coverage instructions   ◆ Not covered or valid by Medicare   ✳ Carrier discretion

◆ **TE**   LPN/LVN

◆ **TF**   Intermediate level of care

◆ **TG**   Complex/high tech level of care

◆ **TH**   Obstetrical treatment/services, prenatal or postpartum

◆ **TJ**   Program group, child and/or adolescent

◆ **TK**   Extra patient or passenger, non-ambulance

◆ **TL**   Early intervention/individualized family service plan (IFSP)

◆ **TM**   Individualized education program (IEP)

◆ **TN**   Rural/outside providers' customary service area

◆ **TP**   Medical transport, unloaded vehicle

◆ **TQ**   Basic life support transport by a volunteer ambulance provider

◆ **TR**   School-based individual education program (IEP) services provided outside the public school district responsible for the student

✻ **TS**   Follow-up service

◆ **TT**   Individualized service provided to more than one patient in same setting

◆ **TU**   Special payment rate, overtime

◆ **TV**   Special payment rates, holidays/weekends

◆ **TW**   Back-up equipment

◆ **U1**   Medicaid Level of Care 1, as defined by each State

◆ **U2**   Medicaid Level of Care 2, as defined by each State

◆ **U3**   Medicaid Level of Care 3, as defined by each State

◆ **U4**   Medicaid Level of Care 4, as defined by each State

◆ **U5**   Medicaid Level of Care 5, as defined by each State

◆ **U6**   Medicaid Level of Care 6, as defined by each State

◆ **U7**   Medicaid Level of Care 7, as defined by each State

◆ **U8**   Medicaid Level of Care 8, as defined by each State

◆ **U9**   Medicaid Level of Care 9, as defined by each State

◆ **UA**   Medicaid Level of Care 10, as defined by each State

◆ **UB**   Medicaid Level of Care 11, as defined by each State

◆ **UC**   Medicaid Level of Care 12, as defined by each State

◆ **UD**   Medicaid Level of Care 13, as defined by each State

✻ **UE**   Used durable medical equipment

◆ **UF**   Services provided in the morning

◆ **UG**   Services provided in the afternoon

◆ **UH**   Services provided in the evening

◆ **UJ**   Services provided at night

◆ **UK**   Services provided on behalf of the client to someone other than the client (collateral relationship)

✻ **UN**   Two patients served

✻ **UP**   Three patients served

✻ **UQ**   Four patients served

✻ **UR**   Five patients served

✻ **US**   Six or more patients served

✻ **V5**   Vascular catheter (alone or with any other vascular access)

✻ **V6**   Arteriovenous graft (or other vascular access not including a vascular catheter)

✻ **V7**   Arteriovenous fistula only (in use with two needles)

~~V8~~   ~~Infection present~~   ✖

~~V9~~   ~~No infection present~~   ✖

✻ **VP**   Aphakic patient

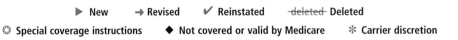

▶ New   → Revised   ✔ Reinstated   ~~deleted~~ Deleted
☺ Special coverage instructions   ◆ Not covered or valid by Medicare   ✻ Carrier discretion

Ambulance Modifiers

Modifiers that are used on claims for ambulance services are created by combining two alpha characters. Each alpha character, with the exception of X, represents an origin (source) code or a destination code. The pair of alpha codes creates one modifier. The first position alpha-code = origin; the second position alpha-code = destination. On form CMS-1491, used to report ambulance services, Item 12 should contain the origin code and Item 13 should contain the destination code. Origin and destination codes and their descriptions are as follows:

D	Diagnostic or therapeutic site other than P or H when these are used as origin codes
E	Residential, domiciliary, custodial facility (other than an 1819 facility)
G	Hospital-based dialysis facility (hospital or hospital related)
H	Hospital
I	Site of transfer (e.g., airport or helicopter pad) between modes of ambulance transport
J	Non–hospital-based dialysis facility
N	Skilled nursing facility (SNF) (1819 facility)
P	Physician's office (includes HMO non-hospital facility, clinic, etc.)
R	Residence
S	Scene of accident or acute event
X	Destination code only. Intermediate stop at physician's office en route to the hospital (includes non-hospital facility, clinic, etc.)

TRANSPORT SERVICES INCLUDING AMBULANCE (A0000-A0999)

A0021-A099: Bill local carrier

◆ **A0021** Ambulance service, outside state per mile, transport (Medicaid only)

Cross Reference A0030

◆ **A0080** Non-emergency transportation, per mile - vehicle provided by volunteer (individual or organization), with no vested interest

◆ **A0090** Non-emergency transportation, per mile - vehicle provided by individual (family member, self, neighbor) with vested interest

◆ **A0100** Non-emergency transportation; taxi

◆ **A0110** Non-emergency transportation and bus, intra or inter state carrier

◆ **A0120** Non-emergency transportation: mini-bus, mountain area transports, or other transportation systems

◆ **A0130** Non-emergency transportation: wheel chair van

◆ **A0140** Non-emergency transportation and air travel (private or commercial), intra or inter state

◆ **A0160** Non-emergency transportation: per mile - caseworker or social worker

◆ **A0170** Transportation: ancillary: parking fees, tolls, other

◆ **A0180** Non-emergency transportation: ancillary: lodging - recipient

◆ **A0190** Non-emergency transportation: ancillary: meals - recipient

◆ **A0200** Non-emergency transportation: ancillary: lodging - escort

◆ **A0210** Non-emergency transportation: ancillary: meals - escort

◆ **A0225** Ambulance service, neonatal transport, base rate, emergency transport, one way

◆ **A0380** BLS mileage (per mile)

Cross Reference A0425

✳ **A0382** BLS routine disposable supplies

✳ **A0384** BLS specialized service disposable supplies; defibrillation (used by ALS ambulances and BLS ambulances in jurisdictions where defibrillation is permitted in BLS ambulances)

◆ **A0390** ALS mileage (per mile)

Cross Reference A0425

✳ **A0392** ALS specialized service disposable supplies; defibrillation (to be used only in jurisdictions where defibrillation cannot be performed in BLS ambulances)

✳ **A0394** ALS specialized service disposable supplies; IV drug therapy

✳ **A0396** ALS specialized service disposable supplies; esophageal intubation

✳ **A0398** ALS routine disposable supplies

▶ New   → Revised   ✔ Reinstated   ~~deleted~~ Deleted

☺ Special coverage instructions   ◆ Not covered or valid by Medicare   ✳ Carrier discretion

* **A0420** Ambulance waiting time (ALS or BLS), one half (½) hour increments

Waiting Time Table			
UNITS	TIME	UNITS	TIME
1	½ to 1 hr.	6	3 to 3½ hrs.
2	1 to 1½ hrs.	7	3½ to 4 hrs.
3	1½ to 2 hrs.	8	4 to 4½ hrs.
4	2 to 2½ hrs.	9	4½ to 5 hrs.
5	2½ to 3 hrs.	10	5 to 5½ hrs.

* **A0422** Ambulance (ALS or BLS) oxygen and oxygen supplies, life sustaining situation

* **A0424** Extra ambulance attendant, ground (ALS or BLS) or air (fixed or rotary winged); (requires medical review)

* **A0425** Ground mileage, per statute mile

* **A0426** Ambulance service, advanced life support, non-emergency transport, Level 1 (ALS1)

* **A0427** Ambulance service, advanced life support, emergency transport, Level 1 (ALS1-Emergency)

* **A0428** Ambulance service, basic life support, non-emergency transport (BLS)

* **A0429** Ambulance service, basic life support, emergency transport (BLS-Emergency)

* **A0430** Ambulance service, conventional air services, transport, one way (fixed wing)

* **A0431** Ambulance service, conventional air services, transport, one way (rotary wing)

* **A0432** Paramedic intercept (PI), rural area, transport furnished by a volunteer ambulance company, which is prohibited by state law from billing third party payers

* **A0433** Advanced life support, Level 2 (ALS2)

* **A0434** Specialty care transport (SCT)

* **A0435** Fixed wing air mileage, per statute mile

* **A0436** Rotary wing air mileage, per statute mile

◆ **A0888** Noncovered ambulance mileage, per mile (e.g., for miles traveled beyond closest appropriate facility)
MCM 2125

◆ **A0998** Ambulance response and treatment, no transport
IOM: 100-02, 10, 20

○ **A0999** Unlisted ambulance service
IOM: 100-02, 10, 20

MEDICAL AND SURGICAL SUPPLIES (A4000-A9999)

* **A4206** Syringe with needle, sterile 1cc or less, each
If "incident to" a physician's service, do not bill; otherwise, bill DME/MAC.

* **A4207** Syringe with needle, sterile 2cc, each
If "incident to" a physician's service, do not bill; otherwise, bill DME/MAC.

* **A4208** Syringe with needle, sterile 3cc, each
If "incident to" a physician's service, do not bill; otherwise, bill DME/MAC.

* **A4209** Syringe with needle, sterile 5cc or greater, each
If "incident to" a physician's service, do not bill; otherwise, bill DME/MAC.

◆ **A4210** Needle-free injection device, each
IOM: 100-03, 4, 280.1
Bill DME/MAC

○ **A4211** Supplies for self-administered injections
If "incident to" a physican service, do not bill; otherwise, bill DME/MAC.
IOM: 100-02, 15, 50

* **A4212** Non-coring needle or stylet with or without catheter
Bill local carrier

* **A4213** Syringe, sterile, 20 cc or greater, each
If "incident to" a physican service, do not bill; otherwise, bill DME/MAC.

* **A4215** Needle, sterile, any size, each
If "incident to" a physican service, do not bill; otherwise, bill DME/MAC.

○ **A4216** Sterile water, saline and/or dextrose diluent/flush, 10 ml
If "incident to" a physican service, do not bill; otherwise, bill DME/MAC.
Other: Broncho Saline, Hyper-Sal, Monoject Prefill advanced, Sodium Chloride, Sodium Chloride Bacteriostatic, Syrex, Vasceze Sodium Chloride, Water for Injection Bacteriostatic
IOM: 100-02, 15, 50

○ **A4217** Sterile water/saline, 500 ml
If "incident to" a physican service, do not bill; otherwise, bill DME/MAC.
Other: Sodium Chloride
IOM: 100-02, 15, 50

▶ New	→ Revised	✔ Reinstated	~~deleted~~ Deleted

○ Special coverage instructions ◆ Not covered or valid by Medicare * Carrier discretion

✻ **A4218** Sterile saline or water, metered dose dispenser, 10 ml

If "incident to" a physican service, do not bill; otherwise, bill DME/MAC.

✻ **A4220** Refill kit for implantable infusion pump

Bill local carrier. Do not report with 95990 or 95991 since Medicare payment for these codes includes the refill kit.

IOM: 100-03, 4, 280.1

✳ **A4221** Supplies for maintenance of drug infusion catheter, per week (list drug separately)

If "incident to" a physican service, do not bill; otherwise, bill DME/MAC. Includes dressings for catheter site and flush solutions not directly related to drug infusion

✳ **A4222** Infusion supplies for external drug infusion pump, per cassette or bag (list drug separately)

If "incident to" physician service, do not bill; otherwise bill DME/MAC. Includes cassette or bag, diluting solutions, tubing and/or administration supplies, port cap changes, compounding charges, and preparation charges.

✳ **A4223** Infusion supplies not used with external infusion pump, per cassette or bag (list drugs separately)

If "incident to" physician service, do not bill; otherwise bill DME/MAC

IOM: 100-03, 4, 280.1

✻ **A4230** Infusion set for external insulin pump, non-needle cannula type

If "incident to" physician service, do not bill; otherwise bill DME/MAC. Requires prior authorization and copy of invoice

IOM: 100-03, 4, 280.1

✻ **A4231** Infusion set for external insulin pump, needle type

If "incident to" physician service, do not bill; otherwise bill DME/MAC. Requires prior authorization and copy of invoice

IOM: 100-03, 4, 280.1

◆ **A4232** Syringe with needle for external insulin pump, sterile, 3cc

If "incident to" physician service, do not bill; otherwise bill DME/MAC. Reports insulin reservoir for use with external insulin infusion pump (E0784); may be glass or plastic; includes needle for drawing up insulin. Does not include insulin for use in reservoir

IOM: 100-03, 4, 280.1

✳ **A4233** Replacement battery, alkaline (other than J cell), for use with medically necessary home blood glucose monitor owned by patient, each

If "incident to" physician service, do not bill; otherwise bill DME/MAC

✳ **A4234** Replacement battery, alkaline, J cell, for use with medically necessary home blood glucose monitor owned by patient, each

If "incident to" a physician's service, do not bill; otherwise, bill DME/MAC.

✳ **A4235** Replacement battery, lithium, for use with medically necessary home blood glucose monitor owned by patient, each

If "incident to" a physician's service, do not bill; otherwise, bill DME/MAC.

✳ **A4236** Replacement battery, silver oxide, for use with medically necessary home blood glucose monitor owned by patient, each

If "incident to" a physician's service, do not bill; otherwise, bill DME/MAC.

✳ **A4244** Alcohol or peroxide, per pint

If "incident to" a physician's service, do not bill; otherwise, bill DME/MAC.

✳ **A4245** Alcohol wipes, per box

If "incident to" a physician's service, do not bill; otherwise, bill DME/MAC.

✳ **A4246** Betadine or pHisoHex solution, per pint

If "incident to" a physician's service, do not bill; otherwise, bill DME/MAC.

✳ **A4247** Betadine or iodine swabs/wipes, per box

If "incident to" a physician's service, do not bill; otherwise, bill DME/MAC.

✳ **A4248** Chlorhexidine containing antiseptic, 1 ml

If "incident to" a physician's service, do not bill; otherwise, bill DME/MAC.

▶ New   → Revised   ✔ Reinstated   ~~deleted~~ Deleted

✪ Special coverage instructions   ◆ Not covered or valid by Medicare   ✳ Carrier discretion

◆ **A4250** Urine test or reagent strips or tablets (100 tablets or strips)

If "incident to" a physician's service, do not bill; otherwise, bill DME/MAC.

IOM: 100-02, 15, 110

◆ **A4252** Blood ketone test or reagent strip, each

Bill DME/MAC

Medicare Statute 1861(n)

☺ **A4253** Blood glucose test or reagent strips for home blood glucose monitor, per 50 strips

Bill DME/MAC. Test strips (1 unit = 50 strips); non-insulin treated (every 3 months) 100 test strips (1×/day testing), 100 lancets (1×/day testing); modifier KS

IOM: 100-03, 1, 40.2

☺ **A4255** Platforms for home blood glucose monitor, 50 per box

Bill DME/MAC

IOM: 100-03, 1, 40.2

☺ **A4256** Normal, low and high calibrator solution/chips

Bill DME/MAC

IOM: 100-03, 1, 40.2

✳ **A4257** Replacement lens shield cartridge for use with laser skin piercing device, each

Bill DME/MAC

☺ **A4258** Spring-powered device for lancet, each

Bill DME/MAC

IOM: 100-03, 1, 40.2

☺ **A4259** Lancets, per box of 100

Bill DME/MAC

IOM: 100-03, 1, 40.2

◆ **A4261** Cervical cap for contraceptive use

Bill local carrier

Medicare Statute 1862A1

☺ **A4262** Temporary, absorbable lacrimal duct implant, each

Bill local carrier

☺ **A4263** Permanent, long term, non-dissolvable lacrimal duct implant, each

Bill local carrier

Bundled if performed in physician office.

IOM: 100-04, 12, 30.4

◆ **A4264** Permanent implantable contraceptive intratubal occlusion device(s) and delivery system

Reports the Essure device.

☺ **A4265** Paraffin, per pound

If "incident to" a physician's service, do not bill; otherwise, bill DME/MAC.

IOM: 100-03, 4, 280.1

◆ **A4266** Diaphragm for contraceptive use

Bill local carrier

◆ **A4267** Contraceptive supply, condom, male, each

Bill local carrier

◆ **A4268** Contraceptive supply, condom, female, each

Bill local carrier

◆ **A4269** Contraceptive supply, spermicide (e.g., foam, gel), each

Bill local carrier

✳ **A4270** Disposable endoscope sheath, each

Bill local carrier

✳ **A4280** Adhesive skin support attachment for use with external breast prosthesis, each

Bill DME/MAC

✳ **A4281** Tubing for breast pump, replacement

Bill DME/MAC

✳ **A4282** Adapter for breast pump, replacement

Bill DME/MAC

✳ **A4283** Cap for breast pump bottle, replacement

Bill DME/MAC

✳ **A4284** Breast shield and splash protector for use with breast pump, replacement

Bill DME/MAC

✳ **A4285** Polycarbonate bottle for use with breast pump, replacement

Bill DME/MAC

✳ **A4286** Locking ring for breast pump, replacement

Bill DME/MAC

✳ **A4290** Sacral nerve stimulation test lead, each

Bill local carrier

Vascular Catheters

☺ **A4300** Implantable access catheter, (e.g., venous, arterial, epidural subarachnoid, or peritoneal, etc.) external access

Bill local carrier

IOM: 100-02, 15, 120

▶ **New** → **Revised** ✔ **Reinstated** ~~deleted~~ **Deleted**

☺ **Special coverage instructions** ◆ **Not covered or valid by Medicare** ✳ **Carrier discretion**

✳ **A4301** Implantable access total; catheter, port/reservoir (e.g., venous, arterial, epidural, subarachnoid, peritoneal, etc.)

Bill local carrier

✳ **A4305** Disposable drug delivery system, flow rate of 50 ml or greater per hour

If "incident to" a physician's service, do not bill; otherwise, bill DME/MAC.

✳ **A4306** Disposable drug delivery system, flow rate of less than 50 ml per hour

If "incident to" a physician's service, do not bill; otherwise, bill DME/MAC.

Incontinence Appliances and Care Supplies

A4310-A4355: If provided in the physician's office for a temporary condition, the item is incident to the physician's service and billed to the local carrier. If provided in the physician's office or other place of service for a permanent condition, the item is a prosthetic device and billed to the DME/MAC.

⊛ **A4310** Insertion tray without drainage bag and without catheter (accessories only)

IOM: 100-02, 15, 120

⊛ **A4311** Insertion tray without drainage bag with indwelling catheter, Foley type, two-way latex with coating (Teflon, silicone, silicone elastomer, or hydrophilic, etc.)

IOM: 100-02, 15, 120

⊛ **A4312** Insertion tray without drainage bag with indwelling catheter, Foley type, two-way, all silicone

IOM: 100-02, 15, 120

⊛ **A4313** Insertion tray without drainage bag with indwelling catheter, Foley type, three-way, for continuous irrigation

IOM: 100-02, 15, 120

⊛ **A4314** Insertion tray with drainage bag with indwelling catheter, Foley type, two-way latex with coating (Teflon, silicone, silicone elastomer or hydrophilic, etc.)

IOM: 100-02, 15, 120

⊛ **A4315** Insertion tray with drainage bag with indwelling catheter, Foley type, two-way, all silicone

IOM: 100-02, 15, 120

⊛ **A4316** Insertion tray with drainage bag with indwelling catheter, Foley type, three-way, for continuous irrigation

IOM: 100-02, 15, 120

⊛ **A4320** Irrigation tray with bulb or piston syringe, any purpose

IOM: 100-02, 15, 120

⊛ **A4321** Therapeutic agent for urinary catheter irrigation

⊛ **A4322** Irrigation syringe, bulb, or piston, each

IOM: 100-02, 15, 120

⊛ **A4326** Male external catheter with integral collection chamber, any type, each

IOM: 100-02, 15, 120

⊛ **A4327** Female external urinary collection device; meatal cup, each

IOM: 100-02, 15, 120

⊛ **A4328** Female external urinary collection device; pouch, each

IOM: 100-02, 15, 120

⊛ **A4330** Perianal fecal collection pouch with adhesive, each

IOM: 100-02, 15, 120

⊛ **A4331** Extension drainage tubing, any type, any length, with connector/adaptor, for use with urinary leg bag or urostomy pouch, each

IOM: 100-02, 15, 120

⊛ **A4332** Lubricant, individual sterile packet, each

IOM: 100-02, 15, 120

⊛ **A4333** Urinary catheter anchoring device, adhesive skin attachment, each

IOM: 100-02, 15, 120

⊛ **A4334** Urinary catheter anchoring device, leg strap, each

IOM: 100-02, 15, 120

⊛ **A4335** Incontinence supply; miscellaneous

IOM: 100-02, 15, 120

⊛ **A4336** Incontinence supply, urethral insert, any type, each

⊛ **A4338** Indwelling catheter; Foley type, two-way latex with coating (Teflon, silicone, silicone elastomer, or hydrophilic, etc.), each

IOM: 100-02, 15, 120

⊛ **A4340** Indwelling catheter; specialty type (e.g., coude, mushroom, wing, etc.), each

IOM: 100-02, 15, 120

⊛ **A4344** Indwelling catheter, Foley type, two-way, all silicone, each

IOM: 100-02, 15, 120

▶ New → Revised ✔ Reinstated ~~deleted~~ Deleted

⊛ Special coverage instructions ◆ Not covered or valid by Medicare ✳ Carrier discretion

⊕ **A4346** Indwelling catheter; Foley type, three way for continuous irrigation, each

IOM: 100-02, 15, 120

⊕ **A4349** Male external catheter, with or without adhesive, disposable, each

IOM: 100-02, 15, 120

⊕ **A4351** Intermittent urinary catheter; straight tip, with or without coating (Teflon, silicone, silicone elastomer, or hydrophilic, etc.), each

IOM: 100-02, 15, 120

⊕ **A4352** Intermittent urinary catheter; coude (curved) tip, with or without coating (Teflon, silicone, silicone elastomeric, or hydrophilic, etc.), each

IOM: 100-02, 15, 120

⊕ **A4353** Intermittent urinary catheter, with insertion supplies

IOM: 100-02, 15, 120

⊕ **A4354** Insertion tray with drainage bag but without catheter

IOM: 100-02, 15, 120

⊕ **A4355** Irrigation tubing set for continuous bladder irrigation through a three-way indwelling Foley catheter, each

IOM: 100-02, 15, 120

External Urinary Supplies

⊕ **A4356** External urethral clamp or compression device (not to be used for catheter clamp), each

If provided in the physician's office for a temporary condition, the item is incident to the physician's service and billed to the local carrier. If provided in the physician's office or other place of service for a permanent condition, the item is a prosthetic device and billed to the DME/MAC.

IOM: 100-02, 15, 120

⊕ **A4357** Bedside drainage bag, day or night, with or without anti-reflux device, with or without tube, each

If provided in the physician's office for a temporary condition, the item is incident to the physician's service and billed to the local carrier. If provided in the physician's office or other place of service for a permanent condition, the item is a prosthetic device and billed to the DME/MAC.

IOM: 100-02, 15, 120

⊕ **A4358** Urinary drainage bag, leg or abdomen, vinyl, with or without tube, with straps, each

If provided in the physician's office for a temporary condition, the item is incident to the physician's service and billed to the local carrier. If provided in the physician's office or other place of service for a permanent condition, the item is a prosthetic device and billed to the DME/MAC.

IOM: 100-02, 15, 120

⊕ **A4360** Disposable external urethral clamp or compression device, with pad and/or pouch, each

Ostomy Supplies

A4361-A4434: If provided in the physician's office for a temporary condition, the item is incident to the physician's service and billed to the local carrier. If provided in the physician's office or other place of service for a permanent condition, the item is a prosthetic device and billed to the DME/MAC.

⊕ **A4361** Ostomy faceplate, each

IOM: 100-02, 15, 120

⊕ **A4362** Skin barrier; solid, 4 × 4 or equivalent; each

IOM: 100-02, 15, 120

⊕ **A4363** Ostomy clamp, any type, replacement only, each

⊕ **A4364** Adhesive, liquid or equal, any type, per oz

Fee schedule category: Ostomy, tracheostomy, and urologicals items.

IOM: 100-02, 15, 120

✳ **A4366** Ostomy vent, any type, each

⊕ **A4367** Ostomy belt, each

IOM: 100-02, 15, 120

✳ **A4368** Ostomy filter, any type, each

⊕ **A4369** Ostomy skin barrier, liquid (spray, brush, etc), per oz

IOM: 100-02, 15, 120

⊕ **A4371** Ostomy skin barrier, powder, per oz

IOM: 100-02, 15, 120

▶ New → Revised ✔ Reinstated ~~deleted~~ Deleted

⊕ Special coverage instructions ◆ Not covered or valid by Medicare ✳ Carrier discretion

⊗ **A4372** Ostomy skin barrier, solid 4 × 4 or equivalent, standard wear, with built-in convexity, each

IOM: 100-02, 15, 120

⊗ **A4373** Ostomy skin barrier, with flange (solid, flexible, or accordian), with built-in convexity, any size, each

IOM: 100-02, 15, 120

⊗ **A4375** Ostomy pouch, drainable, with faceplate attached, plastic, each

IOM: 100-02, 15, 120

⊗ **A4376** Ostomy pouch, drainable, with faceplate attached, rubber, each

IOM: 100-02, 15, 120

⊗ **A4377** Ostomy pouch, drainable, for use on faceplate, plastic, each

IOM: 100-02, 15, 120

⊗ **A4378** Ostomy pouch, drainable, for use on faceplate, rubber, each

IOM: 100-02, 15, 120

⊗ **A4379** Ostomy pouch, urinary, with faceplate attached, plastic, each

IOM: 100-02, 15, 120

⊗ **A4380** Ostomy pouch, urinary, with faceplate attached, rubber, each

IOM: 100-02, 15, 120

⊗ **A4381** Ostomy pouch, urinary, for use on faceplate, plastic, each

IOM: 100-02, 15, 120

⊗ **A4382** Ostomy pouch, urinary, for use on faceplate, heavy plastic, each

IOM: 100-02, 15, 120

⊗ **A4383** Ostomy pouch, urinary, for use on faceplate, rubber, each

IOM: 100-02, 15, 120

⊗ **A4384** Ostomy faceplate equivalent, silicone ring, each

IOM: 100-02, 15, 120

⊗ **A4385** Ostomy skin barrier, solid 4 × 4 or equivalent, extended wear, without built-in convexity, each

IOM: 100-02, 15, 120

⊗ **A4387** Ostomy pouch closed, with barrier attached, with built-in convexity (1 piece), each

IOM: 100-02, 15, 120

⊗ **A4388** Ostomy pouch, drainable, with extended wear barrier attached (1 piece), each

IOM: 100-02, 15, 120

⊗ **A4389** Ostomy pouch, drainable, with barrier attached, with built-in convexity (1 piece), each

IOM: 100-02, 15, 120

⊗ **A4390** Ostomy pouch, drainable, with extended wear barrier attached, with built-in convexity (1 piece), each

IOM: 100-02, 15, 120

⊗ **A4391** Ostomy pouch, urinary, with extended wear barrier attached (1 piece), each

IOM: 100-02, 15, 120

⊗ **A4392** Ostomy pouch, urinary, with standard wear barrier attached, with built-in convexity (1 piece), each

IOM: 100-02, 15, 120

⊗ **A4393** Ostomy pouch, urinary, with extended wear barrier attached, with built-in convexity (1 piece), each

IOM: 100-02, 15, 120

⊗ **A4394** Ostomy deodorant, with or without lubricant, for use in ostomy pouch, per fluid ounce

IOM: 100-02, 15, 20

⊗ **A4395** Ostomy deodorant for use in ostomy pouch, solid, per tablet

IOM: 100-02, 15, 20

⊗ **A4396** Ostomy belt with peristomal hernia support

IOM: 100-02, 15, 120

⊗ **A4397** Irrigation supply; sleeve, each

IOM: 100-02, 15, 120

⊗ **A4398** Ostomy irrigation supply; bag, each

IOM: 100-02, 15, 120

⊗ **A4399** Ostomy irrigation supply; cone/catheter, with or without brush

IOM: 100-02, 15, 120

⊗ **A4400** Ostomy irrigation set

IOM: 100-02, 15, 120

⊗ **A4402** Lubricant, per ounce

IOM: 100-02, 15, 120

⊗ **A4404** Ostomy ring, each

IOM: 100-02, 15, 120

⊗ **A4405** Ostomy skin barrier, non-pectin based, paste, per ounce

IOM: 100-02, 15, 120

⊗ **A4406** Ostomy skin barrier, pectin-based, paste, per ounce

IOM: 100-02, 15, 120

▶ New   → Revised   ✔ Reinstated   deleted Deleted

⊗ Special coverage instructions   ◆ Not covered or valid by Medicare   ✱ Carrier discretion

⊕ **A4407** Ostomy skin barrier, with flange (solid, flexible, or accordion), extended wear, with built-in convexity, 4 × 4 inches or smaller, each

IOM: 100-02, 15, 120

⊕ **A4408** Ostomy skin barrier, with flange (solid, flexible, or accordion), extended wear, with built-in convexity, larger than 4 × 4 inches, each

IOM: 100-02, 15, 120

⊕ **A4409** Ostomy skin barrier, with flange (solid, flexible, or accordion), extended wear, without built-in convexity, 4 × 4 inches or smaller, each

IOM: 100-02, 15, 120

⊕ **A4410** Ostomy skin barrier, with flange (solid, flexible, or accordion), extended wear, without built-in convexity, larger than 4 × 4 inches, each

IOM: 100-02, 15, 120

⊕ **A4411** Ostomy skin barrier, solid 4 × 4 or equivalent, extended wear, with built-in convexity, each

⊕ **A4412** Ostomy pouch, drainable, high output, for use on a barrier with flange (2 piece system), without filter, each

IOM: 100-02, 15, 120

⊕ **A4413** Ostomy pouch, drainable, high output, for use on a barrier with flange (2 piece system), with filter, each

IOM: 100-02, 15, 120

⊕ **A4414** Ostomy skin barrier, with flange (solid, flexible, or accordion), without built-in convexity, 4 × 4 inches or smaller, each

IOM: 100-02, 15, 120

⊕ **A4415** Ostomy skin barrier, with flange (solid, flexible, or accordion), without built-in convexity, larger than 4 × 4 inches, each

IOM: 100-02, 15, 120

✳ **A4416** Ostomy pouch, closed, with barrier attached, with filter (1 piece), each

✳ **A4417** Ostomy pouch, closed, with barrier attached, with built-in convexity, with filter (1 piece), each

✳ **A4418** Ostomy pouch, closed; without barrier attached, with filter (1 piece), each

✳ **A4419** Ostomy pouch, closed; for use on barrier with non-locking flange, with filter (2 piece), each

✳ **A4420** Ostomy pouch, closed; for use on barrier with locking flange (2 piece), each

✳ **A4421** Ostomy supply; miscellaneous

⊕ **A4422** Ostomy absorbent material (sheet/pad/crystal packet) for use in ostomy pouch to thicken liquid stomal output, each

IOM: 100-02, 15, 120

✳ **A4423** Ostomy pouch, closed; for use on barrier with locking flange, with filter (2 piece), each

✳ **A4424** Ostomy pouch, drainable, with barrier attached, with filter (1 piece), each

✳ **A4425** Ostomy pouch, drainable; for use on barrier with non-locking flange, with filter (2 piece system), each

✳ **A4426** Ostomy pouch, drainable; for use on barrier with locking flange (2 piece system), each

✳ **A4427** Ostomy pouch, drainable; for use on barrier with locking flange, with filter (2 piece system), each

✳ **A4428** Ostomy pouch, urinary, with extended wear barrier attached, with faucet-type tap with valve (1 piece), each

✳ **A4429** Ostomy pouch, urinary, with barrier attached, with built-in convexity, with faucet-type tap with valve (1 piece), each

✳ **A4430** Ostomy pouch, urinary, with extended wear barrier attached, with built-in convexity, with faucet-type tap with valve (1 piece), each

✳ **A4431** Ostomy pouch, urinary; with barrier attached, with faucet-type tap with valve (1 piece), each

✳ **A4432** Ostomy pouch, urinary; for use on barrier with non-locking flange, with faucet-type tap with valve (2 piece), each

✳ **A4433** Ostomy pouch, urinary; for use on barrier with locking flange (2 piece), each

✳ **A4434** Ostomy pouch, urinary; for use on barrier with locking flange, with faucet-type tap with valve (2 piece), each

▶ ✳ **A4435** Ostomy pouch, drainable, high output, with extended wear barrier (one-piece system), with or without filter, each

Miscellaneous Supplies

⊕ **A4450** Tape, non-waterproof, per 18 square inches

If "incident to" physician service, do not bill separately; otherwise bill DME/MAC. If used with surgical dressings, billed with AW modifier (in addition to appropriate A1-A9 modifier).

IOM: 100-02, 15, 120

▶ **New** → **Revised** ✔ **Reinstated** ~~deleted~~ **Deleted**
⊕ **Special coverage instructions** ◆ **Not covered or valid by Medicare** ✳ **Carrier discretion**

✪ **A4452** Tape, waterproof, per 18 square inches

If "incident to" physician service, do not bill separately; otherwise, bill DME/MAC. If used with surgical dressings, billed with AW modifier (in addition to appropriate A1-A9 modifier).

IOM: 100-02, 15, 120

✪ **A4455** Adhesive remover or solvent (for tape, cement or other adhesive), per ounce

If "incident to" a physician service, do not bill; otherwise, bill DME/MAC.

IOM: 100-02, 15, 120

✪ **A4456** Adhesive remover, wipes, any type, each

May be reimbursed for male or female clients to home health DME providers and DME medical suppliers in the home setting.

✳ **A4458** Enema bag with tubing, reusable

Bill DME/MAC

✳ **A4461** Surgical dressing holder, non-reusable, each

If "incident to" a physician's service, do not bill; otherwise, bill DME/MAC.

✳ **A4463** Surgical dressing holder, reusable, each

If "incident to" a physician's service, do not bill; otherwise, bill DME/MAC.

✳ **A4465** Non-elastic binder for extremity

Bill DME/MAC

◆ **A4466** Garment, belt, sleeve or other covering, elastic or similar stretchable material, any type, each

✪ **A4470** Gravlee jet washer

Bill local carrier. Symptoms suggestive of endometrial disease must be present for this disposable diagnostic tool to be covered.

IOM: 100-02, 16, 90; 100-03, 4, 230.5

✪ **A4480** VABRA aspirator

Bill local carrier. Symptoms suggestive of endometrial disease must be present for this disposable diagnostic tool to be covered.

IOM: 100-02, 16, 90; 100-03, 4, 230.6

✪ **A4481** Tracheostoma filter, any type, any size, each

If "incident to" a physician's service, do not bill; otherwise, bill DME/MAC.

IOM: 100-02, 15, 120

✪ **A4483** Moisture exchanger, disposable, for use with invasive mechanical ventilation

Bill DME/MAC

IOM: 100-02, 15, 120

◆ **A4490** Surgical stockings above knee length, each

Bill DME/MAC

IOM: 100-02, 15, 100; 100-02, 15, 110; 100-03, 4, 280.1

◆ **A4495** Surgical stockings thigh length, each

Bill DME/MAC

IOM: 100-02, 15, 100; 100-02, 15, 110; 100-03, 4, 280.1

◆ **A4500** Surgical stockings below knee length, each

Bill DME/MAC

IOM: 100-02, 15, 100; 100-02, 15, 110; 100-03, 4, 280.1

◆ **A4510** Surgical stockings full length, each

Bill DME/MAC

IOM: 100-02, 15, 100; 100-02, 15, 110; 100-03, 4, 280.1

◆ **A4520** Incontinence garment, any type, (e.g. brief, diaper), each

Bill DME/MAC

IOM: 100-03, 4, 280.1

✪ **A4550** Surgical trays

Bill local carrier. No longer payable by Medicare; included in practice expense for procedures. Some private payers may pay, most private payers follow Medicare guidelines

IOM: 100-04, 12, 20.3, 30.4

◆ **A4554** Disposable underpads, all sizes

Bill DME/MAC

IOM: 100-02, 15, 120; 100-03, 4, 280.1

✳ **A4556** Electrodes, (e.g., apnea monitor), per pair

If "incident to" a physician's service, do not bill; otherwise, bill DME/MAC.

✳ **A4557** Lead wires, (e.g., apnea monitor), per pair

If "incident to" a physician's service, do not bill; otherwise, bill DME/MAC.

✳ **A4558** Conductive gel or paste, for use with electrical device (e.g., TENS, NMES), per oz

If "incident to" a physician's service, do not bill; otherwise, bill DME/MAC.

▶ New → Revised ✔ Reinstated ~~deleted~~ Deleted

✪ Special coverage instructions ◆ Not covered or valid by Medicare ✳ Carrier discretion

* **A4559**   Coupling gel or paste, for use with ultrasound device, per oz

   If "incident to" a physician's service, do not bill; otherwise, bill DME/MAC.

* **A4561**   Pessary, rubber, any type

   Bill local carrier

* **A4562**   Pessary, non rubber, any type

   Bill local carrier

* **A4565**   Slings

   Bill local carrier

◆ **A4566**   Shoulder sling or vest design, abduction restrainer, with or without swathe control, prefabricated, includes fitting and adjustment

◆ **A4570**   Splint

   Bill local carrier

   IOM: 100-02, 6, 10; 100-02, 15, 100; 100-04, 4, 240

◆ **A4575**   Topical hyperbaric oxygen chamber, disposable

   Bill DME/MAC

   IOM: 100-03, 1, 20.29

◆ **A4580**   Cast supplies (e.g. plaster)

   Bill local carrier

   IOM: 100-02, 6, 10; 100-02, 15, 100; 100-04, 4, 240

◆ **A4590**   Special casting material (e.g. fiberglass)

   Bill local carrier

   IOM: 100-02, 6, 10; 100-02, 15, 100; 100-04, 4, 240

☼ **A4595**   Electrical stimulator supplies, 2 lead, per month, (e.g. TENS, NMES)

   If "incident to" a physician's service, do not bill; otherwise, bill DME/MAC.

   IOM: 100-03, 2, 160.13

* **A4600**   Sleeve for intermittent limb compression device, replacement only, each

   Bill DME/MAC

* **A4601**   Lithium ion battery for non-prosthetic use, replacement

   Bill DME/MAC

* **A4604**   Tubing with integrated heating element for use with positive airway pressure device

   Bill DME/MAC

* **A4605**   Tracheal suction catheter, closed system, each

   Bill DME/MAC

* **A4606**   Oxygen probe for use with oximeter device, replacement

   Bill DME/MAC

* **A4608**   Transtracheal oxygen catheter, each

   Bill DME/MAC

Supplies for Respiratory and Oxygen Equipment

* **A4611**   Battery, heavy duty; replacement for patient owned ventilator

   Bill DME/MAC

* **A4612**   Battery cables; replacement for patient-owned ventilator

   Bill DME/MAC

* **A4613**   Battery charger; replacement for patient-owned ventilator

   Bill DME/MAC

* **A4614**   Peak expiratory flow rate meter, hand held

   If "incident to" a physician's service, do not bill; otherwise, bill DME/MAC.

☼ **A4615**   Cannula, nasal

   If "incident to" a physician's service, do not bill; otherwise, bill DME/MAC.

   IOM: 100-03, 2, 160.6; 100-04, 20, 100.2

☼ **A4616**   Tubing (oxygen), per foot

   If "incident to" a physician's service, do not bill; otherwise, bill DME/MAC.

   IOM: 100-03, 2, 160.6; 100-04, 20, 100.2

☼ **A4617**   Mouth piece

   If "incident to" a physician's service, do not bill; otherwise, bill DME/MAC.

   IOM: 100-03, 2, 160.6; 100-04, 20, 100.2

☼ **A4618**   Breathing circuits

   If "incident to" a physician's service, do not bill; otherwise, bill DME/MAC.

   IOM: 100-03, 2, 160.6; 100-04, 20, 100.2

→ ☼ **A4619**   Face tent

   If "incident to" a physician's service, do not bill; otherwise, bill DME/MAC.

   IOM: 100-03, 2, 160.6; 100-04, 20, 100.2

☼ **A4620**   Variable concentration mask

   If "incident to" a physician's service, do not bill; otherwise, bill DME/MAC.

   IOM: 100-03, 2, 160.6; 100-04, 20, 100.2

☼ **A4623**   Tracheostomy, inner cannula

   If "incident to" a physician's service, do not bill; otherwise, bill DME/MAC.

   IOM: 100-02, 15, 120; 100-03, 1, 20.9

▶ New   → Revised   ✔ Reinstated   ~~deleted~~ Deleted

☼ Special coverage instructions   ◆ Not covered or valid by Medicare   * Carrier discretion

✳ **A4624** Tracheal suction catheter, any type, other than closed system, each

If "incident to" a physician's service, do not bill; otherwise, bill DME/MAC.

Sterile suction catheters are medically necessary only for tracheostomy suctioning. Limitations include three suction catheters per day when covered for medically necessary tracheostomy suctioning. Assign DX V44.0 or V55.0 on the claim form. (CMS Manual System, Pub. 100-3, NCD manual, Chapter 1, Section 280-1)

❂ **A4625** Tracheostomy care kit for new tracheostomy

If "incident to" a physician's service, do not bill; otherwise, bill DME/MAC.

IOM: 100-02, 15, 120

Dressings used with tracheostomies are included in the allowance for the code. This starter kit is covered after a surgical tracheostomy. (https://www.noridianmedicare.com/dme/coverage/docs/lcds/current_lcds/tracheostomy_care_supplies.htm)

❂ **A4626** Tracheostomy cleaning brush, each

If "incident to" a physician's service, do not bill; otherwise, bill DME/MAC.

IOM: 100-02, 15, 120

◆ **A4627** Spacer, bag, or reservoir, with or without mask, for use with metered dose inhaler

If "incident to" a physician's service, do not bill; otherwise, bill DME/MAC.

IOM: 100-02, 15, 110

✳ **A4628** Oropharyngeal suction catheter, each

If "incident to" a physician's service, do not bill; otherwise, bill DME/MAC.

No more than three catheters per week are covered for medically necessary oropharyngeal suctioning because the catheters can be reused if cleansed and disinfected. (MS Manual System, Pub. 100-3, NCD manual, Chapter 1, Section 280-1)

❂ **A4629** Tracheostomy care kit for established tracheostomy

If "incident to" a physician's service, do not bill; otherwise, bill DME/MAC.

IOM: 100-02, 15, 120

Supplies for Other Durable Medical Equipment

A4630-A4640: Bill DME/MAC

❂ **A4630** Replacement batteries, medically necessary, transcutaneous electrical stimulator, owned by patient

IOM: 100-03, 3, 160.7

✳ **A4633** Replacement bulb/lamp for ultraviolet light therapy system, each

✳ **A4634** Replacement bulb for therapeutic light box, tabletop model

❂ **A4635** Underarm pad, crutch, replacement, each

IOM: 100-03, 4, 280.1

❂ **A4636** Replacement, handgrip, cane, crutch, or walker, each

IOM: 100-03, 4, 280.1

❂ **A4637** Replacement, tip, cane, crutch, walker, each

IOM: 100-03, 4, 280.1

✳ **A4638** Replacement battery for patient-owned ear pulse generator, each

✳ **A4639** Replacement pad for infrared heating pad system, each

❂ **A4640** Replacement pad for use with medically necessary alternating pressure pad owned by patient

IOM: 100-03, 4, 280.1; 100-08, 5, 5.2.3

Supplies for Radiological Procedures

✳ **A4641** Radiopharmaceutical, diagnostic, not otherwise classified

Bill local carrier. Is not an applicable tracer for PET scans

✳ **A4642** Indium In-111 satumomab pendetide, diagnostic, per study dose, up to 6 millicuries

Bill local carrier

Miscellaneous Supplies

✳ **A4648** Tissue marker, implantable, any type, each

Bill local carrier

✳ **A4649** Surgical supply; miscellaneous

Bill local carrier if incident to a physician's service (not separately payable) or if supply for implanted prosthetic device or implanted DME. If other, bill DME/MAC.

▶ New   → Revised   ✔ Reinstated   deleted Deleted

❂ Special coverage instructions   ◆ Not covered or valid by Medicare   ✳ Carrier discretion

✳ **A4650**   Implantable radiation dosimeter, each
Bill local carrier

✿ **A4651**   Calibrated microcapillary tube, each
Bill DME/MAC
IOM: 100-04, 3, 40.3

✿ **A4652**   Microcapillary tube sealant
Bill DME/MAC
IOM: 100-04, 3, 40.3

Supplies for Dialysis

A4653-A4932:   Bill DME/MAC

✳ **A4653**   Peritoneal dialysis catheter anchoring device, belt, each

✿ **A4657**   Syringe, with or without needle, each
IOM: 100-04, 8, 90.3.2

✿ **A4660**   Sphygmomanometer/blood pressure apparatus with cuff and stethoscope
IOM: 100-04, 8, 90.3.2

✿ **A4663**   Blood pressure cuff only
IOM: 100-04, 8, 90.3.2

◆ **A4670**   Automatic blood pressure monitor
IOM: 100-04, 8, 90.3.2

✿ **A4671**   Disposable cycler set used with cycler dialysis machine, each
IOM: 100-04, 8, 90.3.2

✿ **A4672**   Drainage extension line, sterile, for dialysis, each
IOM: 100-04, 8, 90.3.2

✿ **A4673**   Extension line with easy lock connectors, used with dialysis
IOM: 100-04, 8, 90.3.2

✿ **A4674**   Chemicals/antiseptics solution used to clean/sterilize dialysis equipment, per 8 oz
IOM: 100-04, 8, 90.3.2

✿ **A4680**   Activated carbon filters for hemodialysis, each
IOM: 100-04, 8, 90.3.2

✿ **A4690**   Dialyzers (artificial kidneys), all types, all sizes, for hemodialysis, each
IOM: 100-04, 8, 90.3.2

✿ **A4706**   Bicarbonate concentrate, solution, for hemodialysis, per gallon
IOM: 100-04, 8, 90.3.2

✿ **A4707**   Bicarbonate concentrate, powder, for hemodialysis, per packet
IOM: 100-04, 8, 90.3.2

✿ **A4708**   Acetate concentrate solution, for hemodialysis, per gallon
IOM: 100-04, 8, 90.3.2

✿ **A4709**   Acid concentrate, solution, for hemodialysis, per gallon
IOM: 100-04, 8, 90.3.2

✿ **A4714**   Treated water (deionized, distilled, or reverse osmosis) for peritoneal dialysis, per gallon
IOM: 100-03, 4, 230.7; 100-04, 3, 40.3

✿ **A4719**   "Y set" tubing for peritoneal dialysis
IOM: 100-04, 8, 90.3.2

✿ **A4720**   Dialysate solution, any concentration of dextrose, fluid volume greater than 249cc, but less than or equal to 999cc, for peritoneal dialysis
Do not use AX modifier
IOM: 100-04, 8, 90.3.2

✿ **A4721**   Dialysate solution, any concentration of dextrose, fluid volume greater than 999cc but less than or equal to 1999cc, for peritoneal dialysis
IOM: 100-04, 8, 90.3.2

✿ **A4722**   Dialysate solution, any concentration of dextrose, fluid volume greater than 1999cc but less than or equal to 2999cc, for peritoneal dialysis
IOM: 100-04, 8, 90.3.2

✿ **A4723**   Dialysate solution, any concentration of dextrose, fluid volume greater than 2999cc but less than or equal to 3999cc, for peritoneal dialysis
IOM: 100-04, 8, 90.3.2

✿ **A4724**   Dialysate solution, any concentration of dextrose, fluid volume greater than 3999cc but less than or equal to 4999cc for peritoneal dialysis
IOM: 100-04, 8, 90.3.2

✿ **A4725**   Dialysate solution, any concentration of dextrose, fluid volume greater than 4999cc but less than or equal to 5999cc, for peritoneal dialysis
IOM: 100-04, 8, 90.3.2

✿ **A4726**   Dialysate solution, any concentration of dextrose, fluid volume greater than 5999cc, for peritoneal dialysis
IOM: 100-04, 8, 90.3.2

✳ **A4728**   Dialysate solution, non-dextrose containing, 500 ml

---

▶ New   → Revised   ✔ Reinstated   ~~deleted~~ Deleted

✿ Special coverage instructions   ◆ Not covered or valid by Medicare   ✳ Carrier discretion

✪ **A4730** Fistula cannulation set for hemodialysis, each

IOM: 100-04, 8, 90.3.2

✪ **A4736** Topical anesthetic, for dialysis, per gram

IOM: 100-04, 8, 90.3.2

✪ **A4737** Injectable anesthetic, for dialysis, per 10 ml

IOM: 100-04, 8, 90.3.2

✪ **A4740** Shunt accessory, for hemodialysis, any type, each

IOM: 100-04, 8, 90.3.2

✪ **A4750** Blood tubing, arterial or venous, for hemodialysis, each

IOM: 100-04, 8, 90.3.2

✪ **A4755** Blood tubing, arterial and venous combined, for hemodialysis, each

IOM: 100-04, 8, 90.3.2

✪ **A4760** Dialysate solution test kit, for peritoneal dialysis, any type, each

IOM: 100-04, 8, 90.3.2

✪ **A4765** Dialysate concentrate, powder, additive for peritoneal dialysis, per packet

IOM: 100-04, 8, 90.3.2

✪ **A4766** Dialysate concentrate, solution, additive for peritoneal dialysis, per 10 ml

IOM: 100-04, 8, 90.3.2

✪ **A4770** Blood collection tube, vacuum, for dialysis, per 50

IOM: 100-04, 8, 90.3.2

✪ **A4771** Serum clotting time tube, for dialysis, per 50

IOM: 100-04, 8, 90.3.2

✪ **A4772** Blood glucose test strips, for dialysis, per 50

IOM: 100-04, 8, 90.3.2

✪ **A4773** Occult blood test strips, for dialysis, per 50

IOM: 100-04, 8, 90.3.2

✪ **A4774** Ammonia test strips, for dialysis, per 50

IOM: 100-04, 8, 90.3.2

✪ **A4802** Protamine sulfate, for hemodialysis, per 50 mg

IOM: 100-04, 8, 90.3.2

✪ **A4860** Disposable catheter tips for peritoneal dialysis, per 10

IOM: 100-04, 8, 90.3.2

✪ **A4870** Plumbing and/or electrical work for home hemodialysis equipment

IOM: 100-04, 8, 90.3.2

✪ **A4890** Contracts, repair and maintenance, for hemodialysis equipment

IOM: 100-02, 15, 110.2

✪ **A4911** Drain bag/bottle, for dialysis, each

✪ **A4913** Miscellaneous dialysis supplies, not otherwise specified

Items not related to dialysis must not be billed with the miscellaneous codes A4913 or E1699.

✪ **A4918** Venous pressure clamp, for hemodialysis, each

✪ **A4927** Gloves, non-sterile, per 100

✪ **A4928** Surgical mask, per 20

✪ **A4929** Tourniquet for dialysis, each

✪ **A4930** Gloves, sterile, per pair

✳ **A4931** Oral thermometer, reusable, any type, each

✳ **A4932** Rectal thermometer, reusable, any type, each

Additional Ostomy Supplies

A5051-A5093: If provided in the physician's office for a temporary condition, the item is incident to the physician's service and billed to the local carrier. If provided in the physician's office or other place of service for a permanent condition, the item is a prosthetic device and billed to the DME/MAC.

✪ **A5051** Ostomy pouch, closed; with barrier attached (1 piece), each

IOM: 100-02, 15, 120

✪ **A5052** Ostomy pouch, closed; without barrier attached (1 piece), each

IOM: 100-02, 15, 120

✪ **A5053** Ostomy pouch, closed; for use on faceplate, each

IOM: 100-02, 15, 120

✪ **A5054** Ostomy pouch, closed; for use on barrier with flange (2 piece), each

IOM: 100-02, 15, 120

✪ **A5055** Stoma cap

IOM: 100-02, 15, 120

✪ **A5056** Ostomy pouch, drainable, with extended wear barrier attached, with filter, (1 piece), each

IOM: 100-02, 15, 120

▶ New   → Revised   ✔ Reinstated   ~~deleted~~ Deleted

✪ Special coverage instructions   ◆ Not covered or valid by Medicare   ✳ Carrier discretion

© **A5057** Ostomy pouch, drainable, with extended wear barrier attached, with built in convexity, with filter, (1 piece), each

IOM: 100-02, 15, 120

✳ **A5061** Ostomy pouch, drainable; with barrier attached, (1 piece), each

IOM: 100-02, 15, 120

© **A5062** Ostomy pouch, drainable; without barrier attached (1 piece), each

IOM: 100-02, 15, 120

© **A5063** Ostomy pouch, drainable; for use on barrier with flange (2 piece system), each

IOM: 100-02, 15, 120

© **A5071** Ostomy pouch, urinary; with barrier attached (1 piece), each

IOM: 100-02, 15, 120

© **A5072** Ostomy pouch, urinary; without barrier attached (1 piece), each

IOM: 100-02, 15, 120

© **A5073** Ostomy pouch, urinary; for use on barrier with flange (2 piece), each

IOM: 100-02, 15, 120

© **A5081** Continent device; plug for continent stoma

IOM: 100-02, 15, 120

© **A5082** Continent device; catheter for continent stoma

IOM: 100-02, 15, 120

✳ **A5083** Continent device, stoma absorptive cover for continent stoma

© **A5093** Ostomy accessory; convex insert

IOM: 100-02, 15, 120

Additional Incontinence Appliances/Supplies

A5102-A5114: If provided in the physician's office for a temporary condition, the item is incident to the physician's service and billed to the local carrier. If provided in the physician's office or other place of service for a permanent condition, the item is a prosthetic device and billed to the DME/MAC.

© **A5102** Bedside drainage bottle with or without tubing, rigid or expandable, each

IOM: 100-02, 15, 120

© **A5105** Urinary suspensory, with leg bag, with or without tube, each

IOM: 100-02, 15, 120

© **A5112** Urinary drainage bag, leg bag, leg or abdomen, latex, with or without tube, with straps, each

IOM: 100-02, 15, 120

© **A5113** Leg strap; latex, replacement only, per set

IOM: 100-02, 15, 120

© **A5114** Leg strap; foam or fabric, replacement only, per set

IOM: 100-02, 15, 120

Supplies for Either Incontinence or Ostomy Appliances

A5120-A5200: If provided in the physician's office for a temporary condition, the item is incident to the physician's service and billed to the local carrier. If provided in the physician's office or other place of service for a permanent condition, the item is a prosthetic device and billed to the DME/MAC.

© **A5120** Skin barrier, wipes or swabs, each

IOM: 100-02, 15, 120

© **A5121** Skin barrier; solid, 6 × 6 or equivalent, each

IOM: 100-02, 15, 120

© **A5122** Skin barrier; solid, 8 × 8 or equivalent, each

IOM: 100-02, 15, 120

© **A5126** Adhesive or non-adhesive; disk or foam pad

IOM: 100-02, 15, 120

© **A5131** Appliance cleaner, incontinence and ostomy appliances, per 16 oz

IOM: 100-02, 15, 120

© **A5200** Percutaneous catheter/tube anchoring device, adhesive skin attachment

IOM: 100-02, 15, 120

Diabetic Shoes, Fitting, and Modifications

A5500-A5513: Bill DME/MAC

© **A5500** For diabetics only, fitting (including follow-up), custom preparation and supply of off-the-shelf depth-inlay shoe manufactured to accommodate multi-density insert(s), per shoe

IOM: 100-02, 15, 140

▶ New → Revised ✔ Reinstated ~~deleted~~ Deleted

© Special coverage instructions ◆ Not covered or valid by Medicare ✳ Carrier discretion

⊛ **A5501** For diabetics only, fitting (including follow-up), custom preparation and supply of shoe molded from cast(s) of patient's foot (custom-molded shoe), per shoe

The diabetic patient must have at least one of the following conditions: peripheral neuropathy with evidence of callus formation, pre-ulcerative calluses, previous ulceration, foot deformity, previous amputation or poor circulation

IOM: 100-02, 15, 140

⊛ **A5503** For diabetics only, modification (including fitting) of off-the-shelf depth-inlay shoe or custom-molded shoe with roller or rigid rocker bottom, per shoe

IOM: 100-02, 15, 140

⊛ **A5504** For diabetics only, modification (including fitting) of off-the-shelf depth-inlay shoe or custom-molded shoe with wedge(s), per shoe

IOM: 100-02, 15, 140

⊛ **A5505** For diabetics only, modification (including fitting) of off-the-shelf depth-inlay shoe or custom-molded shoe with metatarsal bar, per shoe

IOM: 100-02, 15, 140

⊛ **A5506** For diabetics only, modification (including fitting) of off-the-shelf depth-inlay shoe or custom-molded shoe with off-set heel(s), per shoe

IOM: 100-02, 15, 140

⊛ **A5507** For diabetics only, not otherwise specified modification (including fitting) of off-the-shelf depth-inlay shoe or custom-molded shoe, per shoe

Only used for not otherwise specified therapeutic modifications to shoe or for repairs to a diabetic shoe(s)

IOM: 100-02, 15, 140

⊛ **A5508** For diabetics only, deluxe feature of off-the-shelf depth-inlay shoe or custom-molded shoe, per shoe

⊛ **A5510** For diabetics only, direct formed, compression molded to patient's foot without external heat source, multiple-density insert(s) prefabricated, per shoe

IOM: 100-02, 15, 140

✳ **A5512** For diabetics only, multiple density insert, direct formed, molded to foot after external heat source of 230 degrees Fahrenheit or higher, total contact with patient's foot, including arch, base layer minimum of 1/4 inch material of shore a 35 durometer or 3/16 inch material of shore a 40 durometer (or higher), prefabricated, each

✳ **A5513** For diabetics only, multiple density insert, custom molded from model of patient's foot, total contact with patient's foot, including arch, base layer minimum of 3/16 inch material of shore a 35 durometer (or higher), includes arch filler and other shaping material, custom fabricated, each

Dressings

A6010-A6512: Bill local carrier if incident to a physician's service (not separately payable) or if supply for implanted prosthetic device or implanted DME. If other, bill DME/MAC.

◆ **A6000** Non-contact wound warming wound cover for use with the non-contact wound warming device and warming card

Bill DME/MAC

IOM: 100-02, 16, 20

⊛ **A6010** Collagen based wound filler, dry form, sterile, per gram of collagen

IOM: 100-02, 15, 100

⊛ **A6011** Collagen based wound filler, gel/paste, per gram of collagen

IOM: 100-02, 15, 100

➜ ⊛ **A6021** Collagen dressing, sterile, size 16 sq. in. or less, each

IOM: 100-02, 15, 100

➜ ⊛ **A6022** Collagen dressing, sterile, size more than 16 sq. in. but less than or equal to 48 sq. in., each

IOM: 100-02, 15, 100

➜ ⊛ **A6023** Collagen dressing, sterile, size more than 48 sq. in., each

IOM: 100-02, 15, 100

⊛ **A6024** Collagen dressing wound filler, sterile, per 6 inches

IOM: 100-02, 15, 100

▶ **New** ➜ **Revised** ✔ **Reinstated** ~~deleted~~ **Deleted**

⊛ **Special coverage instructions** ◆ **Not covered or valid by Medicare** ✳ **Carrier discretion**

✳ **A6025** Gel sheet for dermal or epidermal application, (e.g., silicone, hydrogel, other), each

Only for gel sheets for treatment of keloids or other scars

If used for the treatment of keloids or other scars, a silicone gel sheet will not meet the definition of the surgical dressing benefit and will be denied as noncovered.

✼ **A6154** Wound pouch, each

Waterproof collection device with drainable port that adheres to skin around wound. Usual dressing change is up to 3 × per week.

IOM: 100-02, 15, 100

✼ **A6196** Alginate or other fiber gelling dressing, wound cover, sterile, pad size 16 sq. in. or less, each dressing

IOM: 100-02, 15, 100

✼ **A6197** Alginate or other fiber gelling dressing, wound cover, sterile, pad size more than 16 sq. in., but less than or equal to 48 sq. in., each dressing

IOM: 100-02, 15, 100

✼ **A6198** Alginate or other fiber gelling dressing, wound cover, sterile, pad size more than 48 sq. in., each dressing

IOM: 100-02, 15, 100

✼ **A6199** Alginate or other fiber gelling dressing, wound filler, sterile, per 6 inches

IOM: 100-02, 15, 100

✼ **A6203** Composite dressing, sterile, pad size 16 sq. in. or less, with any size adhesive border, each dressing

Usual composite dressing change is up to 3 times per week, one wound cover per dressing change.

IOM: 100-02, 15, 100

✼ **A6204** Composite dressing, sterile, pad size more than 16 sq. in. but less than or equal to 48 sq. in., with any size adhesive border, each dressing

Usual composite dressing change is up to 3 times per week, one wound cover per dressing change.

IOM: 100-02, 15, 100

✼ **A6205** Composite dressing, sterile, pad size more than 48 sq. in., with any size adhesive border, each dressing

Usual composite dressing change is up to 3 times per week, one wound cover per dressing change.

IOM: 100-02, 15, 100

✼ **A6206** Contact layer, sterile, 16 sq. in. or less, each dressing

Contact layers are porous to allow wound fluid to pass through for absorption by separate overlying dressing and are not intended to be changed with each dressing change. Usual dressing change is up to once per week.

IOM: 100-02, 15, 100

✼ **A6207** Contact layer, sterile, more than 16 sq. in. but less than or equal to 48 sq. in., each dressing

Contact layer dressings are used to line the entire wound; they are not intended to be changed with each dressing change. Usual dressing change is up to once per week.

IOM: 100-02, 15, 100

✼ **A6208** Contact layer, sterile, more than 48 sq. in., each dressing

Contact layer dressings are used to line the entire wound; they are not intended to be changed with each dressing change. Usual dressing change is up to once per week.

IOM: 100-02, 15, 100

✼ **A6209** Foam dressing, wound cover, sterile, pad size 16 sq. in. or less, without adhesive border, each dressing

Made of open cell, medical grade expanded polymer; with nonadherent property over wound site

IOM: 100-02, 15, 100

✼ **A6210** Foam dressing, wound cover, sterile, pad size more than 16 sq. in. but less than or equal to 48 sq. in., without adhesive border, each dressing

Foam dressings are covered items when used on full thickness wounds (e.g., stage III or IV ulcers) with moderate to heavy exudates. Usual dressing change for a foam wound cover when used as primary dressing is up to 3 times per week. When foam wound cover is used as a secondary dressing for wounds with very heavy exudates, dressing change may be up to 3 times per week. Usual dressing change for foam wound fillers is up to once per day (A6209-A6215).

IOM: 100-02, 15, 100

✼ **A6211** Foam dressing, wound cover, sterile, pad size more than 48 sq. in., without adhesive border, each dressing

IOM: 100-02, 15, 100

▶ New　→ Revised　✔ Reinstated　~~deleted~~ Deleted

✼ Special coverage instructions　◆ Not covered or valid by Medicare　✳ Carrier discretion

⚙ **A6212** Foam dressing, wound cover, sterile, pad size 16 sq. in. or less, with any size adhesive border, each dressing

IOM: 100-02, 15, 100

⚙ **A6213** Foam dressing, wound cover, sterile, pad size more than 16 sq. in. but less than or equal to 48 sq. in., with any size adhesive border, each dressing

IOM: 100-02, 15, 100

⚙ **A6214** Foam dressing, wound cover, sterile, pad size more than 48 sq. in., with any size adhesive border, each dressing

IOM: 100-02, 15, 100

⚙ **A6215** Foam dressing, wound filler, sterile, per gram

IOM: 100-02, 15, 100

⚙ **A6216** Gauze, non-impregnated, non-sterile, pad size 16 sq. in. or less, without adhesive border, each dressing

IOM: 100-02, 15, 100

⚙ **A6217** Gauze, non-impregnated, non-sterile, pad size more than 16 sq. in. but less than or equal to 48 sq. in., without adhesive border, each dressing

IOM: 100-02, 15, 100

⚙ **A6218** Gauze, non-impregnated, non-sterile, pad size more than 48 sq. in., without adhesive border, each dressing

IOM: 100-02, 15, 100

⚙ **A6219** Gauze, non-impregnated, sterile, pad size 16 sq. in. or less, with any size adhesive border, each dressing

IOM: 100-02, 15, 100

⚙ **A6220** Gauze, non-impregnated, sterile, pad size more than 16 sq. in. but less than or equal to 48 sq. in., with any size adhesive border, each dressing

IOM: 100-02, 15, 100

⚙ **A6221** Gauze, non-impregnated, sterile, pad size more than 48 sq. in., with any size adhesive border, each dressing

IOM: 100-02, 15, 100

⚙ **A6222** Gauze, impregnated with other than water, normal saline, or hydrogel, sterile, pad size 16 sq. in. or less, without adhesive border, each dressing

Substances may have been incorporated into dressing material (i.e., iodinated agents, petrolatum, zinc paste, crystalline sodium chloride, chlorhexadine gluconate [CHG], bismuth tribromophenate [BTP], water, aqueous saline, hydrogel, or agents)

IOM: 100-02, 15, 100

⚙ **A6223** Gauze, impregnated with other than water, normal saline, or hydrogel, sterile, pad size more than 16 sq. in. but less than or equal to 48 sq. in., without adhesive border, each dressing

IOM: 100-02, 15, 100

⚙ **A6224** Gauze, impregnated with other than water, normal saline, or hydrogel, sterile, pad size more than 48 square inches, without adhesive border, each dressing

IOM: 100-02, 15, 100

⚙ **A6228** Gauze, impregnated, water or normal saline, sterile, pad size 16 sq. in. or less, without adhesive border, each dressing

IOM: 100-02, 15, 100

⚙ **A6229** Gauze, impregnated, water or normal saline, sterile, pad size more than 16 sq. in. but less than or equal to 48 sq. in., without adhesive border, each dressing

IOM: 100-02, 15, 100

⚙ **A6230** Gauze, impregnated, water or normal saline, sterile, pad size more than 48 sq. in., without adhesive border, each dressing

IOM: 100-02, 15, 100

⚙ **A6231** Gauze, impregnated, hydrogel, for direct wound contact, sterile, pad size 16 sq. in. or less, each dressing

IOM: 100-02, 15, 100

⚙ **A6232** Gauze, impregnated, hydrogel, for direct wound contact, sterile, pad size greater than 16 sq. in., but less than or equal to 48 sq. in., each dressing

IOM: 100-02, 15, 100

⚙ **A6233** Gauze, impregnated, hydrogel, for direct wound contact, sterile, pad size more than 48 sq. in., each dressing

IOM: 100-02, 15, 100

⚙ **A6234** Hydrocolloid dressing, wound cover, sterile, pad size 16 sq. in. or less, without adhesive border, each dressing

This type of dressing is usually used on wounds with light to moderate exudate with an average of three dressing changes a week.

IOM: 100-02, 15, 100

⚙ **A6235** Hydrocolloid dressing, wound cover, sterile, pad size more than 16 sq. in. but less than or equal to 48 sq. in., without adhesive border, each dressing

IOM: 100-02, 15, 100

▶ New   → Revised   ✔ Reinstated   ~~deleted~~ Deleted

⚙ Special coverage instructions   ◆ Not covered or valid by Medicare   ✳ Carrier discretion

⊕ **A6236** Hydrocolloid dressing, wound cover, sterile, pad size more than 48 sq. in., without adhesive border, each dressing

IOM: 100-02, 15, 100

⊕ **A6237** Hydrocolloid dressing, wound cover, sterile, pad size 16 sq. in. or less, with any size adhesive border, each dressing

IOM: 100-02, 15, 100

⊕ **A6238** Hydrocolloid dressing, wound cover, sterile, pad size more than 16 sq. in. but less than or equal to 48 sq. in., with any size adhesive border, each dressing

IOM: 100-02, 15, 100

⊕ **A6239** Hydrocolloid dressing, wound cover, sterile, pad size more than 48 sq. in., with any size adhesive border, each dressing

IOM: 100-02, 15, 100

⊕ **A6240** Hydrocolloid dressing, wound filler, paste, sterile, per ounce

IOM: 100-02, 15, 100

⊕ **A6241** Hydrocolloid dressing, wound filler, dry form, sterile, per gram

IOM: 100-02, 15, 100

⊕ **A6242** Hydrogel dressing, wound cover, sterile, pad size 16 sq. in. or less, without adhesive border, each dressing

Considered medically necessary when used on full thickness wounds with minimal or no exudate (e.g., stage III or IV ulcers)

Usually up to one dressing change per day is considered medically necessary, but if well documented and medically necessary, the payer may allow more frequent dressing changes.

IOM: 100-02, 15, 100

⊕ **A6243** Hydrogel dressing, wound cover, sterile, pad size more than 16 sq. in. but less than or equal to 48 sq. in., without adhesive border, each dressing

IOM: 100-02, 15, 100

⊕ **A6244** Hydrogel dressing, wound cover, sterile, pad size more than 48 sq. in., without adhesive border, each dressing

IOM: 100-02, 15, 100

⊕ **A6245** Hydrogel dressing, wound cover, sterile, pad size 16 sq. in. or less, with any size adhesive border, each dressing

Coverage of a non-elastic gradient compression wrap is limited to one per 6 months per leg.

IOM: 100-02, 15, 100

⊕ **A6246** Hydrogel dressing, wound cover, sterile, pad size more than 16 sq. in. but less than or equal to 48 sq. in., with any size adhesive border, each dressing

IOM: 100-02, 15, 100

⊕ **A6247** Hydrogel dressing, wound cover, sterile, pad size more than 48 sq. in., with any size adhesive border, each dressing

IOM: 100-02, 15, 100

⊕ **A6248** Hydrogel dressing, wound filler, gel, per fluid ounce

IOM: 100-02, 15, 100

⊕ **A6250** Skin sealants, protectants, moisturizers, ointments, any type, any size

IOM: 100-02, 15, 100

⊕ **A6251** Specialty absorptive dressing, wound cover, sterile, pad size 16 sq. in. or less, without adhesive border, each dressing

IOM: 100-02, 15, 100

⊕ **A6252** Specialty absorptive dressing, wound cover, sterile, pad size more than 16 sq. in. but less than or equal to 48 sq. in., without adhesive border, each dressing

IOM: 100-02, 15, 100

⊕ **A6253** Specialty absorptive dressing, wound cover, sterile, pad size more than 48 sq. in., without adhesive border, each dressing

IOM: 100-02, 15, 100

⊕ **A6254** Specialty absorptive dressing, wound cover, sterile, pad size 16 sq. in. or less, with any size adhesive border, each dressing

IOM: 100-02, 15, 100

⊕ **A6255** Specialty absorptive dressing, wound cover, sterile, pad size more than 16 sq. in. but less than or equal to 48 sq. in., with any size adhesive border, each dressing

IOM: 100-02, 15, 100

⊕ **A6256** Specialty absorptive dressing, wound cover, sterile, pad size more than 48 sq. in., with any size adhesive border, each dressing

Considered medically necessary when used for moderately or highly exudative wounds (e.g., stage III or IV ulcers)

IOM: 100-02, 15, 100

▶ New   → Revised   ✔ Reinstated   ~~deleted~~ Deleted
⊕ Special coverage instructions   ◆ Not covered or valid by Medicare   ✳ Carrier discretion

⊛ **A6257** Transparent film, sterile, 16 sq. in. or less, each dressing

Considered medically necessary when used on open partial thickness wounds with minimal exudate or closed wounds

IOM: 100-02, 15, 100

⊛ **A6258** Transparent film, sterile, more than 16 sq. in. but less than or equal to 48 sq. in., each dressing

IOM: 100-02, 15, 100

⊛ **A6259** Transparent film, sterile, more than 48 sq. in., each dressing

IOM: 100-02, 15, 100

⊛ **A6260** Wound cleansers, any type, any size

IOM: 100-02, 15, 100

⊛ **A6261** Wound filler, gel/paste, per fluid ounce, not otherwise specified

Units of service for wound fillers are 1 gram, 1 fluid ounce, 6 inch length, or 1 yard depending on product

IOM: 100-02, 15, 100

⊛ **A6262** Wound filler, dry form, per gram, not otherwise specified

Dry forms (e.g., powder, granules, beads) are used to eliminate dead space in an open wound.

IOM: 100-02, 15, 100

⊛ **A6266** Gauze, impregnated, other than water, normal saline, or zinc paste, sterile, any width, per linear yard

IOM: 100-02, 15, 100

⊛ **A6402** Gauze, non-impregnated, sterile, pad size 16 sq. in. or less, without adhesive border, each dressing

IOM: 100-02, 15, 100

⊛ **A6403** Gauze, non-impregnated, sterile, pad size more than 16 sq. in., less than or equal to 48 sq. in., without adhesive border, each dressing

IOM: 100-02, 15, 100

⊛ **A6404** Gauze, non-impregnated, sterile, pad size more than 48 sq. in., without adhesive border, each dressing

IOM: 100-02, 15, 100

✳ **A6407** Packing strips, non-impregnated, sterile, up to 2 inches in width, per linear yard

IOM: 100-02, 15, 100

⊛ **A6410** Eye pad, sterile, each

IOM: 100-02, 15, 100

⊛ **A6411** Eye pad, non-sterile, each

IOM: 100-02, 15, 100

✳ **A6412** Eye patch, occlusive, each

◆ **A6413** Adhesive bandage, first-aid type, any size, each

First aid type bandage is a wound cover with a pad size of less than 4 square inches.

Medicare Statute 1861(s)(5)

✳ **A6441** Padding bandage, non-elastic, non-woven/non-knitted, width greater than or equal to three inches and less than five inches, per yard

✳ **A6442** Conforming bandage, non-elastic, knitted/woven, non-sterile, width less than three inches, per yard

Non-elastic, moderate or high compression that is typically sustained for one week

✳ **A6443** Conforming bandage, non-elastic, knitted/woven, non-sterile, width greater than or equal to three inches and less than five inches, per yard

✳ **A6444** Conforming bandage, non-elastic, knitted/woven, non-sterile, width greater than or equal to five inches, per yard

✳ **A6445** Conforming bandage, non-elastic, knitted/woven, sterile, width less than three inches, per yard

✳ **A6446** Conforming bandage, non-elastic, knitted/woven, sterile, width greater than or equal to three inches and less than five inches, per yard

✳ **A6447** Conforming bandage, non-elastic, knitted/woven, sterile, width greater than or equal to five inches, per yard

✳ **A6448** Light compression bandage, elastic, knitted/woven, width less than three inches, per yard

Used to hold wound cover dressings in place over a wound. Example is an ACE type elastic bandage.

✳ **A6449** Light compression bandage, elastic, knitted/woven, width greater than or equal to three inches and less than five inches, per yard

✳ **A6450** Light compression bandage, elastic, knitted/woven, width greater than or equal to five inches, per yard

---

▶ New → Revised ✔ Reinstated ~~deleted~~ Deleted

⊛ Special coverage instructions ◆ Not covered or valid by Medicare ✳ Carrier discretion

✳ **A6451** Moderate compression bandage, elastic, knitted/woven, load resistance of 1.25 to 1.34 foot pounds at 50% maximum stretch, width greater than or equal to three inches and less than five inches, per yard

Elastic bandages that produce moderate compression that is typically sustained for one week

Medicare considers coverage if part of a multi-layer compression bandage system for the treatment of a venous stasis ulcer. Do not assign for strains or sprains.

✳ **A6452** High compression bandage, elastic, knitted/woven, load resistance greater than or equal to 1.35 foot pounds at 50% maximum stretch, width greater than or equal to three inches and less than five inches, per yard

Elastic bandages that produce high compression that is typically sustained for one week

✳ **A6453** Self-adherent bandage, elastic, non-knitted/non-woven, width less than three inches, per yard

✳ **A6454** Self-adherent bandage, elastic, non-knitted/non-woven, width greater than or equal to three inches and less than five inches, per yard

✳ **A6455** Self-adherent bandage, elastic, non-knitted/non-woven, width greater than or equal to five inches, per yard

✳ **A6456** Zinc paste impregnated bandage, non-elastic, knitted/woven, width greater than or equal to three inches and less than five inches, per yard

✳ **A6457** Tubular dressing with or without elastic, any width, per linear yard

⊛ **A6501** Compression burn garment, bodysuit (head to foot), custom fabricated

Garments used to reduce hypertrophic scarring and joint contractures following burn injury

IOM: 100-02, 15, 100

⊛ **A6502** Compression burn garment, chin strap, custom fabricated

IOM: 100-02, 15, 100

⊛ **A6503** Compression burn garment, facial hood, custom fabricated

IOM: 100-02, 15, 100

⊛ **A6504** Compression burn garment, glove to wrist, custom fabricated

IOM: 100-02, 15, 100

⊛ **A6505** Compression burn garment, glove to elbow, custom fabricated

IOM: 100-02, 15, 100

⊛ **A6506** Compression burn garment, glove to axilla, custom fabricated

IOM: 100-02, 15, 100

⊛ **A6507** Compression burn garment, foot to knee length, custom fabricated

IOM: 100-02, 15, 100

⊛ **A6508** Compression burn garment, foot to thigh length, custom fabricated

IOM: 100-02, 15, 100

⊛ **A6509** Compression burn garment, upper trunk to waist including arm openings (vest), custom fabricated

IOM: 100-02, 15, 100

⊛ **A6510** Compression burn garment, trunk, including arms down to leg openings (leotard), custom fabricated

IOM: 100-02, 15, 100

⊛ **A6511** Compression burn garment, lower trunk including leg openings (panty), custom fabricated

IOM: 100-02, 15, 100

⊛ **A6512** Compression burn garment, not otherwise classified

IOM: 100-02, 15, 100

✳ **A6513** Compression burn mask, face and/or neck, plastic or equal, custom fabricated

Bill DME/MAC

GRADIENT COMPRESSION STOCKINGS (A6530-A6549)

A6530-A6549: Bill DME/MAC

◆ **A6530** Gradient compression stocking, below knee, 18–30 mmHg, each

IOM: 100-03, 4, 280.1

⊛ **A6531** Gradient compression stocking, below knee, 30–40 mmHg, each

Covered when used in treatment of open venous stasis ulcer. Modifiers A1-A9 are not assigned. Must be billed with AW, RT, or LT

IOM: 100-02, 15, 100

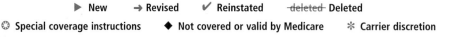

▶ New   → Revised   ✔ Reinstated   ~~deleted~~ Deleted
⊛ Special coverage instructions   ◆ Not covered or valid by Medicare   ✳ Carrier discretion

RESPIRATORY DURABLE MEDICAL EQUIPMENT, INEXPENSIVE AND ROUTINELY PURCHASED

⚙ **A6532**   Gradient compression stocking, below knee, 40–50 mmHg, each

Covered when used in treatment of open venous stasis ulcer. Modifiers A1-A9 are not assigned. Must be billed with AW, RT, or LT

IOM: 100-02, 15, 100

◆ **A6533**   Gradient compression stocking, thigh length, 18–30 mmHg, each

IOM: 100-02, 15, 130; 100-03, 4, 280.1

◆ **A6534**   Gradient compression stocking, thigh length, 30–40 mmHg, each

IOM: 100-02, 15, 130; 100-03, 4, 280.1

◆ **A6535**   Gradient compression stocking, thigh length, 40–50 mmHg, each

IOM: 100-02, 15, 130; 100-03, 4, 280.1

◆ **A6536**   Gradient compression stocking, full length/chap style, 18–30 mmHg, each

IOM: 100-02, 15, 130; 100-03, 4, 280.1

◆ **A6537**   Gradient compression stocking, full length/chap style, 30–40 mmHg, each

IOM: 100-02, 15, 130; 100-03, 4, 280.1

◆ **A6538**   Gradient compression stocking, full length/chap style, 40–50 mmHg, each

IOM: 100-02, 15, 130; 100-03, 4, 280.1

◆ **A6539**   Gradient compression stocking, waist length, 18–30 mmHg, each

IOM: 100-02, 15, 130; 100-03, 4, 280.1

◆ **A6540**   Gradient compression stocking, waist length, 30–40 mmHg, each

IOM: 100-02, 15, 130; 100-03, 4, 280.1

◆ **A6541**   Gradient compression stocking, waist length, 40–50 mmHg, each

IOM: 100-02, 15, 130; 100-03, 4, 280.1

◆ **A6544**   Gradient compression stocking, garter belt

IOM: 100-02, 15, 130; 100-03, 4, 280.1

⚙ **A6545**   Gradient compression wrap, non-elastic, below knee, 30-50 mm hg, each

Modifiers -RT and/or -LT must be appended. When assigned for bilateral items (left/right) on the same date of service, bill both items on the same claim line using -RT/-LT modifiers and 2 units of service.

IOM: 10-02, 15, 100

◆ **A6549**   Gradient compression stocking/sleeve, not otherwise specified

IOM: 100-02, 15, 130; 100-03, 4, 280.1

WOUND CARE (A6550)

✳ **A6550**   Wound care set, for negative pressure wound therapy electrical pump, includes all supplies and accessories

Bill DME/MAC

RESPIRATORY DURABLE MEDICAL EQUIPMENT, INEXPENSIVE AND ROUTINELY PURCHASED (A7000-A7509)

✳ **A7000**   Canister, disposable, used with suction pump, each

Bill DME/MAC

✳ **A7001**   Canister, non-disposable, used with suction pump, each

Bill DME/MAC

✳ **A7002**   Tubing, used with suction pump, each

Bill DME/MAC

✳ **A7003**   Administration set, with small volume nonfiltered pneumatic nebulizer, disposable

Bill DME/MAC

✳ **A7004**   Small volume nonfiltered pneumatic nebulizer, disposable

Bill DME/MAC

✳ **A7005**   Administration set, with small volume nonfiltered pneumatic nebulizer, non-disposable

Bill DME/MAC

✳ **A7006**   Administration set, with small volume filtered pneumatic nebulizer

Bill DME/MAC

✳ **A7007**   Large volume nebulizer, disposable, unfilled, used with aerosol compressor

Bill DME/MAC

✳ **A7008**   Large volume nebulizer, disposable, prefilled, used with aerosol compressor

Bill DME/MAC

✳ **A7009**   Reservoir bottle, nondisposable, used with large volume ultrasonic nebulizer

Bill DME/MAC

✳ **A7010**   Corrugated tubing, disposable, used with large volume nebulizer, 100 feet

Bill DME/MAC

✳ **A7011**   Corrugated tubing, non-disposable, used with large volume nebulizer, 10 feet

Bill DME/MAC

▶ New   → Revised   ✔ Reinstated   ~~deleted~~ Deleted
⚙ Special coverage instructions   ◆ Not covered or valid by Medicare   ✳ Carrier discretion

109

* **A7012** Water collection device, used with large volume nebulizer

  Bill DME/MAC

* **A7013** Filter, disposable, used with aerosol compressor or ultrasonic generator

  Bill DME/MAC

* **A7014** Filter, non-disposable, used with aerosol compressor or ultrasonic generator

  Bill DME/MAC

* **A7015** Aerosol mask, used with DME nebulizer

  Bill DME/MAC

* **A7016** Dome and mouthpiece, used with small volume ultrasonic nebulizer

  Bill DME/MAC

☼ **A7017** Nebulizer, durable, glass or autoclavable plastic, bottle type, not used with oxygen

  Bill DME/MAC

  IOM: 100-03, 4, 280.1

* **A7018** Water, distilled, used with large volume nebulizer, 1000 ml

  Bill DME/MAC

* **A7020** Interface for cough stimulating device, includes all components, replacement only

  Bill DME/MAC

* **A7025** High frequency chest wall oscillation system vest, replacement for use with patient owned equipment, each

  Bill DME/MAC

* **A7026** High frequency chest wall oscillation system hose, replacement for use with patient owned equipment, each

  Bill DME/MAC

* **A7027** Combination oral/nasal mask, used with continuous positive airway pressure device, each

  Bill DME/MAC

* **A7028** Oral cushion for combination oral/nasal mask, replacement only, each

  Bill DME/MAC

* **A7029** Nasal pillows for combination oral/nasal mask, replacement only, pair

  Bill DME/MAC

* **A7030** Full face mask used with positive airway pressure device, each

  Bill DME/MAC

* **A7031** Face mask interface, replacement for full face mask, each

  Bill DME/MAC

* **A7032** Cushion for use on nasal mask interface, replacement only, each

  Bill DME/MAC

* **A7033** Pillow for use on nasal cannula type interface, replacement only, pair

  Bill DME/MAC

* **A7034** Nasal interface (mask or cannula type) used with positive airway pressure device, with or without head strap

  Bill DME/MAC

* **A7035** Headgear used with positive airway pressure device

  Bill DME/MAC

* **A7036** Chinstrap used with positive airway pressure device

  Bill DME/MAC

* **A7037** Tubing used with positive airway pressure device

  Bill DME/MAC

* **A7038** Filter, disposable, used with positive airway pressure device

  Bill DME/MAC

* **A7039** Filter, non disposable, used with positive airway pressure device

  Bill DME/MAC

* **A7040** One way chest drain valve

  Bill local carrier

* **A7041** Water seal drainage container and tubing for use with implanted chest tube

  Bill local carrier

* **A7042** Implanted pleural catheter, each

  Bill local carrier

* **A7043** Vacuum drainage bottle and tubing for use with implanted catheter

  Bill local carrier

* **A7044** Oral interface used with positive airway pressure device, each

  Bill DME/MAC

☼ **A7045** Exhalation port with or without swivel used with accessories for positive airway devices, replacement only

  Bill DME/MAC

  IOM: 100-03, 4, 230.17

▶ New → Revised ✔ Reinstated ~~deleted~~ Deleted

☼ Special coverage instructions ◆ Not covered or valid by Medicare * Carrier discretion

⊛ **A7046** Water chamber for humidifier, used with positive airway pressure device, replacement, each

Bill DME/MAC

IOM: 100-03, 4, 230.17

⊛ **A7501** Tracheostoma valve, including diaphragm, each

Bill DME/MAC

IOM: 100-02, 15, 120

⊛ **A7502** Replacement diaphragm/faceplate for tracheostoma valve, each

Bill DME/MAC

IOM: 100-02, 15, 120

⊛ **A7503** Filter holder or filter cap, reusable, for use in a tracheostoma heat and moisture exchange system, each

Bill DME/MAC

IOM: 100-02, 15, 120

⊛ **A7504** Filter for use in a tracheostoma heat and moisture exchange system, each

Bill DME/MAC

IOM: 100-02, 15, 120

⊛ **A7505** Housing, reusable without adhesive, for use in a heat and moisture exchange system and/or with a tracheostoma valve, each

Bill DME/MAC

IOM: 100-02, 15, 120

⊛ **A7506** Adhesive disc for use in a heat and moisture exchange system and/or with tracheostoma valve, any type, each

Bill DME/MAC

IOM: 100-02, 15, 120

⊛ **A7507** Filter holder and integrated filter without adhesive, for use in a tracheostoma heat and moisture exchange system, each

Bill DME/MAC

IOM: 100-02, 15, 120

⊛ **A7508** Housing and integrated adhesive, for use in a tracheostoma heat and moisture exchange system and/or with a tracheostoma valve, each

Bill DME/MAC

IOM: 100-02, 15, 120

⊛ **A7509** Filter holder and integrated filter housing, and adhesive, for use as a tracheostoma heat and moisture exchange system, each

Bill DME/MAC

IOM: 100-02, 15, 120

＊ **A7520** Tracheostomy/laryngectomy tube, non-cuffed, polyvinylchloride (PVC), silicone or equal, each

Bill DME/MAC

＊ **A7521** Tracheostomy/laryngectomy tube, cuffed, polyvinylchloride (PVC), silicone or equal, each

Bill DME/MAC

＊ **A7522** Tracheostomy/laryngectomy tube, stainless steel or equal (sterilizable and reusable), each

Bill DME/MAC

＊ **A7523** Tracheostomy shower protector, each

Bill DME/MAC

＊ **A7524** Tracheostoma stent/stud/button, each

Bill DME/MAC

＊ **A7525** Tracheostomy mask, each

Bill DME/MAC

＊ **A7526** Tracheostomy tube collar/holder, each

Bill DME/MAC

＊ **A7527** Tracheostomy/laryngectomy tube plug/stop, each

Bill DME/MAC

HELMETS (A8000-A8004)

A8000-8004: Bill DME/MAC

＊ **A8000** Helmet, protective, soft, prefabricated, includes all components and accessories

＊ **A8001** Helmet, protective, hard, prefabricated, includes all components and accessories

＊ **A8002** Helmet, protective, soft, custom fabricated, includes all components and accessories

＊ **A8003** Helmet, protective, hard, custom fabricated, includes all components and accessories

＊ **A8004** Soft interface for helmet, replacement only

▶ New   → Revised   ✔ Reinstated   ~~deleted~~ Deleted

⊛ Special coverage instructions   ◆ Not covered or valid by Medicare   ＊ Carrier discretion

ADMINISTRATIVE, MISCELLANEOUS, AND INVESTIGATIONAL (A9000-A9999)

NOTE: The following codes do not imply that codes in other sections are necessarily covered.

⊚ **A9150** Non-prescription drugs

Bill local carrier

IOM: 100-02, 15, 50

◆ **A9152** Single vitamin/mineral/trace element, oral, per dose, not otherwise specified

Bill local carrier

◆ **A9153** Multiple vitamins, with or without minerals and trace elements, oral, per dose, not otherwise specified

Bill local carrier

✳ **A9155** Artificial saliva, 30 ml

Bill local carrier

◆ **A9180** Pediculosis (lice infestation) treatment, topical, for administration by patient/ caretaker

Bill local carrier

◆ **A9270** Non-covered item or service

Bill DME/MAC

IOM: 100-02, 16, 20

◆ **A9272** Mechanical wound suction, disposable, includes dressing, all accessories and components, each

◆ **A9273** Hot water bottle, ice cap or collar, heat and/or cold wrap, any type

◆ **A9274** External ambulatory insulin delivery system, disposable, each, includes all supplies and accessories

Bill DME/MAC

◆ **A9275** Home glucose disposable monitor, includes test strips

Bill DME/MAC

◆ **A9276** Sensor; invasive (e.g. subcutaneous), disposable, for use with interstitial continuous glucose monitoring system, one unit = 1 day supply

Bill DME/MAC

Medicare Statute 1861(n)

◆ **A9277** Transmitter; external, for use with interstitial continuous glucose monitoring system

Bill DME/MAC

Medicare Statute 1861(n)

◆ **A9278** Receiver (monitor); external, for use with interstitial continuous glucose monitoring system

Bill DME/MAC

Medicare Statute 1861(n)

◆ **A9279** Monitoring feature/device, stand-alone or integrated, any type, includes all accessories, components and electronics, not otherwise classified

Bill DME/MAC

◆ **A9280** Alert or alarm device, not otherwise classified

Bill DME/MAC

Medicare Statute 1861

◆ **A9281** Reaching/grabbing device, any type, any length, each

Bill DME/MAC

Medicare Statute 1862 SSA

◆ **A9282** Wig, any type, each

Bill DME/MAC

Medicare Statute 1862 SSA

◆ **A9283** Foot pressure off loading/supportive device, any type, each

Bill DME/MAC

Medicare Statute 1862A(i)13

⊚ **A9284** Spirometer, non-electronic, includes all accessories

Bill DME/MAC

◆ **A9300** Exercise equipment

Bill DME/MAC

IOM: 100-02, 15, 110.1; 100-03, 4, 280.1

Supplies for Radiology Procedures (Radiopharmaceuticals)

A9500-9700: Bill local carrier

✳ **A9500** Technetium Tc-99m sestamibi, diagnostic, per study dose

Should be filed on same claim as procedure code reporting radiopharmaceutical. Verify with payer definition of a "study."

✳ **A9501** Technetium Tc-99m teboroxime, diagnostic, per study dose

✳ **A9502** Technetium Tc-99m tetrofosmin, diagnostic, per study dose

✳ **A9503** Technetium Tc-99m medronate, diagnostic, per study dose, up to 30 millicuries

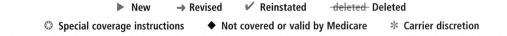

▶ New → Revised ✔ Reinstated ~~deleted~~ Deleted

⊚ Special coverage instructions ◆ Not covered or valid by Medicare ✳ Carrier discretion

✳ **A9504**   Technetium Tc-99m apcitide, diagnostic, per study dose, up to 20 millicuries

✳ **A9505**   Thallium Tl-201 thallous chloride, diagnostic, per millicurie

✳ **A9507**   Indium In-111 capromab pendetide, diagnostic, per study dose, up to 10 millicuries

✳ **A9508**   Iodine I-131 iobenguane sulfate, diagnostic, per 0.5 millicurie

✳ **A9509**   Iodine I-123 sodium iodide, diagnostic, per millicurie

✳ **A9510**   Technetium Tc-99m disofenin, diagnostic, per study dose, up to 15 millicuries

✳ **A9512**   Technetium Tc-99m pertechnetate, diagnostic, per millicurie

✳ **A9516**   Iodine I-123 sodium iodide, diagnostic, per 100 microcuries, up to 999 microcuries

✳ **A9517**   Iodine I-131 sodium iodide capsule(s), therapeutic, per millicurie

✳ **A9521**   Technetium Tc-99m exametazime, diagnostic, per study dose, up to 25 millicuries

✳ **A9524**   Iodine I-131 iodinated serum albumin, diagnostic, per 5 microcuries

✳ **A9526**   Nitrogen N-13 ammonia, diagnostic, per study dose, up to 40 millicuries

✳ **A9527**   Iodine I-125, sodium iodide solution, therapeutic, per millicurie

✳ **A9528**   Iodine I-131 sodium iodide capsule(s), diagnostic, per millicurie

✳ **A9529**   Iodine I-131 sodium iodide solution, diagnostic, per millicurie

✳ **A9530**   Iodine I-131 sodium iodide solution, therapeutic, per millicurie

✳ **A9531**   Iodine I-131 sodium iodide, diagnostic, per microcurie (up to 100 microcuries)

✳ **A9532**   Iodine I-125 serum albumin, diagnostic, per 5 microcuries

✳ **A9536**   Technetium Tc-99m depreotide, diagnostic, per study dose, up to 35 millicuries

✳ **A9537**   Technetium Tc-99m mebrofenin, diagnostic, per study dose, up to 15 millicuries

✳ **A9538**   Technetium Tc-99m pyrophosphate, diagnostic, per study dose, up to 25 millicuries

✳ **A9539**   Technetium Tc-99m pentetate, diagnostic, per study dose, up to 25 millicuries

✳ **A9540**   Technetium Tc-99m macroaggregated albumin, diagnostic, per study dose, up to 10 millicuries

✳ **A9541**   Technetium Tc-99m sulfur colloid, diagnostic, per study dose, up to 20 millicuries

✳ **A9542**   Indium In-111 ibritumomab tiuxetan, diagnostic, per study dose, up to 5 millicuries

Specifically for diagnostic use.

✳ **A9543**   Yttrium Y-90 ibritumomab tiuxetan, therapeutic, per treatment dose, up to 40 millicuries

Specifically for therapeutic use.

✳ **A9544**   Iodine I-131 tositumomab, diagnostic, per study dose

✳ **A9545**   Iodine I-131 tositumomab, therapeutic, per treatment dose

✳ **A9546**   Cobalt Co-57/58, cyanocobalamin, diagnostic, per study dose, up to 1 microcurie

✳ **A9547**   Indium In-111 oxyquinoline, diagnostic, per 0.5 millicurie

✳ **A9548**   Indium In-111 pentetate, diagnostic, per 0.5 millicurie

✳ **A9550**   Technetium Tc-99m sodium gluceptate, diagnostic, per study dose, up to 25 millicuries

✳ **A9551**   Technetium Tc-99m succimer, diagnostic, per study dose, up to 10 millicuries

✳ **A9552**   Fluorodeoxyglucose F-18 FDG, diagnostic, per study dose, up to 45 millicuries

✳ **A9553**   Chromium Cr-51 sodium chromate, diagnostic, per study dose, up to 250 microcuries

✳ **A9554**   Iodine I-125 sodium Iothalamate, diagnostic, per study dose, up to 10 microcuries

✳ **A9555**   Rubidium Rb-82, diagnostic, per study dose, up to 60 millicuries

✳ **A9556**   Gallium Ga-67 citrate, diagnostic, per millicurie

✳ **A9557**   Technetium Tc-99m bicisate, diagnostic, per study dose, up to 25 millicuries

✳ **A9558**   Xenon Xe-133 gas, diagnostic, per 10 millicuries

✳ **A9559**   Cobalt Co-57 cyanocobalamin, oral, diagnostic, per study dose, up to 1 microcurie

✳ **A9560**   Technetium Tc-99m labeled red blood cells, diagnostic, per study dose, up to 30 millicuries

▶ New   → Revised   ✔ Reinstated   ~~deleted~~ Deleted

☼ Special coverage instructions   ◆ Not covered or valid by Medicare   ✳ Carrier discretion

* A9561 Technetium Tc-99m oxidronate, diagnostic, per study dose, up to 30 millicuries

* A9562 Technetium Tc-99m mertiatide, diagnostic, per study dose, up to 15 millicuries

* A9563 Sodium phosphate P-32, therapeutic, per millicurie

* A9564 Chromic phosphate P-32 suspension, therapeutic, per millicurie

* A9566 Technetium Tc-99m fanolesomab, diagnostic, per study dose, up to 25 millicuries

* A9567 Technetium Tc-99m pentetate, diagnostic, aerosol, per study dose, up to 75 millicuries

* A9568 Technetium TC-99m arcitumomab, diagnostic, per study dose, up to 45 millicuries

* A9569 Technetium Tc-99m exametazime labeled autologous white blood cells, diagnostic, per study dose

* A9570 Indium In-111 labeled autologous white blood cells, diagnostic, per study dose

* A9571 Indium In-111 labeled autologous platelets, diagnostic, per study dose

* A9572 Indium In-111 pentetreotide, diagnostic, per study dose, up to 6 millicuries

* A9576 Injection, gadoteridol, (ProHance Multipack), per ml

* A9577 Injection, gadobenate dimeglumine (MultiHance), per ml

* A9578 Injection, gadobenate dimeglumine (MultiHance Multipack), per ml

* A9579 Injection, gadolinium-based magnetic resonance contrast agent, not otherwise specified (NOS), per ml

   NDC: Magnevist, Omniscan, Optimark, Prohance

* A9580 Sodium fluoride F-18, diagnostic, per study dose, up to 30 millicuries

* A9581 Injection, gadoxetate disodium, 1 ml

   Local Medicare contractors may require the use of modifier JW to identify unused product from single-dose vials that are appropriately discarded.

* A9582 Iodine I-123 iobenguane, diagnostic, per study dose, up to 15 millicuries

   Molecular imaging agent that assists in the identification of rare neuroendocrine tumors.

* A9583 Injection, gadofosveset trisodium, 1 ml

   NDC: Ablavar

* A9584 Iodine 1-123 ioflupane, diagnostic, per study dose, up to 5 millicuries

* A9585 Injection, gadobutrol, 0.1 ml

   NDC: Gadavist

▶ ◆ A9586 Florbetapir F18, diagnostic, per study dose, up to 10 millicuries

* A9600 Strontium Sr-89 chloride, therapeutic, per millicurie

* A9604 Samarium SM-153 lexidronam, therapeutic, per treatment dose, up to 150 millicuries

☺ A9698 Non-radioactive contrast imaging material, not otherwise classified, per study

   IOM: 100-04, 12, 70; 100-04, 13, 20

* A9699 Radiopharmaceutical, therapeutic, not otherwise classified

☺ A9700 Supply of injectable contrast material for use in echocardiography, per study

   IOM: 100-04, 12, 30.4

Miscellaneous Service Component

* A9900 Miscellaneous DME supply, accessory, and/or service component of another HCPCS code

   Local carrier if used with implanted DME. If other, bill DME/MAC.

   On DMEPOS fee schedule as a payable replacement for miscellaneous implanted or non-implanted items.

* A9901 DME delivery, set up, and/or dispensing service component of another HCPCS code

   Bill DME/MAC

* A9999 Miscellaneous DME supply or accessory, not otherwise specified

   Local carrier if used with implanted DME. If other, bill DME/MAC.

   On DMEPOS fee schedule as a payable replacement for miscellaneous implanted or non-implanted items.

▶ New   → Revised   ✔ Reinstated   <del>deleted</del> Deleted
☺ Special coverage instructions   ◆ Not covered or valid by Medicare   * Carrier discretion

ENTERAL AND PARENTERAL THERAPY (B4000-B9999)

Enteral Formulae and Enteral Medical Supplies

B4034-B4162: Bill DME/MAC

⚙ **B4034** Enteral feeding supply kit; syringe fed, per day, includes but not limited to feeding/flushing syringe, administration set tubing, dressings, tape

Dressings used with gastrostomy tubes for enteral nutrition (covered under the prosthetic device benefit) are included in the payment.

IOM: 100-02, 15, 120; 100-03, 3, 180.2; 100-04, 20, 100.2.2

⚙ **B4035** Enteral feeding supply kit; pump fed, per day, includes but not limited to feeding/flushing syringe, administration set tubing, dressings, tape

IOM: 100-02, 15, 120; 100-03, 3, 180.2; 100-04, 20, 100.2.2

⚙ **B4036** Enteral feeding supply kit; gravity fed, per day, includes but not limited to feeding/flushing syringe, administration set tubing, dressings, tape

IOM: 100-02, 15, 120; 100-03, 3, 180.2; 100-04, 20, 100.2.2

⚙ **B4081** Nasogastric tubing with stylet

More than 3 nasogastric tubes (B4081-B4083), or 1 gastrostomy/jejunostomy tube (B4087-B4088) every three months is rarely medically necessary

IOM: 100-02, 15, 120; 100-03, 3, 180.2; 100-04, 20, 100.2.2

⚙ **B4082** Nasogastric tubing without stylet

IOM: 100-02, 15, 120; 100-03, 3, 180.2; 100-04, 20, 100.2.2

⚙ **B4083** Stomach tube - Levine type

IOM: 100-02, 15, 120; 100-03, 3, 180.2; 100-04, 20, 100.2.2

✳ **B4087** Gastrostomy/jejunostomy tube, standard, any material, any type, each

✳ **B4088** Gastrostomy/jejunostomy tube, low-profile, any material, any type, each

◆ **B4100** Food thickener, administered orally, per ounce

⚙ **B4102** Enteral formula, for adults, used to replace fluids and electrolytes (e.g. clear liquids), 500 ml = 1 unit

IOM: 100-03, 3, 180.2

⚙ **B4103** Enteral formula, for pediatrics, used to replace fluids and electrolytes (e.g. clear liquids), 500 ml = 1 unit

IOM: 100-03, 3, 180.2

⚙ **B4104** Additive for enteral formula (e.g. fiber)

IOM: 100-03, 3, 180.2

⚙ **B4149** Enteral formula, manufactured blenderized natural foods with intact nutrients, includes proteins, fats, carbohydrates, vitamins and minerals, may include fiber, administered through an enteral feeding tube, 100 calories = 1 unit

Produced to meet unique nutrient needs for specific disease conditions; medical record must document specific condition and need for special nutrient

IOM: 100-02, 15, 120; 100-03, 3, 180.2; 100-04, 20, 100.2.2

⚙ **B4150** Enteral formulae, nutritionally complete with intact nutrients, includes proteins, fats, carbohydrates, vitamins, and minerals, may include fiber, administered through an enteral feeding tube, 100 calories = 1 unit

IOM: 100-02, 15, 120; 100-03, 3, 180.2; 100-04, 20, 100.2.2

⚙ **B4152** Enteral formula, nutritionally complete, calorically dense (equal to or greater than 1.5 kcal/ml) with intact nutrients, includes proteins, fats, carbohydrates, vitamins and minerals, may include fiber, administered through an enteral feeding tube, 100 calories = 1 unit

IOM: 100-02, 15, 120; 100-03, 3, 180.2; 100-04, 20, 100.2.2

⚙ **B4153** Enteral formula, nutritionally complete, hydrolyzed proteins (amino acids and peptide chain), includes fats, carbohydrates, vitamins and minerals, may include fiber, administered through an enteral feeding tube, 100 calories = 1 unit

If 2 enteral nutrition products described by same HCPCS code and provided at same time billed on single claim line with units of service reflecting total calories of both nutrients

IOM: 100-02, 15, 120; 100-03, 3, 180.2; 100-04, 20, 100.2.2

⊗ **B4154**   Enteral formula, nutritionally complete, for special metabolic needs, excludes inherited disease of metabolism, includes altered composition of proteins, fats, carbohydrates, vitamins and/or minerals, may include fiber, administered through an enteral feeding tube, 100 calories = 1 unit

IOM: 100-02, 15, 120; 100-03, 3, 180.2; 100-04, 20, 100.2.2

⊗ **B4155**   Enteral formula, nutritionally incomplete/modular nutrients, includes specific nutrients, carbohydrates (e.g. glucose polymers), proteins/amino acids (e.g. glutamine, arginine), fat (e.g. medium chain triglycerides) or combination, administered through an enteral feeding tube, 100 calories = 1 unit

IOM: 100-02, 15, 120; 100-03, 3, 180.2; 100-04, 20, 100.2.2

⊗ **B4157**   Enteral formula, nutritionally complete, for special metabolic needs for inherited disease of metabolism, includes proteins, fats, carbohydrates, vitamins and minerals, may include fiber, administered through an enteral feeding tube, 100 calories = 1 unit

IOM: 100-03, 3, 180.2

⊗ **B4158**   Enteral formula, for pediatrics, nutritionally complete with intact nutrients, includes proteins, fats, carbohydrates, vitamins and minerals, may include fiber and/or iron, administered through an enteral feeding tube, 100 calories = 1 unit

Bill DME/MAC

IOM: 100-03, 3, 180.2

⊗ **B4159**   Enteral formula, for pediatrics, nutritionally complete soy based with intact nutrients, includes proteins, fats, carbohydrates, vitamins and minerals, may include fiber and/or iron, administered through an enteral feeding tube, 100 calories = 1 unit

IOM: 100-03, 3, 180.2

⊗ **B4160**   Enteral formula, for pediatrics, nutritionally complete calorically dense (equal to or greater than 0.7 kcal/ml) with intact nutrients, includes proteins, fats, carbohydrates, vitamins and minerals, may include fiber, administered through an enteral feeding tube, 100 calories = 1 unit

IOM: 100-03, 3, 180.2

⊗ **B4161**   Enteral formula, for pediatrics, hydrolyzed/amino acids and peptide chain proteins, includes fats, carbohydrates, vitamins and minerals, may include fiber, administered through an enteral feeding tube, 100 calories = 1 unit

IOM: 100-03, 3, 180.2

⊗ **B4162**   Enteral formula, for pediatrics, special metabolic needs for inherited disease of metabolism, includes proteins, fats, carbohydrates, vitamins and minerals, may include fiber, administered through an enteral feeding tube, 100 calories = 1 unit

IOM: 100-03, 3, 180.2

Parenteral Nutritional Solutions and Supplies

B4164-B5200:   Bill DME/MAC

⊗ **B4164**   Parenteral nutrition solution: carbohydrates (dextrose), 50% or less (500 ml = 1 unit) - homemix

IOM: 100-02, 15, 120; 100-03, 3, 180.2; 100-04, 20, 100.2.2

⊗ **B4168**   Parenteral nutrition solution; amino acid, 3.5%, (500 ml = 1 unit) - homemix

IOM: 100-02, 15, 120; 100-03, 3, 180.2; 100-04, 20, 100.2.2

➡ ⊗ **B4172**   Parenteral nutrition solution; amino acid, 5.5% through 7%, (500 ml = 1 unit)

IOM: 100-02, 15, 120; 100-03, 3, 180.2; 100-04, 20, 100.2.2

➡ ⊗ **B4176**   Parenteral nutrition solution; amino acid, 7% through 8.5%, (500 ml = 1 unit)

IOM: 100-02, 15, 120; 100-03, 3, 180.2; 100-04, 20, 100.2.2

➡ ⊗ **B4178**   Parenteral nutrition solution: amino acid, greater than 8.5%, (500 ml = 1 unit)

IOM: 100-02, 15, 120; 100-03, 3, 180.2; 100-04, 20, 100.2.2

⊗ **B4180**   Parenteral nutrition solution; carbohydrates (dextrose), greater than 50% (500 ml = 1 unit) - home mix

IOM: 100-02, 15, 120; 100-03, 3, 180.2; 100-04, 20, 100.2.2

⊗ **B4185**   Parenteral nutrition solution, per 10 grams lipids

---

▶ New   ➡ Revised   ✔ Reinstated   ~~deleted~~ Deleted

⊗ Special coverage instructions   ◆ Not covered or valid by Medicare   ✱ Carrier discretion

⚙ **B4189** Parenteral nutrition solution; compounded amino acid and carbohydrates with electrolytes, trace elements, and vitamins, including preparation, any strength, 10 to 51 grams of protein - premix

IOM: 100-02, 15, 120; 100-03, 3, 180.2; 100-04, 20, 100.2.2

⚙ **B4193** Parenteral nutrition solution; compounded amino acid and carbohydrates with electrolytes, trace elements, and vitamins, including preparation, any strength, 52 to 73 grams of protein - premix

IOM: 100-02, 15, 120; 100-03, 3, 180.2; 100-04, 20, 100.2.2

⚙ **B4197** Parenteral nutrition solution; compounded amino acid and carbohydrates with electrolytes, trace elements and vitamins, including preparation, any strength, 74 to 100 grams of protein - premix

IOM: 100-02, 15, 120; 100-03, 3, 180.2; 100-04, 20, 100.2.2

⚙ **B4199** Parenteral nutrition solution; compounded amino acid and carbohydrates with electrolytes, trace elements and vitamins, including preparation, any strength, over 100 grams of protein - premix

IOM: 100-02, 15, 120; 100-03, 3, 180.2; 100-04, 20, 100.2.2

⚙ **B4216** Parenteral nutrition; additives (vitamins, trace elements, heparin, electrolytes) homemix per day

IOM: 100-02, 15, 120; 100-03, 3, 180.2; 100-04, 20, 100.2.2

⚙ **B4220** Parenteral nutrition supply kit; premix, per day

IOM: 100-02, 15, 120; 100-03, 3, 180.2; 100-04, 20, 100.2.2

⚙ **B4222** Parenteral nutrition supply kit; home mix, per day

IOM: 100-02, 15, 120; 100-03, 3, 180.2; 100-04, 20, 100.2.2

⚙ **B4224** Parenteral nutrition administration kit, per day

Dressings used with parenteral nutrition (covered under the prosthetic device benefit) are included in the payment. (www.cms.gov/medicare-coverage-database/)

IOM: 100-02, 15, 120; 100-03, 3, 180.2; 100-04, 20, 100.2.2

⚙ **B5000** Parenteral nutrition solution: compounded amino acid and carbohydrates with electrolytes, trace elements, and vitamins, including preparation, any strength, renal - Amirosyn-RF, NephrAmine, RenAmine - premix

IOM: 100-02, 15, 120; 100-03, 3, 180.2; 100-04, 20, 100.2.2

⚙ **B5100** Parenteral nutrition solution: compounded amino acid and carbohydrates with electrolytes, trace elements, and vitamins, including preparation, any strength, hepatic - FreAmine HBC, HepatAmine - premix

IOM: 100-02, 15, 120; 100-03, 3, 180.2; 100-04, 20, 100.2.2

⚙ **B5200** Parenteral nutrition solution; compounded amino acid and carbohydrates with electrolytes, trace elements, and vitamins, including preparation, any strength, stress - branch chain amino acids - premix

Bill DME/MAC

IOM: 100-02, 15, 120; 100-03, 3, 180.2; 100-04, 20, 100.2.2

Enteral and Parenteral Pumps

B9000-B9999: Bill DME/MAC

⚙ **B9000** Enteral nutrition infusion pump - without alarm

Pump will be denied as not medically necessary if medical necessity of pump is not documented

IOM: 100-02, 15, 120; 100-03, 3, 180.2; 100-04, 20, 100.2.2

▶ New → Revised ✔ Reinstated ~~deleted~~ Deleted

⚙ Special coverage instructions ◆ Not covered or valid by Medicare ✳ Carrier discretion

⚙ **B9002**   Enteral nutrition infusion pump - with alarm

IOM: 100-02, 15, 120; 100-03, 3, 180.2; 100-04, 20, 100.2.2

⚙ **B9004**   Parenteral nutrition infusion pump, portable

IOM: 100-02, 15, 120; 100-03, 3, 180.2; 100-04, 20, 100.2.2

⚙ **B9006**   Parenteral nutrition infusion pump, stationary

IOM: 100-02, 15, 120; 100-03, 3, 180.2; 100-04, 20, 100.2.2

⚙ **B9998**   NOC for enteral supplies

IOM: 100-02, 15, 120; 100-03, 3, 180.2; 100-04, 20, 100.2.2

⚙ **B9999**   NOC for parenteral supplies

Determine if an alternative HCPCS Level II or a CPT code better describes the service being reported. This code should be reported only if a more specific code is unavailable.

IOM: 100-02, 15, 120; 100-03, 3, 180.2; 100-04, 20, 100.2.2

▶ **New**   → **Revised**   ✔ **Reinstated**   ~~deleted~~ **Deleted**

⚙ **Special coverage instructions**   ◆ **Not covered or valid by Medicare**   ✳ **Carrier discretion**

CMS HOSPITAL OUTPATIENT PAYMENT SYSTEM (C1000-C9999)

NOTE: C codes are used ONLY as a part of Hospital Outpatient Prospective Payment System (OPPS) and are not to be used to report other services. C codes are updated quarterly by the Centers for Medicare and Medicaid Services.

◎ **C1300** Hyperbaric oxygen under pressure, full body chamber, per 30-minute interval

Medicare Statute 1833(t)

◎ **C1713** Anchor/Screw for opposing bone-to-bone or soft tissue-to-bone (implantable)

Medicare Statute 1833(t)

◎ **C1714** Catheter, transluminal atherectomy, directional

Medicare Statute 1833(t)

◎ **C1715** Brachytherapy needle

Medicare Statute 1833(t)

◎ **C1716** Brachytherapy source, non-stranded, gold-198, per source

Medicare Statute 1833(t)

◎ **C1717** Brachytherapy source, non-stranded, high dose rate iridium 192, per source

Medicare Statute 1833(t)

◎ **C1719** Brachytherapy source, non-stranded, non-high dose rate iridium-192, per source

Medicare Statute 1833(t)

◎ **C1721** Cardioverter-defibrillator, dual chamber (implantable)

Related CPT codes: 33224, 33240, 33249.

Medicare Statute 1833(t)

◎ **C1722** Cardioverter-defibrillator, single chamber (implantable)

Related CPT codes: 33240, 33249.

Medicare Statute 1833(t)

◎ **C1724** Catheter, transluminal atherectomy, rotational

Medicare Statute 1833(t)

◎ **C1725** Catheter, transluminal angioplasty, non-laser (may include guidance, infusion/perfusion capability)

Medicare Statute 1833(t)

◎ **C1726** Catheter, balloon dilatation, non-vascular

Medicare Statute 1833(t)

◎ **C1727** Catheter, balloon tissue dissector, non-vascular (insertable)

Medicare Statute 1833(t)

◎ **C1728** Catheter, brachytherapy seed administration

Medicare Statute 1833(t)

◎ **C1729** Catheter, drainage

Medicare Statute 1833(t)

◎ **C1730** Catheter, electrophysiology, diagnostic, other than 3D mapping (19 or fewer electrodes)

Medicare Statute 1833(t)

◎ **C1731** Catheter, electrophysiology, diagnostic, other than 3D mapping (20 or more electrodes)

Medicare Statute 1833(t)

◎ **C1732** Catheter, electrophysiology, diagnostic/ablation, 3D or vector mapping

Medicare Statute 1833(t)

◎ **C1733** Catheter, electrophysiology, diagnostic/ablation, other than 3D or vector mapping, other than cool-tip

Medicare Statute 1833(t)

◎ **C1749** Endoscope, retrograde imaging/illumination colonoscope device (implantable)

Medicare Statute 1833(t)

◎ **C1750** Catheter, hemodialysis/peritoneal, long-term

Medicare Statute 1833(t)

◎ **C1751** Catheter, infusion, inserted peripherally, centrally, or midline (other than hemodialysis)

Medicare Statute 1833(t)

◎ **C1752** Catheter, hemodialysis/peritoneal, short-term

Medicare Statute 1833(t)

◎ **C1753** Catheter, intravascular ultrasound

Medicare Statute 1833(t)

◎ **C1754** Catheter, intradiscal

Medicare Statute 1833(t)

◎ **C1755** Catheter, instraspinal

Medicare Statute 1833(t)

◎ **C1756** Catheter, pacing, transesophageal

Medicare Statute 1833(t)

◎ **C1757** Catheter, thrombectomy/embolectomy

Medicare Statute 1833(t)

◎ **C1758** Catheter, ureteral

Medicare Statute 1833(t)

▶ New → Revised ✔ Reinstated ~~deleted~~ Deleted
◎ Special coverage instructions ◆ Not covered or valid by Medicare ✳ Carrier discretion

⊙ **C1759** Catheter, intracardiac echocardiography

Medicare Statute 1833(t)

⊙ **C1760** Closure device, vascular (implantable/insertable)

Medicare Statute 1833(t)

⊙ **C1762** Connective tissue, human (includes fascia lata)

Medicare Statute 1833(t)

⊙ **C1763** Connective tissue, non-human (includes synthetic)

Medicare Statute 1833(t)

⊙ **C1764** Event recorder, cardiac (implantable)

Medicare Statute 1833(t)

⊙ **C1765** Adhesion barrier

Medicare Statute 1833(t)

⊙ **C1766** Introducer/sheath, guiding, intracardiac electrophysiological, steerable, other than peel-away

Medicare Statute 1833(t)

⊙ **C1767** Generator, neurostimulator (implantable), nonrechargeable

Related CPT codes: 61885, 61886, 63685, 64590.

Medicare Statute 1833(t)

⊙ **C1768** Graft, vascular

Medicare Statute 1833(t)

⊙ **C1769** Guide wire

Medicare Statute 1833(t)

⊙ **C1770** Imaging coil, magnetic reasonance (insertable)

Medicare Statute 1833(t)

⊙ **C1771** Repair device, urinary, incontinence, with sling graft

Medicare Statute 1833(t)

⊙ **C1772** Infusion pump, programmable (implantable)

Medicare Statute 1833(t)

⊙ **C1773** Retrieval device, insertable (used to retrieve fractured medical devices)

Medicare Statute 1833(t)

⊙ **C1776** Joint device (implantable)

Medicare Statute 1833(t)

⊙ **C1777** Lead, cardioverter-defibrillator, endocardial single coil (implantable)

Related CPT codes: 33216, 33217, 33249.

Medicare Statute 1833(t)

⊙ **C1778** Lead, neurostimulator (implantable)

Related CPT codes: 43647, 63650, 63655, 63663, 63664, 64553, 64555, 64560, 64561, 64565, 64573, 64575, 64577, 64580, 64581.

Medicare Statute 1833(t)

⊙ **C1779** Lead, pacemaker, trasvenous VDD single pass

Related CPT codes: 33206, 33207, 33208, 33210, 33211, 33214, 33216, 33217, 33249.

Medicare Statute 1833(t)

⊙ **C1780** Lens, intraocular (new technology)

Medicare Statute 1833(t)

⊙ **C1781** Mesh (implantable)

Medicare Statute 1833(t)

⊙ **C1782** Morcellator

Medicare Statute 1833(t)

⊙ **C1783** Ocular implant, aqueous drainage assist device

Medicare Statute 1833(t)

⊙ **C1784** Ocular device, intraoperative, detached retina

Medicare Statute 1833(t)

⊙ **C1785** Pacemaker, dual chamber, rate-responsive (implantable)

Related CPT codes: 33206, 33207, 33208, 33213, 33214, 33224.

Medicare Statute 1833(t)

⊙ **C1786** Pacemaker, single chamber, rate-responsive (implantable)

Related CPT codes: 33206, 33207, 33212.

Medicare Statute 1833(t)

⊙ **C1787** Patient programmer, neurostimulator

Medicare Statute 1833(t)

⊙ **C1788** Port, indwelling (implantable)

Medicare Statute 1833(t)

⊙ **C1789** Prosthesis, breast (implantable)

Medicare Statute 1833(t)

⊙ **C1813** Prosthesis, penile, inflatable

Medicare Statute 1833(t)

⊙ **C1814** Retinal tamponade device, silicone oil

Medicare Statute 1833(t)

⊙ **C1815** Prosthesis, urinary sphincter (implantable)

Medicare Statute 1833(t)

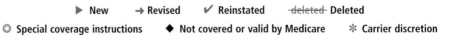

▶ **New**   → **Revised**   ✔ **Reinstated**   deleted **Deleted**
⊙ **Special coverage instructions**   ◆ **Not covered or valid by Medicare**   ✳ **Carrier discretion**

C1759 – C1815   CMS HOSPITAL OUTPATIENT PAYMENT SYSTEM

✪ **C1816** Receiver and/or transmitter, neurostimulator (implantable)

Medicare Statute 1833(t)

✪ **C1817** Septal defect implant system, intracardiac

Medicare Statute 1833(t)

✪ **C1818** Integrated keratoprosthesic

Medicare Statute 1833(t)

✪ **C1819** Surgical tissue localization and excision device (implantable)

Medicare Statute 1833(t)

✪ **C1820** Generator, neurostimulator (implantable), with rechargeable battery and charging system

Related CPT codes: 61885, 61886, 63685, 64590.

Medicare Statute 1833(t)

✪ **C1821** Interspinous process distraction device (implantable)

Medicare Statute 1833(t)

✪ **C1830** Powered bone marrow biopsy needle

Medicare Statute 1833(t)

✪ **C1840** Lens, intraocular (telescopic)

Medicare Statute 1833(t)

✪ **C1874** Stent, coated/covered, with delivery system

Medicare Statute 1833(t)

✪ **C1875** Stent, coated/covered, without delivery system

Medicare Statute 1833(t)

✪ **C1876** Stent, non-coated/non-covered, with delivery system

Medicare Statute 1833(t)

✪ **C1877** Stent, non-coated/non-covered, without delivery system

Medicare Statute 1833(t)

✪ **C1878** Material for vocal cord medialization, synthetic (implantable)

Medicare Statute 1833(t)

✪ **C1879** Tissue marker (implantable)

Medicare Statute 1833(t)

✪ **C1880** Vena cava filter

Medicare Statute 1833(t)

✪ **C1881** Dialysis access system (implantable)

Medicare Statute 1833(t)

✪ **C1882** Cardioverter-defibrillator, other than single or dual chamber (implantable)

Related CPT codes: 33224, 33240, 33249.

Medicare Statute 1833(t)

✪ **C1883** Adaptor/Extension, pacing lead or neurostimulator lead (implantable)

Medicare Statute 1833(t)

✪ **C1884** Embolization protective system

Medicare Statute 1833(t)

✪ **C1885** Catheter, transluminal angioplasty, laser

Medicare Statute 1833(t)

✪ **C1886** Catheter, extravascular tissue ablation, any modality (insertable)

Medicare Statute 1833(t)

✪ **C1887** Catheter, guiding (may include infusion/perfusion capability)

Medicare Statute 1833(t)

✪ **C1888** Catheter, ablation, non-cardiac, endovascular (implantable)

Medicare Statute 1833(t)

✪ **C1891** Infusion pump, non-programmable, permanent (implantable)

Medicare Statute 1833(t)

✪ **C1892** Introducer/sheath, guiding, intracardiac electrophysiological, fixed-curve, peel-away

Medicare Statute 1833(t)

✪ **C1893** Introducer/sheath, guiding, intracardiac electrophysiological, fixed-curve, other than peel-away

Medicare Statute 1833(t)

✪ **C1894** Introducer/sheath, other than guiding, other than intracardiac electrophysiological, non-laser

Medicare Statute 1833(t)

✪ **C1895** Lead, cardioverter-defibrillator, endocardial dual coil (implantable)

Related CPT codes: 33216, 33217, 33249.

Medicare Statute 1833(t)

✪ **C1896** Lead, cardioverter-defibrillator, other than endocardial single or dual coil (implantable)

Related CPT codes: 33216, 33217, 33249.

Medicare Statute 1833(t)

▶ New ➔ Revised ✔ Reinstated ~~deleted~~ Deleted

✪ Special coverage instructions ◆ Not covered or valid by Medicare ✳ Carrier discretion

⊙ **C1897** Lead, neurostimulator test kit (implantable)

Related CPT codes: 43647, 63650, 63655, 63663, 63664, 64553, 64555, 64560, 64561, 64565, 64575, 64577, 64580, 64581.

Medicare Statute 1833(t)

⊙ **C1898** Lead, pacemaker, other than transvenous VDD single pass

Related CPT codes: 33206, 33207, 33208, 33210, 33211, 33214, 33216, 33217, 33249.

Medicare Statute 1833(t)

⊙ **C1899** Lead, pacemaker/cardioverter-defibrillator combination (implantable)

Related CPT codes: 33216, 33217, 33249.

Medicare Statute 1833(t)

⊙ **C1900** Lead, left ventricular coronary venous system

Related CPT codes: 33224, 33225.

Medicare Statute 1833(t)

⊙ **C2614** Probe, percutaneous lumbar discectomy

Medicare Statute 1833(t)

⊙ **C2615** Sealant, pulmonary, liquid

Medicare Statute 1833(t)

⊙ **C2616** Brachytherapy source, non-stranded, yttrium-90, per source

Medicare Statute 1833(t)

⊙ **C2617** Stent, non-coronary, temporary, without delivery system

Medicare Statute 1833(t)

⊙ **C2618** Probe, cryoablation

Medicare Statute 1833(t)

⊙ **C2619** Pacemaker, dual chamber, non rate-responsive (implantable)

Related CPT codes: 33206, 33207, 33208, 33213, 33214, 33224.

Medicare Statute 1833(t)

⊙ **C2620** Pacemaker, single chamber, non rate-responsive (implantable)

Related CPT codes: 33206, 33207, 33212, 33224.

Medicare Statute 1833(t)

⊙ **C2621** Pacemaker, other than single or dual chamber (implantable)

Related CPT codes: 33206, 33207, 33208, 33212, 33213, 33214, 33224.

Medicare Statute 1833(t)

⊙ **C2622** Prosthesis, penile, non-inflatable

Medicare Statute 1833(t)

⊙ **C2625** Stent, non-coronary, temporary, with delivery system

Medicare Statute 1833(t)

⊙ **C2626** Infusion pump, non-programmable, temporary (implantable)

Medicare Statute 1833(t)

⊙ **C2627** Catheter, suprapubic/cystoscopic

Medicare Statute 1833(t)

⊙ **C2628** Catheter, occlusion

Medicare Statute 1833(t)

⊙ **C2629** Introducer/Sheath, other than guiding, intracardiac electrophysiological, laser

Medicare Statute 1833(t)

⊙ **C2630** Catheter, electrophysiology, diagnostic/ablation, other than 3D or vector mapping, cool-tip

Medicare Statute 1833(t)

⊙ **C2631** Repair device, urinary, incontinence, without sling graft

Medicare Statute 1833(t)

⊙ **C2634** Brachytherapy source, non-stranded, high activity, iodine-125, greater than 1.01 mci (NIST), per source

Medicare Statute 1833(t)

⊙ **C2635** Brachytherapy source, non-stranded, high activity, paladium-103, greater than 2.2 mci (NIST), per source

Medicare Statute 1833(t)

⊙ **C2636** Brachytherapy linear source, non-stranded, paladium-103, per 1 mm

⊙ **C2637** Brachytherapy source, non-stranded, Ytterbium-169, per source

Medicare Statute 1833(t)

⊙ **C2638** Brachytherapy source, stranded, iodine-125, per source

Medicare Statute 1833(t)(2)

⊙ **C2639** Brachytherapy source, non-stranded, iodine-125, per source

Medicare Statute 1833(t)(2)

⊙ **C2640** Brachytherapy source, stranded, palladium-103, per source

Medicare Statute 1833(t)(2)

⊙ **C2641** Brachytherapy source, non-stranded, palladium-103, per source

Medicare Statute 1833(t)(2)

⊙ **C2642** Brachytherapy source, stranded, cesium-131, per source

Medicare Statute 1833(t)(2)

▶ New → Revised ✔ Reinstated ~~deleted~~ Deleted

⊙ Special coverage instructions ◆ Not covered or valid by Medicare ✳ Carrier discretion

☼ **C2643** Brachytherapy source, non-stranded, cesium-131, per source

Medicare Statute 1833(t)(2)

☼ **C2698** Brachytherapy source, stranded, not otherwise specified, per source

Medicare Statute 1833(t)(2)

☼ **C2699** Brachytherapy source, non-stranded, not otherwise specified, per source

Medicare Statute 1833(t)(2)

☼ **C8900** Magnetic resonance angiography with contrast, abdomen

Medicare Statute 1833(t)(2)

☼ **C8901** Magnetic resonance angiography without contrast, abdomen

Medicare Statute 1833(t)(2)

☼ **C8902** Magnetic resonance angiography without contrast followed by with contrast, abdomen

Medicare Statute 1833(t)(2)

☼ **C8903** Magnetic resonance imaging with contrast, breast; unilateral

Medicare Statute 1833(t)(2)

☼ **C8904** Magnetic resonance imaging without contrast, breast; unilateral

Medicare Statute 1833(t)(2)

☼ **C8905** Magnetic resonance imaging without contrast followed by with contrast, breast; unilateral

Medicare Statute 1833(t)(2)

☼ **C8906** Magnetic resonance imaging with contrast, breast; bilateral

Medicare Statute 1833(t)(2)

☼ **C8907** Magnetic resonance imaging without contrast, breast; bilateral

Medicare Statute 1833(t)(2)

☼ **C8908** Magnetic resonance imaging without contrast followed by with contrast, breast; bilateral

Medicare Statute 1833(t)(2)

☼ **C8909** Magnetic resonance angiography with contrast, chest (excluding myocardium)

Medicare Statute 1833(t)(2)

☼ **C8910** Magnetic resonance angiography without contrast, chest (excluding myocardium)

Medicare Statute 1833(t)(2)

☼ **C8911** Magnetic resonance angiography without contrast followed by with contrast, chest (excluding myocardium)

Medicare Statute 1833(t)(2)

☼ **C8912** Magnetic resonance angiography with contrast, lower extremity

Medicare Statute 1833(t)(2)

☼ **C8913** Magnetic resonance angiography without contrast, lower extremity

Medicare Statute 1833(t)(2)

☼ **C8914** Magnetic resonance angiography without contrast followed by with contrast, lower extremity

Medicare Statute 1833(t)(2)

☼ **C8918** Magnetic resonance angiography with contrast, pelvis

Medicare Statute 1833(t)(2)

☼ **C8919** Magnetic resonance angiography without contrast, pelvis

Medicare Statute 1833(t)(2)

☼ **C8920** Magnetic resonance angiography without contrast followed by with contrast, pelvis

Medicare Statute 1833(t)(2)

☼ **C8921** Transthoracic echocardiography with contrast, or without contrast followed by with contrast, for congenital cardiac anomalies; complete

Medicare Statute 1833(t)(2)

☼ **C8922** Transthoracic echocardiography with contrast, or without contrast followed by with contrast, for congenital cardiac anomalies; follow-up or limited study

Medicare Statute 1833(t)(2)

☼ **C8923** Transthoracic echocardiography with contrast, or without contrast followed by with contrast, real-time with image documentation (2D), includes M-mode recording, when performed, complete, without spectral or color Doppler echocardiography

Medicare Statute 1833(t)(2)

☼ **C8924** Transthoracic echocardiography with contrast, or without contrast followed by with contrast, real-time with image documentation (2D), includes M-mode recording, when performed, follow-up or limited study

Medicare Statute 1833(t)(2)

☼ **C8925** Transesophageal echocardiography (TEE) with contrast, or without contrast followed by with contrast, real time with image documentation (2D) (with or without M-mode recording); including probe placement, image acquisition, interpretation and report

Medicare Statute 1833(t)(2)

▶ New   → Revised   ✔ Reinstated   ~~deleted~~ Deleted

☼ Special coverage instructions   ◆ Not covered or valid by Medicare   ✳ Carrier discretion

⊛ **C8926** Transesophageal echocardiography (TEE) with contrast, or without contrast followed by with contrast, for congenital cardiac anomalies; including probe placement, image acquisition, interpretation and report

Medicare Statute 1833(t)(2)

⊛ **C8927** Transesophageal echocardiography (TEE) with contrast, or without contrast followed by with contrast, for monitoring purposes, including probe placement, real time 2-dimensional image acquisition and interpretation leading to ongoing (continuous) assessment of (dynamically changing) cardiac pumping function and to therapeutic measures on an immediate time basis

Medicare Statute 1833(t)(2)

⊛ **C8928** Transthoracic echocardiography with contrast, or without contrast followed by with contrast, real-time with image documentation (2D), includes M-mode recording, when performed, during rest and cardiovascular stress test using treadmill, bicycle exercise and/or pharmacologically induced stress, with interpretation and report

Medicare Statute 1833(t)(2)

⊛ **C8929** Transthoracic echocardiography with contrast, or without contrast followed by with contrast, real-time with image documentation (2D), includes M-mode recording, when performed, complete, with spectral Doppler echocardiography, and with color flow Doppler echocardiography

Medicare Statute 1833(t)(2)

⊛ **C8930** Transthoracic echocardiography, with contrast, or without contrast followed by with contrast, real-time with image documentation (2D), includes M-mode recording, when performed, during rest and cardiovascular stress test using treadmill, bicycle exercise and/or pharmacologically induced stress, with interpretation and report; including performance of continuous electrocardiographic monitoring, with physician supervision

Medicare Statute 1833(t)(2)

⊛ **C8931** Magnetic resonance angiography with contrast, spinal canal and contents

Medicare Statute 1833(t)

⊛ **C8932** Magnetic resonance angiography without contrast, spinal canal and contents

Medicare Statute 1833(t)

⊛ **C8933** Magnetic resonance angiography without contrast followed by with contrast, spinal canal and contents

Medicare Statute 1833(t)

⊛ **C8934** Magnetic resonance angiography with contrast, upper extremity

Medicare Statute 1833(t)

⊛ **C8935** Magnetic resonance angiography without contrast, upper extremity

Medicare Statute 1833(t)

⊛ **C8936** Magnetic resonance angiography without contrast followed by with contrast, upper extremity

Medicare Statute 1833(t)

⊛ **C8957** Intravenous infusion for therapy/diagnosis; initiation of prolonged infusion (more than 8 hours), requiring use of portable or implantable pump

Medicare Statute 1833(t)

⊛ **C9113** Injection, pantoprazole sodium, per vial

Medicare Statute 1833(t)

⊛ **C9121** Injection, argatroban, per 5 mg

Medicare Statute 1833(t)

✳ **C9248** Injection, clevidipine butyrate, 1 mg

Medicare Statute 1833(t)

⊛ **C9250** Human plasma fibrin sealant, vapor-heated, solvent-detergent (ARTISS), 2ml

Example of diagnosis codes to be reported with C9250: 941.00–949.5.

Medicare Statute 621MMA

⊛ **C9254** Injection, lacosamide, 1 mg

Medicare Statute 621MMA

⊛ **C9257** injection, bevacizumab, 0.25 mg

Medicare Statute 1833(t)

~~C9270~~ ~~Injection, immune globulin (gammaplex), intravenous, non-lyophilized (e. g. Liquid), 500 mg~~ ✖

Cross Reference: J1741

⊛ **C9275** Injection, hexaminolevulinate hydrochloride, 100 mg, per study dose

Medicare Statute 1833(t)

~~C9279~~ ~~Injection, ibuprofen, 100 mg~~ ✖

Cross Reference: CPT J1741

▶ New   → Revised   ✔ Reinstated   ~~deleted~~ Deleted

⊛ Special coverage instructions   ◆ Not covered or valid by Medicare   ✳ Carrier discretion

✺ **C9285** Lidocaine 70 mg/tetracaine 70 mg, per patch

Medicare Statute 1833(t)

~~C9286~~ ~~Injection, belatacept, 1 mg~~ ✖

Cross Reference: CPT J0485

~~C9287~~ ~~Injection, brentuximab vedotin,~~ ✖
~~1 mg~~

Cross Reference: CPT J9042

~~C9288~~ ~~Injection, centruroides (scorpion)~~ ✖
~~immune f(ab)2 (equine), 1 vial~~

Cross Reference: CPT J7016

~~C9289~~ ~~Injection, asparaginase Erwinia~~ ✖
~~chrysanthemi, 1,000 international~~
~~units (I.U.)~~

Cross Reference: J9019

▶ ✺ **C9290** Injection, bupivacaine liposome, 1 mg

Medicare Statute 1833(t)

~~C9291~~ ~~Mitomycin, 40 mg~~ ✖

Cross Reference: J0178, Q2046

▶ ✺ **C9292** Injection, pertuzumab, 10 mg

Medicare Statute 1833(t)

▶ ✺ **C9293** Injection, glucarpidase, 10 units

Medicare Statute 1833(t)

▶ ✺ **C9294** Injection, taliglucerase alfa, 10 units

Medicare Statute 1833(t)

▶ ✺ **C9295** Injection, carfilzomib, 1 mg

Medicare Statute 1833(t)

▶ ✺ **C9296** Injection, ziv-aflibercept, 1 mg

Medicare Statute 1833(t)

✺ **C9352** Microporous collagen implantable tube (NeuraGen Nerve Guide), per centimeter length

Medicare Statute 621MMA

✺ **C9353** Microporous collagen implantable slit tube (NeuraWrap Nerve Protector), per centimeter length

Medicare Statute 621MMA

✺ **C9354** Acellular pericardial tissue matrix of non-human origin (Veritas), per square centimeter

Medicare Statute 621MMA

✺ **C9355** Collagen nerve cuff (NeuroMatrix), per 0.5 centimeter length

Medicare Statute 621MMA

✺ **C9356** Tendon, porous matrix of cross-linked collagen and glycosaminoglycan matrix (TenoGlide Tendon Protector Sheet), per square centimeter

Medicare Statute 621MMA

✺ **C9358** Dermal substitute, native, non-denatured collagen, fetal bovine origin (SurgiMend Collagen Matrix), per 0.5 square centimeters

Medicare Statute 621MMA

✺ **C9359** Porous purified collagen matrix bone void filler (Integra Mozaik Osteoconductive Scaffold Putty, Integra OS Osteoconductive Scaffold Putty), per 0.5 cc

Medicare Statute 1833(t)

✺ **C9360** Dermal substitute, native, non-denatured collagen, neonatal bovine origin (SurgiMend Collagen Matrix), per 0.5 square centimeters

Medicare Statute 621MMA

✺ **C9361** Collagen matrix nerve wrap (NeuroMend Collagen Nerve Wrap), per 0.5 centimeter length

Medicare Statute 621MMA

✺ **C9362** Porous purified collagen matrix bone void filler (Integra Mozaik Osteoconductive Scaffold Strip), per 0.5 cc

Medicare Statute 621MMA

✺ **C9363** Skin substitute, Integra Meshed Bilayer Wound Matrix, per square centimeter

Medicare Statute 621MMA

✺ **C9364** Porcine implant, Permacol, per square centimeter

Medicare Statute 621MMA

~~C9366~~ ~~Epifix, per square centimeter~~ ✖

Cross Reference: CPT Q4131

✺ **C9367** Skin substitute, endoform dermal template, per square centimeter

Medicare Statute 1833(t)(6)

~~C9368~~ ~~Grafix core, per square centimeter~~ ✖

Cross Reference: Q4132

~~C9369~~ ~~Graffix prime, per square centimeter~~ ✖

Cross Reference: Q4133

✺ **C9399** Unclassified drugs or biologicals

Medicare Statute 621MMA

▶ New   → Revised   ✔ Reinstated   ~~deleted~~ Deleted
✺ Special coverage instructions   ◆ Not covered or valid by Medicare   ✳ Carrier discretion

▶ ✿ **C9600** Percutaneous transcatheter placement of drug eluting intracoronary stent(s), with coronary angioplasty when performed; a single major coronary artery or branch

Medicare Statute 1833(t)

▶ ✿ **C9601** Percutaneous transcatheter placement of drug-eluting intracoronary stent(s), with coronary angioplasty when performed; each additional branch of a major coronary artery (list separately in addition to code for primary procedure)

Medicare Statute 1833(t)

▶ ✿ **C9602** Percutaneous transluminal coronary atherectomy, with drug eluting intracoronary stent, with coronary angioplasty when performed; a single major coronary artery or branch

Medicare Statute 1833(t)

▶ ✿ **C9603** Percutaneous transluminal coronary atherectomy, with drug-eluting intracoronary stent, with coronary angioplasty when performed; each additional branch of a major coronary artery (list separately in addition to code for primary procedure)

Medicare Statute 1833(t)

▶ ✿ **C9604** Percutaneous transluminal revascularization of or through coronary artery bypass graft (internal mammary, free arterial, venous), any combination of drug-eluting intracoronary stent, atherectomy and angioplasty, including distal protection when performed; a single vessel

▶ ✿ **C9605** Percutaneous transluminal revascularization of or through coronary artery bypass graft (internal mammary, free arterial, venous), any combination of drug-eluting intracoronary stent, atherectomy and angioplasty, including distal protection when performed; each additional branch subtended by the bypass graft (list separately in addition to code for primary procedure)

Medicare Statute 1833(t)

▶ ✿ **C9606** Percutaneous transluminal revascularization of acute total/subtotal occlusion during acute myocardial infarction, coronary artery or coronary artery bypass graft, any combination of drug-eluting intracoronary stent, atherectomy and angioplasty, including aspiration thrombectomy when performed, single vessel

Medicare Statute 1833(t)

▶ ✿ **C9607** Percutaneous transluminal revascularization of chronic total occlusion, coronary artery, coronary artery branch, or coronary artery bypass graft, any combination of drug-eluting intracoronary stent, atherectomy and angioplasty; a single vessel

Medicare Statute 1833(t)

▶ ✿ **C9608** Percutaneous transluminal revascularization of chronic total occlusion, coronary artery, coronary artery branch, or coronary artery bypass graft, any combination of drug-eluting intracoronary stent, atherectomy and angioplasty; a each additional coronary artery, coronary artery branch, or bypass graft (list separately in addition to code for primary procedure)

Medicare Statute 1833(t)

~~C9716~~ ~~Creations of thermal anal lesions by radiofrequency energy~~ ✖

→ ✿ **C9724** Endoscopic full-thickness plication of the stomach using endoscopic plication system (EPS); includes endoscopy

Medicare Statute 1833(t)

✿ **C9725** Placement of endorectal intracavitary applicator for high intensity brachytherapy

Medicare Statute 1833(t)

✿ **C9726** Placement and removal (if performed) of applicator into breast for radiation therapy

Medicare Statute 1833(t)

✿ **C9727** Insertion of implants into the soft palate; minimum of three implants

Medicare Statute 1833(t)

▶ New	→ Revised	✔ Reinstated	~~deleted~~ Deleted

✿ Special coverage instructions   ◆ Not covered or valid by Medicare   ✳ Carrier discretion

✳ **C9728** Placement of interstitial device(s) for radiation therapy/surgery guidance (e.g., fiducial markers, dosimeter), for other than the following sites (any approach): abdomen, pelvis, prostate, retroperitoneum, thorax, single or multiple

Medicare Statute 1833(t)

~~C9732~~ ~~Insertion of ocular telescope prosthesis including removal of crystalline lens~~ ✖

Cross Reference: CPT 0308T

▶ **C9733** Non-ophthalmic fluorescent vascular angiography

Medicare Statute 1833(t)

☼ **C9800** Dermal injection procedure(s) for facial lipodystrophy syndrome (LDS) and provision of radiesse or sculptra dermal filler, including all items and supplies

Temporary office-based destination

Medicare Statute 1833(t)

☼ **C9898** Radiolabeled product provided during a hospital inpatient stay

☼ **C9899** Implanted prosthetic device, payable only for inpatients who do not have inpatient coverage

Medicare Statute 1833(t)

▶ New   → Revised   ✔ Reinstated   ~~deleted~~ Deleted
☼ Special coverage instructions   ◆ Not covered or valid by Medicare   ✳ Carrier discretion

DURABLE MEDICAL EQUIPMENT (E0100-E9999)

Canes

E0100-E0105 Bill DME/MAC

⊛ **E0100** Cane, includes canes of all materials, adjustable or fixed, with tip

IOM: 100-02, 15, 110.1; 100-03, 4, 280.1; 100-03, 4, 280.2

⊛ **E0105** Cane, quad or three prong, includes canes of all materials, adjustable or fixed, with tips

IOM: 100-02, 15, 110.1; 100-03, 4, 280.1; 100-03, 4, 280.2

Crutches

E0110-E0118: Bill DME/MAC

⊛ **E0110** Crutches, forearm, includes crutches of various materials, adjustable or fixed, pair, complete with tips and handgrips

Crutches are covered when prescribed for a patient who is normally ambulatory but suffers from a condition that impairs ambulation. Provides minimal to moderate weight support while ambulating.

IOM: 100-02, 15, 110.1; 100-03, 4, 280.1

⊛ **E0111** Crutch forearm, includes crutches of various materials, adjustable or fixed, each, with tips and handgrips

IOM: 100-02, 15, 110.1; 100-03, 4, 280.1

⊛ **E0112** Crutches, underarm, wood, adjustable or fixed, pair, with pads, tips, and handgrips

IOM: 100-02, 15, 110.1; 100-03, 4, 280.1

⊛ **E0113** Crutch underarm, wood, adjustable or fixed, each, with pad, tip, and handgrip

IOM: 100-02, 15, 110.1; 100-03, 4, 280.1

⊛ **E0114** Crutches, underarm, other than wood, adjustable or fixed, pair, with pads, tips and handgrips

IOM: 100-02, 15, 110.1; 100-03, 4, 280.1

⊛ **E0116** Crutch, underarm, other than wood, adjustable or fixed, with pad, tip, handgrip, with or without shock absorber, each

IOM: 100-02, 15, 110.1; 100-03, 4, 280.1

⊛ **E0117** Crutch, underarm, articulating, spring assisted, each

IOM: 100-02, 15, 110.1

✳ **E0118** Crutch substitute, lower leg platform, with or without wheels, each

Walkers

E0130-E0155: Bill DME/MAC

⊛ **E0130** Walker, rigid (pickup), adjustable or fixed height

Standard walker criteria for payment: Individual has a mobility limitation that significantly impairs ability to participate in mobility-related activities of daily living that cannot be adequately or safely addressed by a cane. The patient is able to use the walker safely; the functional mobility deficit can be resolved with use of a standard walker.

IOM: 100-02, 15, 110.1; 100-03, 4, 280.1

⊛ **E0135** Walker, folding (pickup), adjustable or fixed height

IOM: 100-02, 15, 110.1; 100-03, 4, 280.1

⊛ **E0140** Walker, with trunk support, adjustable or fixed height, any type

IOM: 100-02, 15, 110.1; 100-03, 4, 280.1

⊛ **E0141** Walker, rigid, wheeled, adjustable or fixed height

IOM: 100-02, 15, 110.1; 100-03, 4, 280.1

⊛ **E0143** Walker, folding, wheeled, adjustable or fixed height

IOM: 100-02, 15, 110.1; 100-03, 4, 280.1

⊛ **E0144** Walker, enclosed, four sided framed, rigid or folding, wheeled, with posterior seat

IOM: 100-02, 15, 110.1; 100-03, 4, 280.1

⊛ **E0147** Walker, heavy duty, multiple braking system, variable wheel resistance

Heavy-duty walker is labeled as capable of supporting more than 300 pounds.

IOM: 100-02, 15, 110.1; 100-03, 4, 280.1

✳ **E0148** Walker, heavy duty, without wheels, rigid or folding, any type, each

Heavy-duty walker is labeled as capable of supporting more than 300 pounds

✳ **E0149** Walker, heavy duty, wheeled, rigid or folding, any type

Heavy-duty walker is labeled as capable of supporting more than 300 pounds

✳ **E0153** Platform attachment, forearm crutch, each

✳ **E0154** Platform attachment, walker, each

▶ New	→ Revised	✔ Reinstated	~~deleted~~ Deleted
⊛ Special coverage instructions	◆ Not covered or valid by Medicare	✳ Carrier discretion	

* **E0155** Wheel attachment, rigid pick-up walker, per pair

Attachments

E0156-E0159: Bill DME/MAC

* **E0156** Seat attachment, walker

* **E0157** Crutch attachment, walker, each

* **E0158** Leg extensions for walker, per set of four (4)

Leg extensions are considered medically necessary DME for patients 6 feet tall or more

* **E0159** Brake attachment for wheeled walker, replacement, each

Commodes

E0160-E0175: Bill DME/MAC

☺ **E0160** Sitz type bath or equipment, portable, used with or without commode

IOM: 100-03, 4, 280.1

☺ **E0161** Sitz type bath or equipment, portable, used with or without commode, with faucet attachment/ s

IOM: 100-03, 4, 280.1

☺ **E0162** Sitz bath chair

IOM: 100-03, 4, 280.1

☺ **E0163** Commode chair, mobile or stationary, with fixed arms

IOM: 100-02, 15, 110.1; 100-03, 4, 280.1

☺ **E0165** Commode chair, mobile or stationary, with detachable arms

IOM: 100-02, 15, 110.1; 100-03, 4, 280.1

☺ **E0167** Pail or pan for use with commode chair, replacement only

IOM: 100-03, 4, 280.1

* **E0168** Commode chair, extra wide and/or heavy duty, stationary or mobile, with or without arms, any type, each

Extra-wide or heavy duty commode chair is labeled as capable of supporting more than 300 pounds

* **E0170** Commode chair with integrated seat lift mechanism, electric, any type

* **E0171** Commode chair with integrated seat lift mechanism, non-electric, any type

◆ **E0172** Seat lift mechanism placed over or on top of toilet, any type

Medicare Statute 1861 SSA

* **E0175** Foot rest, for use with commode chair, each

Decubitus Care Equipment

E0181-E0199: Bill DME/MAC

☺ **E0181** Powered pressure reducing mattress overlay/pad, alternating, with pump, includes heavy duty

Requires the provider to determine medical necessity compliance. To demonstrate the requirements in the medical policy were met, attach -KX.

IOM: 100-03, 4, 280.1; 100-08, 5, 5.2.3

☺ **E0182** Pump for alternating pressure pad, for replacement only

IOM: 100-03, 4, 280.1; 100-08, 5, 5.2.3

☺ **E0184** Dry pressure mattress

IOM: 100-03, 4, 280.1; 100-08, 5, 5.2.3

☺ **E0185** Gel or gel-like pressure pad for mattress, standard mattress length and width

IOM: 100-03, 4, 280.1; 100-08, 5, 5.2.3

☺ **E0186** Air pressure mattress

IOM: 100-03, 4, 280.1

☺ **E0187** Water pressure mattress

IOM: 100-03, 4, 280.1

☺ **E0188** Synthetic sheepskin pad

IOM: 100-03, 4, 280.1; 100-08, 5, 5.2.3

☺ **E0189** Lambswool sheepskin pad, any size

IOM: 100-03, 4, 280.1; 100-08, 5, 5.2.3

☺ **E0190** Positioning cushion/pillow/wedge, any shape or size, includes all components and accessories

IOM: 100-02, 15, 110.1

* **E0191** Heel or elbow protector, each

* **E0193** Powered air flotation bed (low air loss therapy)

☺ **E0194** Air fluidized bed

IOM: 100-03, 4, 280.1

☺ **E0196** Gel pressure mattress

IOM: 100-03, 4, 280.1

☺ **E0197** Air pressure pad for mattress, standard mattress length and width

IOM: 100-03, 4, 280.1

☺ **E0198** Water pressure pad for mattress, standard mattress length and width

IOM: 100-03, 4, 280.1

▶ **New** → **Revised** ✔ **Reinstated** ~~deleted~~ **Deleted**

☺ **Special coverage instructions** ◆ **Not covered or valid by Medicare** * **Carrier discretion**

⊛ **E0199**   Dry pressure pad for mattress, standard mattress length and width

IOM: 100-03, 4, 280.1

Heat/Cold Application

E0200-E0239:   Bill DME/MAC

⊛ **E0200**   Heat lamp, without stand (table model), includes bulb, or infrared element

Covered when medical review determines patient's medical condition is one for which application of heat by heat lamp is therapeutically effective

IOM: 100-02, 15, 110.1; 100-03, 4, 280.1

✳ **E0202**   Phototherapy (bilirubin) light with photometer

◆ **E0203**   Therapeutic lightbox, minimum 10,000 lux, table top model

IOM: 100-03, 4, 280.1

⊛ **E0205**   Heat lamp, with stand, includes bulb, or infrared element

IOM: 100-02, 15, 110.1; 100-03, 4, 280.1

⊛ **E0210**   Electric heat pad, standard

Flexible device containing electric resistive elements producing heat; has fabric cover to prevent burns; with or without timing devices for automatic shut-off

IOM: 100-03, 4, 280.1

⊛ **E0215**   Electric heat pad, moist

Flexible device containing electric resistive elements producing heat. Must have component that will absorb and retain liquid (water)

IOM: 100-03, 4, 280.1

⊛ **E0217**   Water circulating heat pad with pump

Consists of flexible pad containing series of channels through which water is circulated by means of electrical pumping mechanism and heated in external reservoir

IOM: 100-03, 4, 280.1

⊛ **E0218**   Water circulating cold pad with pump

IOM: 100-03, 4, 280.1

✳ **E0221**   Infrared heating pad system

⊛ **E0225**   Hydrocollator unit, includes pads

IOM: 100-02, 15, 230; 100-03, 4, 280.1

◆ **E0231**   Non-contact wound warming device (temperature control unit, AC adapter and power cord) for use with warming card and wound cover

IOM: 100-02, 16, 20

◆ **E0232**   Warming card for use with the non-contact wound warming device and non-contact wound warming wound cover

IOM: 100-02, 16, 20

⊛ **E0235**   Paraffin bath unit, portable (see medical supply code A4265 for paraffin)

Ordered by physician and patient's condition expected to be relieved by long term use of modality

IOM: 100-02, 15, 230; 100-03, 4, 280.1

⊛ **E0236**   Pump for water circulating pad

IOM: 100-03, 4, 280.1

⊛ **E0239**   Hydrocollator unit, portable

IOM: 100-02, 15, 230; 100-03, 4, 280.1

Bath and Toilet Aids

E0240-E0249:   Bill DME/MAC

◆ **E0240**   Bath/shower chair, with or without wheels, any size

IOM: 100-03, 4, 280.1

◆ **E0241**   Bath tub wall rail, each

IOM: 100-02, 15, 110.1; 100-03, 4, 280.1

◆ **E0242**   Bath tub rail, floor base

IOM: 100-02, 15, 110.1; 100-03, 4, 280.1

◆ **E0243**   Toilet rail, each

IOM: 100-02, 15, 110.1; 100-03, 4, 280.1

◆ **E0244**   Raised toilet seat

IOM: 100-03, 4, 280.1

◆ **E0245**   Tub stool or bench

IOM: 100-03, 4, 280.1

✳ **E0246**   Transfer tub rail attachment

⊛ **E0247**   Transfer bench for tub or toilet with or without commode opening

IOM: 100-03, 4, 280.1

⊛ **E0248**   Transfer bench, heavy duty, for tub or toilet with or without commode opening

Heavy duty transfer bench is labeled as capable of supporting more than 300 pounds

IOM: 100-03, 4, 280.1

✳ **E0249**   Pad for water circulating heat unit, for replacement only

Describes durable replacement pad used with water circulating heat pump system

IOM: 100-03, 4, 280.1

▶ New   → Revised   ✔ Reinstated   ~~deleted~~ Deleted

⊛ Special coverage instructions   ◆ Not covered or valid by Medicare   ✳ Carrier discretion

Hospital Beds and Accessories

E0250-E0373: Bill DME/MAC

⊛ **E0250** Hospital bed, fixed height, with any type side rails, with mattress
IOM: 100-02, 15, 110.1; 100-03, 4, 280.7

⊛ **E0251** Hospital bed, fixed height, with any type side rails, without mattress
IOM:100-02, 15, 110.1; 100-03, 4, 280.7

⊛ **E0255** Hospital bed, variable height, hi-lo, with any type side rails, with mattress
IOM: 100-02, 15, 110.1; 100-03, 4, 280.7

⊛ **E0256** Hospital bed, variable height, hi-lo, with any type side rails, without mattress
IOM: 100-02, 15, 110.1; 100-03, 4, 280.7

⊛ **E0260** Hospital bed, semi-electric (head and foot adjustment), with any type side rails, with mattress
IOM: 100-02, 15, 110.1; 100-03, 4, 280.7

⊛ **E0261** Hospital bed, semi-electric (head and foot adjustment), with any type side rails, without mattress
IOM: 100-02, 15, 110.1; 100-03, 4, 280.7

⊛ **E0265** Hospital bed, total electric (head, foot and height adjustments), with any type side rails, with mattress
IOM: 100-02, 15, 110.1; 100-03, 4, 280.7

⊛ **E0266** Hospital bed, total electric (head, foot and height adjustments), with any type side rails, without mattress
IOM: 100-02, 15, 110.1; 100-03, 4, 280.7

◆ **E0270** Hospital bed, institutional type includes: oscillating, circulating and Stryker frame, with mattress
IOM: 100-03, 4, 280.1

⊛ **E0271** Mattress, innerspring
IOM: 100-03, 4, 280.1; 100-03, 4, 280.7

⊛ **E0272** Mattress, foam rubber
IOM: 100-03, 4, 280.1; 100-03, 4, 280.7

◆ **E0273** Bed board
IOM: 100-03, 4, 280.1

◆ **E0274** Over-bed table
IOM: 100-03, 4, 280.1

⊛ **E0275** Bed pan, standard, metal or plastic
IOM: 100-03, 4, 280.1

⊛ **E0276** Bed pan, fracture, metal or plastic
IOM: 100-03, 4, 280.1

⊛ **E0277** Powered pressure-reducing air mattress
IOM: 100-03, 4, 280.1

✳ **E0280** Bed cradle, any type

⊛ **E0290** Hospital bed, fixed height, without side rails, with mattress
IOM: 100-02, 15, 110.1; 100-03, 4, 280.7

⊛ **E0291** Hospital bed, fixed height, without side rails, without mattress
IOM: 100-02, 15, 110.1; 100-03, 4, 280.7

⊛ **E0292** Hospital bed, variable height, hi-lo, without side rails, with mattress
IOM: 100-02, 15, 110.1; 100-03, 4, 280.7

⊛ **E0293** Hospital bed, variable height, hi-lo, without side rails, without mattress
IOM: 100-02, 15, 110.1; 100-03, 4, 280.7

⊛ **E0294** Hospital bed, semi-electric (head and foot adjustment), without side rails, with mattress
IOM: 100-02, 15, 110.1; 100-03, 4, 280.7

⊛ **E0295** Hospital bed, semi-electric (head and foot adjustment), without side rails, without mattress
IOM: 100-02, 15, 110.1; 100-03, 4, 280.7

⊛ **E0296** Hospital bed, total electric (head, foot and height adjustments). Without side rails, with mattress
IOM: 100-02, 15, 110.1; 100-03, 4, 280.7

⊛ **E0297** Hospital bed, total electric (head, foot and height adjustments), without side rails, without mattress
IOM: 100-02, 15, 110.1; 100-03, 4, 280.7

→ ✳ **E0300** Pediatric crib, hospital grade, fully enclosed, with or without top enclosure

⊛ **E0301** Hospital bed, heavy duty, extra wide, with weight capacity greater than 350 pounds, but less than or equal to 600 pounds, with any type side rails, without mattress
IOM: 100-03, 4, 280.7

⊛ **E0302** Hospital bed, extra heavy duty, extra wide, with weight capacity greater than 600 pounds, with any type side rails, without mattress
IOM: 100-03, 4, 280.7

⊛ **E0303** Hospital bed, heavy duty, extra wide, with weight capacity greater than 350 pounds, but less than or equal to 600 pounds, with any type side rails, with mattress
IOM: 100-03, 4, 280.7

▶ New → Revised ✔ Reinstated deleted Deleted
⊛ Special coverage instructions ◆ Not covered or valid by Medicare ✳ Carrier discretion

⊙ **E0304** Hospital bed, extra heavy duty, extra wide, with weight capacity greater than 600 pounds, with any type side rails, with mattress

IOM: 100-03, 4, 280.7

⊙ **E0305** Bed side rails, half length

IOM: 100-03, 4, 280.7

⊙ **E0310** Bed side rails, full length

IOM: 100-03, 4, 280.7

◆ **E0315** Bed accessory: board, table, or support device, any type

IOM: 100-03, 4, 280.1

✳ **E0316** Safety enclosure frame/canopy for use with hospital bed, any type

⊙ **E0325** Urinal; male, jug-type, any material

IOM: 100-03, 4, 280.1

⊙ **E0326** Urinal; female, jug-type, any material

IOM: 100-03, 4, 280.1

✳ **E0328** Hospital bed, pediatric, manual, 360 degree side enclosures, top of headboard, footboard and side rails up to 24 inches above the spring, includes mattress

✳ **E0329** Hospital bed, pediatric, electric or semi-electric, 360 degree side enclosures, top of headboard, footboard and side rails up to 24 inches above the spring, includes mattress

✳ **E0350** Control unit for electronic bowel irrigation/evacuation system

Pulsed Irrigation Enhanced Evacuation (PIEE) is pulsed irrigation of severely impacted fecal material and may be necessary for patients who have not responded to traditional bowel program.

✳ **E0352** Disposable pack (water reservoir bag, speculum, valving mechanism and collection bag/box) for use with the electronic bowel irrigation/evacuation system

Therapy kit includes 1 B-Valve circuit, 2 containment bags, 1 lubricating jelly, 1 bed pad, 1 tray liner-waste disposable bag, and 2 hose clamps

✳ **E0370** Air pressure elevator for heel

✳ **E0371** Non powered advanced pressure reducing overlay for mattress, standard mattress length and width

Patient has at least one large Stage III or Stage IV pressure sore (greater than 2 × 2 cm.) on trunk, with only two turning surfaces on which to lie

✳ **E0372** Powered air overlay for mattress, standard mattress length and width

✳ **E0373** Non powered advanced pressure reducing mattress

Oxygen and Related Respiratory Equipment

E0424-E0487: Bill DME/MAC

⊙ **E0424** Stationary compressed gaseous oxygen system, rental; includes container, contents, regulator, flowmeter, humidifier, nebulizer, cannula or mask, and tubing

IOM: 100-03, 4, 280.1; 100-04, 20, 30.6

⊙ **E0425** Stationary compressed gas system, purchase; includes regulator, flowmeter, humidifier, nebulizer, cannula or mask, and tubing

IOM: 100-03, 4, 280.1; 100-04, 20, 30.6

⊙ **E0430** Portable gaseous oxygen system, purchase; includes regulator, flowmeter, humidifier, cannula or mask, and tubing

IOM: 100-03, 4, 280.1; 100-04, 20, 30.6

⊙ **E0431** Portable gaseous oxygen system, rental; includes portable container, regulator, flowmeter, humidifier, cannula or mask, and tubing

IOM: 100-03, 4, 280.1; 100-04, 20, 30.6

✳ **E0433** Portable liquid oxygen system, rental; home liquefier used to fill portable liquid oxygen containers, includes portable containers, regulator, flowmeter, humidifier, cannula or mask and tubing, with or without supply reservoir and contents gauge

⊙ **E0434** Portable liquid oxygen system, rental; includes portable container, supply reservoir, humidifier, flowmeter, refill adaptor, contents gauge, cannula or mask, and tubing

Fee schedule payments for stationary oxygen system rentals are all-inclusive and represent monthly allowance for beneficiary. Non-Medicare payers may rent device to beneficiaries, or arrange for purchase of device

IOM: 100-03, 4, 280.1; 100-04, 20, 30.6

▶ **New**   → **Revised**   ✔ **Reinstated**   ~~deleted~~ **Deleted**

⊙ **Special coverage instructions**   ◆ **Not covered or valid by Medicare**   ✳ **Carrier discretion**

⚙ **E0435** Portable liquid oxygen system, purchase; includes portable container, supply reservoir, flowmeter, humidifier, contents gauge, cannula or mask, tubing and refill adaptor

IOM: 100-03, 4, 280.1; 100-04, 20, 30.6

⚙ **E0439** Stationary liquid oxygen system, rental; includes container, contents, regulator, flowmeter, humidifier, nebulizer, cannula or mask, & tubing

This allowance includes payment for equipment, contents, and accessories furnished during rental month

IOM: 100-03, 4, 280.1; 100-04, 20, 30.6

⚙ **E0440** Stationary liquid oxygen system, purchase; includes use of reservoir, contents indicator, regulator, flowmeter, humidifier, nebulizer, cannula or mask, and tubing

IOM: 100-03, 4, 280.1; 100-04, 20, 30.6

✳ **E0441** Stationary oxygen contents, gaseous, 1 month's supply = 1 unit

IOM: 100-03, 4, 280.1; 100-04, 20, 30.6

✳ **E0442** Stationary oxygen contents, liquid, 1 month's supply = 1 unit

IOM: 100-03, 4, 280.1; 100-04, 20, 30.6

✳ **E0443** Portable oxygen contents, gaseous, 1 month's supply = 1 unit

IOM: 100-03, 4, 280.1; 100-04, 20, 30.6

✳ **E0444** Portable oxygen contents, liquid, 1 month's supply = 1 unit

IOM: 100-03, 4, 280.1; 100-04, 20, 30.6

✳ **E0445** Oximeter device for measuring blood oxygen levels non-invasively

◆ **E0446** Topical oxygen delivery system, not otherwise specified, includes all supplies and accessories

⚙ **E0450** Volume control ventilator, without pressure support mode, may include pressure control mode, used with invasive interface (e.g., tracheostomy tube)

Patient confined to wheelchair during day may receive reimbursement for 2 ventilators. One ventilator is mounted to wheelchair and second used while in bed

IOM: 100-03, 4, 280.1

⚙ **E0455** Oxygen tent, excluding croup or pediatric tents

IOM: 100-03, 4, 280.1; 100-04, 20, 30.6

✳ **E0457** Chest shell (cuirass)

✳ **E0459** Chest wrap

⚙ **E0460** Negative pressure ventilator; portable or stationary

Noninvasive device, generates airflow into lungs by creating negative pressure around chest by means of interface

IOM: 100-03, 4, 240.2

⚙ **E0461** Volume control ventilator, without pressure support mode, may include pressure control mode, used with non-invasive interface (e.g. mask)

IOM: 100-03, 4, 240.2

✳ **E0462** Rocking bed with or without side rails

✳ **E0463** Pressure support ventilator with volume control mode, may include pressure control mode, used with invasive interface (e.g., tracheostomy tube)

✳ **E0464** Pressure support ventilator with volume control mode, may include pressure control mode, used with non-invasive interface (e.g., mask)

⚙ **E0470** Respiratory assist device, bi-level pressure capability, without backup rate feature, used with noninvasive interface, e.g., nasal or facial mask (intermittent assist device with continuous positive airway pressure device)

IOM: 100-03, 4, 240.2

⚙ **E0471** Respiratory assist device, bi-level pressure capability, with back-up rate feature, used with noninvasive interface, e.g., nasal or facial mask (intermittent assist device with continuous positive airway pressure device)

IOM: 100-03, 4, 240.2

⚙ **E0472** Respiratory assist device, bi-level pressure capability, with backup rate feature, used with invasive interface, e.g., tracheostomy tube (intermittent assist device with continuous positive airway pressure device)

IOM: 100-03, 4, 240.2

⚙ **E0480** Percussor, electric or pneumatic, home model

IOM: 100-03, 4, 240.2

◆ **E0481** Intrapulmonary percussive ventilation system and related accessories

IOM: 100-03, 4, 240.2

✳ **E0482** Cough stimulating device, alternating positive and negative airway pressure

---

▶ **New** → **Revised** ✔ **Reinstated** ~~deleted~~ **Deleted**

⚙ **Special coverage instructions** ◆ **Not covered or valid by Medicare** ✳ **Carrier discretion**

✳ **E0483** High frequency chest wall oscillation air-pulse generator system, (includes hoses and vest), each

✳ **E0484** Oscillatory positive expiratory pressure device, non-electric, any type, each

✳ **E0485** Oral device/appliance used to reduce upper airway collapsibility, adjustable or non-adjustable, prefabricated, includes fitting and adjustment

✳ **E0486** Oral device/appliance used to reduce upper airway collapsibility, adjustable or non-adjustable, custom fabricated, includes fitting and adjustment

☺ **E0487** Spirometer, electronic, includes all accessories

IPPB Machines

☺ **E0500** IPPB machine, all types, with built-in nebulization; manual or automatic valves; internal or external power source

Bill DME/MAC

IOM: 100-03, 4, 240.2

Humidifiers/Nebulizers/Compressors for Use with Oxygen IPPB Equipment

E0550-E0585: Bill DME/MAC

☺ **E0550** Humidifier, durable for extensive supplemental humidification during IPPB treatments or oxygen delivery

IOM: 100-03, 4, 240.2

☺ **E0555** Humidifier, durable, glass or autoclavable plastic bottle type, for use with regulator or flowmeter

IOM: 100-03, 4, 280.1; 100-04, 20, 30.6

☺ **E0560** Humidifier, durable for supplemental humidification during IPPB treatment or oxygen delivery

IOM: 100-03, 4, 280.1

✳ **E0561** Humidifier, non-heated, used with positive airway pressure device

✳ **E0562** Humidifier, heated, used with positive airway pressure device

✳ **E0565** Compressor, air power source for equipment which is not self-contained or cylinder driven

☺ **E0570** Nebulizer, with compressor

IOM: 100-03, 4, 240.2; 100-03, 4, 280.1

✳ **E0572** Aerosol compressor, adjustable pressure, light duty for intermittent use

✳ **E0574** Ultrasonic/electronic aerosol generator with small volume nebulizer

☺ **E0575** Nebulizer, ultrasonic, large volume

IOM: 100-03, 4, 240.2

☺ **E0580** Nebulizer, durable, glass or autoclavable plastic, bottle type, for use with regulator or flowmeter

IOM: 100-03, 4, 240.2; 100-03, 4, 280.1

☺ **E0585** Nebulizer, with compressor and heater

IOM: 100-03, 4, 240.2; 100-03, 4, 280.1

Suction Pump/Room Vaporizers

E0600-E0606: Bill DME/MAC

☺ **E0600** Respiratory suction pump, home model, portable or stationary, electric

IOM: 100-03, 4, 240.2

☺ **E0601** Continuous airway pressure (CPAP) device

IOM: 100-03, 4, 240.4

✳ **E0602** Breast pump, manual, any type

Bill either manual breast pump or breast pump kit

✳ **E0603** Breast pump, electric (AC and/or DC), any type

✳ **E0604** Breast pump, hospital grade, electric (AC and/or DC), any type

☺ **E0605** Vaporizer, room type

IOM: 100-03, 4, 240.2

☺ **E0606** Postural drainage board

IOM: 100-03, 4, 240.2

Monitoring Equipment

☺ **E0607** Home blood glucose monitor

Bill DME/MAC

Document recipient or caregiver is competent to monitor equipment and that device is designed for home rather than clinical use

IOM: 100-03, 4, 280.1; 100-03, 1, 40.2

▶ New   → Revised   ✔ Reinstated   -deleted- Deleted
☺ Special coverage instructions   ◆ Not covered or valid by Medicare   ✳ Carrier discretion

DURABLE MEDICAL EQUIPMENT
E0483 – E0607

Pacemaker Monitor

✪ **E0610** Pacemaker monitor, self-contained, (checks battery depletion, includes audible and visible check systems)

Bill DME/MAC

IOM: 100-03, 1, 20.8

✪ **E0615** Pacemaker monitor, self-contained, checks battery depletion and other pacemaker components, includes digital/visible check systems

Bill DME/MAC

IOM: 100-03, 1, 20.8

✳ **E0616** Implantable cardiac event recorder with memory, activator and programmer

Bill local carrier

Assign when two 30-day pre-symptom external loop recordings fail to establish a definitive diagnosis. Bill to local carrier.

✳ **E0617** External defibrillator with integrated electrocardiogram analysis

Bill DME/MAC

✳ **E0618** Apnea monitor, without recording feature

Bill DME/MAC

✳ **E0619** Apnea monitor, with recording feature

Bill DME/MAC

✳ **E0620** Skin piercing device for collection of capillary blood, laser, each

Bill DME/MAC

Patient Lifts

E0621-E0642: Bill DME/MAC

✪ **E0621** Sling or seat, patient lift, canvas or nylon

IOM: 100-03, 4, 240.2, 280.4

◆ **E0625** Patient lift, bathroom or toilet, not otherwise classified

IOM: 100-03, 4, 240.2

✪ **E0627** Seat lift mechanism incorporated into a combination lift-chair mechanism

IOM: 100-03, 4, 280.4; 100-04, 4, 20

Cross Reference Q0080

✪ **E0628** Separate seat lift mechanism for use with patient owned furniture - electric

IOM: 100-03, 4, 280.4; 100-04, 4, 20

Cross Reference Q0078

✪ **E0629** Separate seat lift mechanism for use with patient owned furniture - non-electric

IOM: 100-04, 4, 20

Cross Reference Q0079

✪ **E0630** Patient lift, hydraulic or mechanical, includes any seat, sling, strap(s) or pad(s)

IOM: 100-03, 4, 240.2

✪ **E0635** Patient lift, electric, with seat or sling

IOM: 100-03, 4, 240.2

✳ **E0636** Multipositional patient support system, with integrated lift, patient accessible controls

◆ **E0637** Combination sit to stand frame/table system, any size including pediatric, with seat lift feature, with or without wheels

IOM: 100-03, 4, 240.2

◆ **E0638** Standing frame/table system, one position (e.g. upright, supine or prone stander), any size including pediatric, with or without wheels

IOM: 100-03, 4, 240.2

✳ **E0639** Patient lift, moveable from room to room with disassembly and reassembly, includes all components/accessories

✳ **E0640** Patient lift, fixed system, includes all components/accessories

◆ **E0641** Standing frame/table system, multi-position (e.g. three-way stander), any size including pediatric, with or without wheels

IOM: 100-03, 4, 240.2

◆ **E0642** Standing frame/table system, mobile (dynamic stander), any size including pediatric

IOM: 100-03, 4, 240.2

Pneumatic Compressor and Appliances

E0650-E0676: Bill DME/MAC

✪ **E0650** Pneumatic compressor, non-segmental home model

Lymphedema pumps are classified as segmented or nonsegmented, depending on whether distinct segments of devices can be inflated sequentially

IOM: 100-03, 4, 280.6

▶ **New** → **Revised** ✔ **Reinstated** ~~deleted~~ **Deleted**

✪ **Special coverage instructions** ◆ **Not covered or valid by Medicare** ✳ **Carrier discretion**

⊘ **E0651** Pneumatic compressor, segmental home model without calibrated gradient pressure

IOM: 100-03, 4, 280.6

⊘ **E0652** Pneumatic compressor, segmental home model with calibrated gradient pressure

IOM: 100-03, 4, 280.6

⊘ **E0655** Non-segmental pneumatic appliance for use with pneumatic compressor, half arm

IOM: 100-03, 4, 280.6

⊘ **E0656** Segmental pneumatic appliance for use with pneumatic compressor, trunk

⊘ **E0657** Segmental pneumatic appliance for use with pneumatic compressor, chest

⊘ **E0660** Non-segmental pneumatic appliance for use with pneumatic compressor, full leg

IOM: 100-03, 4, 280.6

⊘ **E0665** Non-segmental pneumatic appliance for use with pneumatic compressor, full arm

IOM: 100-03, 4, 280.6

⊘ **E0666** Non-segmental pneumatic appliance for use with pneumatic compressor, half leg

IOM: 100-03, 4, 280.6

⊘ **E0667** Segmental pneumatic appliance for use with pneumatic compressor, full leg

IOM: 100-03, 4, 280.6

⊘ **E0668** Segmental pneumatic appliance for use with pneumatic compressor, full arm

IOM: 100-03, 4, 280.6

⊘ **E0669** Segmental pneumatic appliance for use with pneumatic compressor, half leg

IOM: 100-03, 4, 280.6

▶ ⊘ **E0670** Segmental pneumatic appliance for use with pneumatic compressor, integrated, 2 full legs and trunk

IOM 100-03, 4, 280.6

⊘ **E0671** Segmental gradient pressure pneumatic appliance, full leg

IOM: 100-03, 4, 280.6

⊘ **E0672** Segmental gradient pressure pneumatic appliance, full arm

IOM: 100-03, 4, 280.6

⊘ **E0673** Segmental gradient pressure pneumatic appliance, half leg

IOM: 100-03, 4, 280.6

✳ **E0675** Pneumatic compression device, high pressure, rapid inflation/deflation cycle, for arterial insufficiency (unilateral or bilateral system)

✳ **E0676** Intermittent limb compression device (includes all accessories), not otherwise specified

Ultraviolet Cabinet

E0691-E0694: Bill DME/MAC

✳ **E0691** Ultraviolet light therapy system, includes bulbs/lamps, timer and eye protection; treatment area 2 square feet or less

✳ **E0692** Ultraviolet light therapy system panel, includes bulbs/lamps, timer and eye protection, 4 foot panel

✳ **E0693** Ultraviolet light therapy system panel, includes bulbs/lamps, timer and eye protection, 6 foot panel

✳ **E0694** Ultraviolet multidirectional light therapy system in 6 foot cabinet, includes bulbs/lamps, timer and eye protection

Safety Equipment

E0700-E0705: Bill DME/MAC

✳ **E0700** Safety equipment, device or accessory, any type

⊘ **E0705** Transfer device, any type, each

Restraints

✳ **E0710** Restraints, any type (body, chest, wrist or ankle)

Bill DME/MAC

Transcutaneous and/or Neuromuscular Electrical Nerve Stimulators (TENS)

⊘ **E0720** Transcutaneous electrical nerve stimulation (TENS) device, two lead, localized stimulation

Bill DME/MAC

A Certificate of Medical Necessity (CMN) is not needed for a TENS rental, but is needed purchase.

IOM: 100-03, 2, 160.2; 100-03, 4, 280.1

▶ **New**   → **Revised**   ✔ **Reinstated**   ~~deleted~~ **Deleted**

⊘ **Special coverage instructions**   ◆ **Not covered or valid by Medicare**   ✳ **Carrier discretion**

⊕ **E0730** Transcutaneous electrical nerve stimulation (TENS) device, four or more leads, for multiple nerve stimulation

Bill DME/MAC

IOM: 100-03, 2, 160.2; 100-03, 4, 280.1

⊕ **E0731** Form fitting conductive garment for delivery of TENS or NMES (with conductive fibers separated from the patient's skin by layers of fabric)

Bill DME/MAC

IOM: 100-03, 2, 160.13

⊕ **E0740** Incontinence treatment system, pelvic floor stimulator, monitor, sensor and/or trainer

Bill DME/MAC

IOM: 100-03, 4, 230.8

✳ **E0744** Neuromuscular stimulator for scoliosis

Bill DME/MAC

⊕ **E0745** Neuromuscular stimulator, electronic shock unit

Bill DME/MAC

IOM: 100-03, 2, 160.12

⊕ **E0746** Electromyography (EMG), biofeedback device

Bill local carrier

IOM: 100-03, 1, 30.1

⊕ **E0747** Osteogenesis stimulator, electrical, non-invasive, other than spinal applications

Bill DME/MAC

Devices are composed of two basic parts: Coils that wrap around cast and pulse generator that produces electric current

⊕ **E0748** Osteogenesis stimulator, electrical, non-invasive, spinal applications

Bill DME/MAC

Device should be applied within 30 days as adjunct to spinal fusion surgery

⊕ **E0749** Osteogenesis stimulator, electrical, surgically implanted

Bill local carrier

✳ **E0755** Electronic salivary reflex stimulator (intra-oral/non-invasive)

Bill DME/MAC

✳ **E0760** Osteogenesis stimulator, low intensity ultrasound, non-invasive

Bill DME/MAC

Ultrasonic osteogenesis stimulator may not be used concurrently with other noninvasive stimulators

⊕ **E0761** Non-thermal pulsed high frequency radiowaves, high peak power electromagnetic energy treatment device

Bill DME/MAC

✳ **E0762** Transcutaneous electrical joint stimulation device system, includes all accessories

Bill DME/MAC

⊕ **E0764** Functional neuromuscular stimulator, transcutaneous stimulation of sequential muscle groups of ambulation with computer control, used for walking by spinal cord injured, entire system, after completion of training program

Bill DME/MAC

IOM: 100-03, 2, 160.12

✳ **E0765** FDA approved nerve stimulator, with replaceable batteries, for treatment of nausea and vomiting

Bill DME/MAC

⊕ **E0769** Electrical stimulation or electromagnetic wound treatment device, not otherwise classified

Bill DME/MAC

IOM: 100-04, 32, 11.1

⊕ **E0770** Functional electrical stimulator, transcutaneous stimulation of nerve and/or muscle groups, any type, complete system, not otherwise specified

Bill DME/MAC

▶ **New**   → **Revised**   ✔ **Reinstated**   ~~deleted~~ **Deleted**

⊕ **Special coverage instructions**   ◆ **Not covered or valid by Medicare**   ✳ **Carrier discretion**

Infusion Supplies

* **E0776**   IV pole

    Bill DME/MAC

* **E0779**   Ambulatory infusion pump, mechanical, reusable, for infusion 8 hours or greater

    Bill DME/MAC

    Requires prior authorization and copy of invoice

    This is a capped rental infusion pump modifier. The correct monthly modifier (-KH, -KI, -KJ) is used to indicate which month the rental is for (i.e. -KH, month 1; -KI, months 2 and 3; -KJ, months 4 through 13).

* **E0780**   Ambulatory infusion pump, mechanical, reusable, for infusion less than 8 hours

    Bill DME/MAC

    Requires prior authorization and copy of invoice

☺ **E0781**   Ambulatory infusion pump, single or multiple channels, electric or battery operated with administrative equipment, worn by patient

    Billable to both the local carrier and the DME/MAC. This item may be billed to the DME/MAC whenever the infusion is initiated in the physician's office but the patient does not return during the same business day.

    IOM: 100-03, 1, 50.3

☺ **E0782**   Infusion pump, implantable, non-programmable (includes all components, e.g., pump, cathether, connectors, etc.)

    Bill local carrier

    IOM: 100-03, 1, 50.3

☺ **E0783**   Infusion pump system, implantable, programmable (includes all components, e.g., pump, catheter, connectors, etc.)

    Bill local carrier

    IOM: 100-03, 1, 50.3

☺ **E0784**   External ambulatory infusion pump, insulin

    Bill DME/MAC

    IOM: 100-03, 4, 280.14

☺ **E0785**   Implantable intraspinal (epidural/intrathecal) catheter used with implantable infusion pump, replacement

    Bill local carrier

    IOM: 100-03, 1, 50.3

☺ **E0786**   Implantable programmable infusion pump, replacement (excludes implantable intraspinal catheter)

    Bill local carrier

    IOM: 100-03, 1, 50.3

☺ **E0791**   Parenteral infusion pump, stationary, single or multi-channel

    Bill DME/MAC

    IOM: 100-02, 15, 120; 100-03, 3, 180.2; 100-04, 20, 100.2.2

Traction Equipment: All Types and Cervical

E0830-E0856:   Bill DME/MAC

☺ **E0830**   Ambulatory traction device, all types, each

    IOM: 100-03, 4, 280.1

☺ **E0840**   Traction frame, attached to headboard, cervical traction

    IOM: 100-03, 4, 280.1

* **E0849**   Traction equipment, cervical, free-standing stand/frame, pneumatic, applying traction force to other than mandible

☺ **E0850**   Traction stand, free standing, cervical traction

    IOM: 100-03, 4, 280.1

* **E0855**   Cervical traction equipment not requiring additional stand or frame

* **E0856**   Cervical traction device, cervical collar with inflatable air bladder

Traction: Overdoor

☺ **E0860**   Traction equipment, overdoor, cervical

    Bill DME/MAC

    IOM: 100-03, 4, 280.1

Traction: Extremity

E0870-E0880:   Bill DME/MAC

☺ **E0870**   Traction frame, attached to footboard, extremity traction, (e.g., Buck's)

    IOM: 100-03, 4, 280.1

▶ New   → Revised   ✔ Reinstated   ~~deleted~~ Deleted

☺ Special coverage instructions   ◆ Not covered or valid by Medicare   * Carrier discretion

⊛ **E0880** Traction stand, free standing, extremity traction, (e.g., Buck's)

IOM: 100-03, 4, 280.1

Traction: Pelvic

E0890-E0900: Bill DME/MAC

⊛ **E0890** Traction frame, attached to footboard, pelvic traction

IOM: 100-03, 4, 280.1

⊛ **E0900** Traction stand, free standing, pelvic traction, (e.g., Buck's)

IOM: 100-03, 4, 280.1

Trapeze Equipment, Fracture Frame, and Other Orthopedic Devices

E0910-E0948: Bill DME/MAC

⊛ **E0910** Trapeze bars, A/K/A patient helper, attached to bed, with grab bar

IOM: 100-03, 4, 280.1

⊛ **E0911** Trapeze bar, heavy duty, for patient weight capacity greater than 250 pounds, attached to bed, with grab bar

IOM: 100-03, 4, 280.1

⊛ **E0912** Trapeze bar, heavy duty, for patient weight capacity greater than 250 pounds, free standing, complete with grab bar

IOM: 100-03, 4, 280.1

⊛ **E0920** Fracture frame, attached to bed, includes weights

IOM: 100-03, 4, 280.1

⊛ **E0930** Fracture frame, free standing, includes weights

IOM: 100-03, 4, 280.1

⊛ **E0935** Continuous passive motion exercise device for use on knee only

To qualify for coverage, use of device must commence within two days following surgery

IOM: 100-03, 4, 280.1

◆ **E0936** Continuous passive motion exercise device for use other than knee

⊛ **E0940** Trapeze bar, free standing, complete with grab bar

IOM: 100-03, 4, 280.1

⊛ **E0941** Gravity assisted traction device, any type

IOM: 100-03, 4, 280.1

✳ **E0942** Cervical head harness/halter

✳ **E0944** Pelvic belt/harness/boot

✳ **E0945** Extremity belt/harness

⊛ **E0946** Fracture, frame, dual with cross bars, attached to bed, (e.g. Balken, 4 poster)

IOM: 100-03, 4, 280.1

⊛ **E0947** Fracture frame, attachments for complex pelvic traction

IOM: 100-03, 4, 280.1

⊛ **E0948** Fracture frame, attachments for complex cervical traction

IOM: 100-03, 4, 280.1

Wheelchair Accessories

E0950-E1030: Bill DME/MAC

⊛ **E0950** Wheelchair accessory, tray, each

IOM: 100-03, 4, 280.1

✳ **E0951** Heel loop/holder, any type, with or without ankle strap, each

⊛ **E0952** Toe loop/holder, any type, each

IOM: 100-03, 4, 280.1

✳ **E0955** Wheelchair accessory, headrest, cushioned, any type, including fixed mounting hardware, each

✳ **E0956** Wheelchair accessory, lateral trunk or hip support, any type, including fixed mounting hardware, each

✳ **E0957** Wheelchair accessory, medial thigh support, any type, including fixed mounting hardware, each

⊛ **E0958** Manual wheelchair accessory, one-arm drive attachment, each

IOM: 100-03, 4, 280.1

✳ **E0959** Manual wheelchair accessory, adapter for amputee, each

IOM: 100-03, 4, 280.1

✳ **E0960** Wheelchair accessory, shoulder harness/straps or chest strap, including any type mounting hardware

✳ **E0961** Manual wheelchair accessory, wheel lock brake extension (handle), each

IOM: 100-03, 4, 280.1

▶ New	→ Revised	✔ Reinstated	~~deleted~~ Deleted
⊛ Special coverage instructions	◆ Not covered or valid by Medicare	✳ Carrier discretion	

✳ **E0966** Manual wheelchair accessory, headrest extension, each

IOM: 100-03, 4, 280.1

✪ **E0967** Manual wheelchair accessory, hand rim with projections, any type, each

IOM: 100-03, 4, 280.1

✪ **E0968** Commode seat, wheelchair

IOM: 100-03, 4, 280.1

✪ **E0969** Narrowing device, wheelchair

IOM: 100-03, 4, 280.1

◆ **E0970** No.2 footplates, except for elevating leg rest

IOM: 100-03, 4, 280.1

Cross Reference CPT K0037, K0042

✳ **E0971** Manual wheelchair accessory, anti-tipping device, each

IOM: 100-03, 4, 280.1

Cross Reference CPT K0021

✪ **E0973** Wheelchair accessory, adjustable height, detachable armrest, complete assembly, each

IOM: 100-03, 4, 280.1

✪ **E0974** Manual wheelchair accessory, anti-rollback device, each

IOM: 100-03, 4, 280.1

✳ **E0978** Wheelchair accessory, positioning belt/safety belt/pelvic strap, each

✳ **E0980** Safety vest, wheelchair

✳ **E0981** Wheelchair accessory, seat upholstery, replacement only, each

✳ **E0982** Wheelchair accessory, back upholstery, replacement only, each

✳ **E0983** Manual wheelchair accessory, power add-on to convert manual wheelchair to motorized wheelchair, joystick control

✳ **E0984** Manual wheelchair accessory, power add-on to convert manual wheelchair to motorized wheelchair, tiller control

✳ **E0985** Wheelchair accessory, seat lift mechanism

✳ **E0986** Manual wheelchair accessory, push activated power assist, each

✳ **E0988** Manual wheelchair accessory, lever-activated, wheel drive, pair

✳ **E0990** Wheelchair accessory, elevating leg rest, complete assembly, each

IOM: 100-03, 4, 280.1

✳ **E0992** Manual wheelchair accessory, solid seat insert

✪ **E0994** Arm rest, each

IOM: 100-03, 4, 280.1

✳ **E0995** Wheelchair accessory, calf rest/pad, each

IOM: 100-03, 4, 280.1

✳ **E1002** Wheelchair accessory, power seating system, tilt only

✳ **E1003** Wheelchair accessory, power seating system, recline only, without shear reduction

✳ **E1004** Wheelchair accessory, power seating system, recline only, with mechanical shear reduction

✳ **E1005** Wheelchair accessory, power seating system, recline only, with power shear reduction

✳ **E1006** Wheelchair accessory, power seating system, combination tilt and recline, without shear reduction

✳ **E1007** Wheelchair accessory, power seating system, combination tilt and recline, with mechanical shear reduction

✳ **E1008** Wheelchair accessory, power seating system, combination tilt and recline, with power shear reduction

✳ **E1009** Wheelchair accessory, addition to power seating system, mechanically linked leg elevation system, including pushrod and leg rest, each

✳ **E1010** Wheelchair accessory, addition to power seating system, power leg elevation system, including leg rest, pair

✪ **E1011** Modification to pediatric size wheelchair, width adjustment package (not to be dispensed with initial chair)

IOM: 100-03, 4, 280.1

✪ **E1014** Reclining back, addition to pediatric size wheelchair

IOM: 100-03, 4, 280.1

✪ **E1015** Shock absorber for manual wheelchair, each

IOM: 100-03, 4, 280.1

✪ **E1016** Shock absorber for power wheelchair, each

IOM: 100-03, 4, 280.1

✪ **E1017** Heavy duty shock absorber for heavy duty or extra heavy duty manual wheelchair, each

IOM: 100-03, 4, 280.1

▶ New   → Revised   ✔ Reinstated   ~~deleted~~ Deleted
✪ Special coverage instructions   ◆ Not covered or valid by Medicare   ✳ Carrier discretion

⚙ **E1018** Heavy duty shock absorber for heavy duty or extra heavy duty power wheelchair, each

IOM: 100-03, 4, 280.1

➜ ⚙ **E1020** Residual limb support system for wheelchair, any type

IOM: 100-03, 3, 280.3

✳ **E1028** Wheelchair accessory, manual swingaway, retractable or removable mounting hardware for joystick, other control interface or positioning accessory

✳ **E1029** Wheelchair accessory, ventilator tray, fixed

✳ **E1030** Wheelchair accessory, ventilator tray, gimbaled

Rollabout Chair and Transfer System

E1031-E1039: Bill DME/MAC

⚙ **E1031** Rollabout chair, any and all types with castors 5" or greater

IOM: 100-03, 4, 280.1

✳ **E1035** Multi-positional patient transfer system, with integrated seat, operated by care giver, patient weight capacity up to and including 300 lbs

IOM: 100-02, 15, 110

✳ **E1036** Multi-positional patient transfer system, extra-wide, with integrated seat, operated by caregiver, patient weight capacity greater than 300 lbs

⚙ **E1037** Transport chair, pediatric size

IOM: 100-03, 4, 280.1

⚙ **E1038** Transport chair, adult size, patient weight capacity up to and including 300 pounds

IOM: 100-03, 4, 280.1

✳ **E1039** Transport chair, adult size, heavy duty, patient weight capacity greater than 300 pounds

Wheelchair: Fully Reclining

E1050-E1093: Bill DME/MAC

⚙ **E1050** Fully-reclining wheelchair, fixed full length arms, swing away detachable elevating leg rests

IOM: 100-03, 4, 280.1

⚙ **E1060** Fully-reclining wheelchair, detachable arms, desk or full length, swing away detachable elevating legrests

IOM: 100-03, 4, 280.1

⚙ **E1070** Fully-reclining wheelchair, detachable arms (desk or full length) swing away detachable footrests

IOM: 100-03, 4, 280.1

⚙ **E1083** Hemi-wheelchair, fixed full length arms, swing away detachable elevating leg rest

IOM: 100-03, 4, 280.1

⚙ **E1084** Hemi-wheelchair, detachable arms desk or full length arms, swing away detachable elevating leg rests

IOM: 100-03, 4, 280.1

◆ **E1085** Hemi-wheelchair, fixed full length arms, swing away detachable foot rests

IOM: 100-03, 4, 280.1

Cross Reference CPT K0002

◆ **E1086** Hemi-wheelchair, detachable arms desk or full length, swing away detachable footrests

IOM: 100-03, 4, 280.1

Cross Reference CPT K0002

⚙ **E1087** High strength lightweight wheelchair, fixed full length arms, swing away detachable elevating leg rests

IOM: 100-03, 4, 280.1

⚙ **E1088** High strength lightweight wheelchair, detachable arms desk or full length, swing away detachable elevating leg rests

IOM: 100-03, 4, 280.1

◆ **E1089** High strength lightweight wheelchair, fixed length arms, swing away detachable footrest

IOM: 100-03, 4, 280.1

Cross Reference CPT K0004

◆ **E1090** High strength lightweight wheelchair, detachable arms desk or full length, swing away detachable foot rests

IOM: 100-03, 4, 280.1

Cross Reference CPT K0004

⚙ **E1092** Wide heavy duty wheelchair, detachable arms (desk or full length) swing away detachable elevating leg rests

IOM: 100-03, 4, 280.1

▶ **New**   ➜ **Revised**   ✔ **Reinstated**   ~~deleted~~ **Deleted**
⚙ **Special coverage instructions**   ◆ **Not covered or valid by Medicare**   ✳ **Carrier discretion**

⊛ **E1093** Wide heavy duty wheelchair, detachable arms (desk or full length arms), swing away detachable foot rests

IOM: 100-03, 4, 280.1

Wheelchair: Semi-reclining

E1100-E1110: Bill DME/MAC

⊛ **E1100** Semi-reclining wheelchair, fixed full length arms, swing away detachable elevating leg rests

IOM: 100-03, 4, 280.1

⊛ **E1110** Semi-reclining wheelchair, detachable arms (desk or full length), elevating leg rest

IOM: 100-03, 4, 280.1

Wheelchair: Standard

E1130-E1161: Bill DME/MAC

◆ **E1130** Standard wheelchair, fixed full length arms, fixed or swing away detachable footrests

IOM: 100-03, 4, 280.1

Cross Reference CPT K0001

◆ **E1140** Wheelchair, detachable arms, desk or full length, swing away detachable footrests

IOM: 100-03, 4, 280.1

Cross Reference CPT K0001

⊛ **E1150** Wheelchair, detachable arms, desk or full length, swing away detachable elevating legrests

IOM: 100-03, 4, 280.1

⊛ **E1160** Wheelchair, fixed full length arms, swing away detachable elevating legrests

IOM: 100-03, 4, 280.1

✳ **E1161** Manual adult size wheelchair, includes tilt in space

Wheelchair: Amputee

E1170-E1200: Bill DME/MAC

⊛ **E1170** Amputee wheelchair, fixed full length arms, swing away detachable elevating legrests

IOM: 100-03, 4, 280.1

⊛ **E1171** Amputee wheelchair, fixed full length arms, without footrests or legrest

IOM: 100-03, 4, 280.1

⊛ **E1172** Amputee wheelchair, detachable arms (desk or full length) without footrests or legrest

IOM: 100-03, 4, 280.1

⊛ **E1180** Amputee wheelchair, detachable arms (desk or full length) swing away detachable footrests

IOM: 100-03, 4, 280.1

⊛ **E1190** Amputee wheelchair, detachable arms (desk or full length), swing away detachable elevating legrests

IOM: 100-03, 4, 280.1

⊛ **E1195** Heavy duty wheelchair, fixed full length arms, swing away detachable elevating legrests

IOM: 100-03, 4, 280.1

⊛ **E1200** Amputee wheelchair, fixed full length arms, swing away detachable footrest

IOM: 100-03, 4, 280.1

Wheelchair: Special Size

E1220-E1239: Bill DME/MAC

⊛ **E1220** Wheelchair; specially sized or constructed, (indicate brand name, model number, if any) and justification

IOM: 100-03, 4, 280.3

⊛ **E1221** Wheelchair with fixed arm, footrests

IOM: 100-03, 4, 280.3

⊛ **E1222** Wheelchair with fixed arm, elevating legrests

IOM: 100-03, 4, 280.3

⊛ **E1223** Wheelchair with detachable arms, footrests

IOM: 100-03, 4, 280.3

⊛ **E1224** Wheelchair with detachable arms, elevating legrests

IOM: 100-03, 4, 280.3

⊛ **E1225** Wheelchair accessory, manual semi-reclining back, (recline greater than 15 degrees, but less than 80 degrees), each

IOM: 100-03, 4, 280.3

⊛ **E1226** Wheelchair accessory, manual fully reclining back, (recline greater than 80 degrees), each

IOM: 100-03, 4, 280.1

⊛ **E1227** Special height arms for wheelchair

IOM: 100-03, 4, 280.3

⊛ **E1228** Special back height for wheelchair

IOM: 100-03, 4, 280.3

▶ New → Revised ✔ Reinstated ~~deleted~~ Deleted

⊛ Special coverage instructions ◆ Not covered or valid by Medicare ✳ Carrier discretion

✳ **E1229** Wheelchair, pediatric size, not otherwise specified

✪ **E1230** Power operated vehicle (three or four wheel non-highway), specify brand name and model number

Patient is unable to operate manual wheelchair; patient capable of safely operating controls for scooter; patient can transfer safely in and out of scooter

IOM: 100-08, 5, 5.2.3

✪ **E1231** Wheelchair, pediatric size, tilt-in-space, rigid, adjustable, with seating system

IOM: 100-03, 4, 280.1

✪ **E1232** Wheelchair, pediatric size, tilt-in-space, folding, adjustable, with seating system

IOM: 100-03, 4, 280.1

✪ **E1233** Wheelchair, pediatric size, tilt-in-space, rigid, adjustable, without seating system

IOM: 100-03, 4, 280.1

✪ **E1234** Wheelchair, pediatric size, tilt-in-space, folding, adjustable, without seating system

IOM: 100-03, 4, 280.1

✪ **E1235** Wheelchair, pediatric size, rigid, adjustable, with seating system

IOM: 100-03, 4, 280.1

✪ **E1236** Wheelchair, pediatric size, folding, adjustable, with seating system

IOM: 100-03, 4, 280.1

✪ **E1237** Wheelchair, pediatric size, rigid, adjustable, without seating system

IOM: 100-03, 4, 280.1

✪ **E1238** Wheelchair, pediatric size, folding, adjustable, without seating system

IOM: 100-03, 4, 280.1

✳ **E1239** Power wheelchair, pediatric size, not otherwise specified

Wheelchair: Lightweight

E1240-E1270: Bill DME/MAC

✪ **E1240** Lightweight wheelchair, detachable arms, (desk or full length) swing away detachable, elevating leg rests

IOM: 100-03, 4, 280.1

◆ **E1250** Lightweight wheelchair, fixed full length arms, swing away detachable footrest

IOM: 100-03, 4, 280.1

Cross Reference CPT K0003

◆ **E1260** Lightweight wheelchair, detachable arms (desk or full length) swing away detachable footrest

IOM: 100-03, 4, 280.1

Cross Reference CPT K0003

✪ **E1270** Lightweight wheelchair, fixed full length arms, swing away detachable elevating legrests

IOM: 100-03, 4, 280.1

Wheelchair: Heavy Duty

E1280-E1298: Bill DME/MAC

✪ **E1280** Heavy duty wheelchair, detachable arms (desk or full length), elevating legrests

IOM: 100-03, 4, 280.1

◆ **E1285** Heavy duty wheelchair, fixed full length arms, swing away detachable footrest

IOM: 100-03, 4, 280.1

Cross Reference CPT K0006

◆ **E1290** Heavy duty wheelchair, detachable arms (desk or full length) swing away detachable footrest

IOM: 100-03, 4, 280.1

Cross Reference CPT K0006

✪ **E1295** Heavy duty wheelchair, fixed full length arms, elevating legrest

IOM: 100-03, 4, 280.1

✪ **E1296** Special wheelchair seat height from floor

IOM: 100-03, 4, 280.3

✪ **E1297** Special wheelchair seat depth, by upholstery

IOM: 100-03, 4, 280.3

✪ **E1298** Special wheelchair seat depth and/or width, by construction

IOM: 100-03, 4, 280.3

Whirlpool Equipment

E1300-E1310: Bill DME/MAC

◆ **E1300** Whirlpool, portable (overtub type)

IOM: 100-03, 4, 280.1

✪ **E1310** Whirlpool, non-portable (built-in type)

IOM: 100-03, 4, 280.1

▶ **New** → **Revised** ✔ **Reinstated** ~~deleted~~ **Deleted**

✪ **Special coverage instructions** ◆ **Not covered or valid by Medicare** ✳ **Carrier discretion**

Additional Oxygen Related Equipment

⚙ **E1353** Regulator

Bill DME/MAC

IOM: 100-03, 4, 240.2

✳ **E1354** Oxygen accessory, wheeled cart for portable cylinder or portable concentrator, any type, replacement only, each

Bill DME/MAC

⚙ **E1355** Stand/rack

Bill DME/MAC

IOM: 100-03, 4, 240.2

✳ **E1356** Oxygen accessory, battery pack/ cartridge for portable concentrator, any type, replacement only, each

Bill DME/MAC

✳ **E1357** Oxygen accessory, battery charger for portable concentrator, any type, replacement only, each

Bill DME/MAC

◆ **E1358** Oxygen accessory, DC power adapter for portable concentrator, any type, replacement only, each

Bill DME/MAC

⚙ **E1372** Immersion external heater for nebulizer

Bill DME/MAC

IOM: 100-03, 4, 240.2

⚙ **E1390** Oxygen concentrator, single delivery port, capable of delivering 85 percent or greater oxygen concentration at the prescribed flow rate

Bill DME/MAC

IOM: 100-03, 4, 240.2

⚙ **E1391** Oxygen concentrator, dual delivery port, capable of delivering 85 percent or greater oxygen concentration at the prescribed flow rate, each

Bill DME/MAC

IOM: 100-03, 4, 240.2

⚙ **E1392** Portable oxygen concentrator, rental

Bill DME/MAC

IOM: 100-03, 4, 240.2

✳ **E1399** Durable medical equipment, miscellaneous

Local carrier if used with implanted DME. If other, bill DME/MAC.

Example: Therapeutic exercise putty; rubber exercise tubing; anti-vibration gloves

On DMEPOS fee schedule as a payable replacement for miscellaneous implanted or non-implanted items.

⚙ **E1405** Oxygen and water vapor enriching system with heated delivery

Bill DME/MAC

IOM: 100-03, 4, 240.2

⚙ **E1406** Oxygen and water vapor enriching system without heated delivery

Bill DME/MAC

IOM: 100-03, 4, 240.2

Artificial Kidney Machines and Accessories

E1500-E1699: Bill DME/MAC

⚙ **E1500** Centrifuge, for dialysis

⚙ **E1510** Kidney, dialysate delivery syst. kidney machine, pump recirculating, air removal syst. flowrate meter, power off, heater and temperature control with alarm, I.V. poles, pressure gauge, concentrate container

⚙ **E1520** Heparin infusion pump for hemodialysis

⚙ **E1530** Air bubble detector for hemodialysis, each, replacement

⚙ **E1540** Pressure alarm for hemodialysis, each, replacement

✳ **E1550** Bath conductivity meter for hemodialysis, each

⚙ **E1560** Blood leak detector for hemodialysis, each, replacement

⚙ **E1570** Adjustable chair, for ESRD patients

⚙ **E1575** Transducer protectors/fluid barriers for hemodialysis, any size, per 10

⚙ **E1580** Unipuncture control system for hemodialysis

⚙ **E1590** Hemodialysis machine

⚙ **E1592** Automatic intermittent peritoneal dialysis system

⚙ **E1594** Cycler dialysis machine for peritoneal dialysis

⚙ **E1600** Delivery and/or installation charges for hemodialysis equipment

---

▶ New → Revised ✔ Reinstated ~~deleted~~ Deleted

⚙ Special coverage instructions ◆ Not covered or valid by Medicare ✳ Carrier discretion

☺ **E1610** Reverse osmosis water purification system, for hemodialysis

IOM: 100-03, 4, 230.7

☺ **E1615** Deionizer water purification system, for hemodialysis

IOM: 100-03, 4, 230.7

☺ **E1620** Blood pump for hemodialysis replacement

☺ **E1625** Water softening system, for hemodialysis

IOM: 100-03, 4, 230.7

✳ **E1630** Reciprocating peritoneal dialysis system

☺ **E1632** Wearable artificial kidney, each

☺ **E1634** Peritoneal dialysis clamps, each

IOM: 100-04, 8, 60.4.2; 100-04, 8, 90.1; 100-04, 18, 80; 100-04, 18, 90

☺ **E1635** Compact (portable) travel hemodialyzer system

☺ **E1636** Sorbent cartridges, for hemodialysis, per 10

☺ **E1637** Hemostats, each

☺ **E1639** Scale, each

☺ **E1699** Dialysis equipment, not otherwise specified

Jaw Motion Rehabilitation System and Accessories

E1700-E1702: Bill DME/MAC

✳ **E1700** Jaw motion rehabilitation system

Must be prescribed by physician

✳ **E1701** Replacement cushions for jaw motion rehabilitation system, pkg. of 6

✳ **E1702** Replacement measuring scales for jaw motion rehabilitation system, pkg. of 200

Other Orthopedic Devices

E1800-E1841: Bill DME/MAC

✳ **E1800** Dynamic adjustable elbow extension/ flexion device, includes soft interface material

✳ **E1801** Static progressive stretch elbow device, extension and/or flexion, with or without range of motion adjustment, includes all components and accessories

✳ **E1802** Dynamic adjustable forearm pronation/ supination device, includes soft interface material

✳ **E1805** Dynamic adjustable wrist extension/ flexion device, includes soft interface material

✳ **E1806** Static progressive stretch wrist device, flexion and/or extension, with or without range of motion adjustment, includes all components and accessories

✳ **E1810** Dynamic adjustable knee extension/ flexion device, includes soft interface material

✳ **E1811** Static progressive stretch knee device, extension and/or flexion, with or without range of motion adjustment, includes all components and accessories

✳ **E1812** Dynamic knee, extension/flexion device with active resistance control

✳ **E1815** Dynamic adjustable ankle extension/ flexion device, includes soft interface material

✳ **E1816** Static progressive stretch ankle device, flexion and/or extension, with or without range of motion adjustment, includes all components and accessories

✳ **E1818** Static progressive stretch forearm pronation/supination device with or without range of motion adjustment, includes all components and accessories

✳ **E1820** Replacement soft interface material, dynamic adjustable extension/flexion device

✳ **E1821** Replacement soft interface material/ cuffs for bi-directional static progressive stretch device

✳ **E1825** Dynamic adjustable finger extension/ flexion device, includes soft interface material

✳ **E1830** Dynamic adjustable toe extension/ flexion device, includes soft interface material

✳ **E1831** Static progressive stretch toe device, extension and/or flexion, with or without range of motion adjustment, includes all components and accessories

✳ **E1840** Dynamic adjustable shoulder flexion/ abduction/rotation device, includes soft interface material

＊ **E1841**   Static progressive stretch shoulder device, with or without range of motion adjustment, includes all components and accessories

MISCELLANEOUS (E1902-E2120)

＊ **E1902**   Communication board, non-electronic augmentative or alternative communication device

＊ **E2000**   Gastric suction pump, home model, portable or stationary, electric

⊙ **E2100**   Blood glucose monitor with integrated voice synthesizer

    IOM: 100-03, 4, 230.16

⊙ **E2101**   Blood glucose monitor with integrated lancing/blood sample

    IOM: 100-03, 4, 230.16

＊ **E2120**   Pulse generator system for tympanic treatment of inner ear endolymphatic fluid

Wheelchair Assessories

E2201-E2397:   Bill DME/MAC

＊ **E2201**   Manual wheelchair accessory, nonstandard seat frame, width greater than or equal to 20 inches and less than 24 inches

＊ **E2202**   Manual wheelchair accessory, nonstandard seat frame width, 24-27 inches

＊ **E2203**   Manual wheelchair accessory, nonstandard seat frame depth, 20 to less than 22 inches

＊ **E2204**   Manual wheelchair accessory, nonstandard seat frame depth, 22 to 25 inches

＊ **E2205**   Manual wheelchair accessory, handrim without projections (includes ergonomic or contoured), any type, replacement only, each

＊ **E2206**   Manual wheelchair accessory, wheel lock assembly, complete, each

＊ **E2207**   Wheelchair accessory, crutch and cane holder, each

＊ **E2208**   Wheelchair accessory, cylinder tank carrier, each

＊ **E2209**   Accessory arm trough, with or without hand support, each

＊ **E2210**   Wheelchair accessory, bearings, any type, replacement only, each

＊ **E2211**   Manual wheelchair accessory, pneumatic propulsion tire, any size, each

＊ **E2212**   Manual wheelchair accessory, tube for pneumatic propulsion tire, any size, each

＊ **E2213**   Manual wheelchair accessory, insert for pneumatic propulsion tire (removable), any type, any size, each

＊ **E2214**   Manual wheelchair accessory, pneumatic caster tire, any size, each

＊ **E2215**   Manual wheelchair accessory, tube for pneumatic caster tire, any size, each

＊ **E2216**   Manual wheelchair accessory, foam filled propulsion tire, any size, each

＊ **E2217**   Manual wheelchair accessory, foam filled caster tire, any size, each

＊ **E2218**   Manual wheelchair accessory, foam propulsion tire, any size, each

＊ **E2219**   Manual wheelchair accessory, foam caster tire, any size, each

＊ **E2220**   Manual wheelchair accessory, solid (rubber/plastic) propulsion tire, any size, each

＊ **E2221**   Manual wheelchair accessory, solid (rubber/plastic) caster tire (removable), any size, each

＊ **E2222**   Manual wheelchair accessory, solid (rubber/plastic) caster tire with integrated wheel, any size, each

＊ **E2224**   Manual wheelchair accessory, propulsion wheel excludes tire, any size, each

＊ **E2225**   Manual wheelchair accessory, caster wheel excludes tire, any size, replacement only, each

＊ **E2226**   Manual wheelchair accessory, caster fork, any size, replacement only, each

＊ **E2227**   Manual wheelchair accessory, gear reduction drive wheel, each

＊ **E2228**   Manual wheelchair accessory, wheel braking system and lock, complete, each

◆ **E2230**   Manual wheelchair accessory, manual standing system

＊ **E2231**   Manual wheelchair accessory, solid seat support base (replaces sling seat), includes any type mounting hardware

＊ **E2291**   Back, planar, for pediatric size wheelchair including fixed attaching hardware

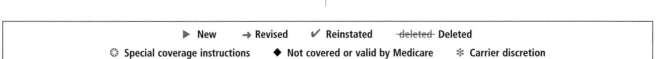

▶ **New**   → **Revised**   ✔ **Reinstated**   ~~deleted~~ **Deleted**

⊙ **Special coverage instructions**   ◆ **Not covered or valid by Medicare**   ＊ **Carrier discretion**

✳ **E2292** Seat, planar, for pediatric size wheelchair including fixed attaching hardware

✳ **E2293** Back, contoured, for pediatric size wheelchair including fixed attaching hardware

✳ **E2294** Seat, contoured, for pediatric size wheelchair including fixed attaching hardware

✳ **E2295** Manual wheelchair accessory, for pediatric size wheelchair, dynamic seating frame, allows coordinated movement of multiple positioning features

✳ **E2300** Power wheelchair accessory, power seat elevation system

✳ **E2301** Power wheelchair accessory, power standing system

✳ **E2310** Power wheelchair accessory, electronic connection between wheelchair controller and one power seating system motor, including all related electronics, indicator feature, mechanical function selection switch, and fixed mounting hardware

✳ **E2311** Power wheelchair accessory, electronic connection between wheelchair controller and two or more power seating system motors, including all related electronics, indicator feature, mechanical function selection switch, and fixed mounting hardware

✳ **E2312** Power wheelchair accessory, hand or chin control interface, mini-proportional remote joystick, proportional, including fixed mounting hardware

✳ **E2313** Power wheelchair accessory, harness for upgrade to expandable controller, including all fasteners, connectors and mounting hardware, each

✳ **E2321** Power wheelchair accessory, hand control interface, remote joystick, nonproportional, including all related electronics, mechanical stop switch, and fixed mounting hardware

✳ **E2322** Power wheelchair accessory, hand control interface, multiple mechanical switches, nonproportional, including all related electronics, mechanical stop switch, and fixed mounting hardware

✳ **E2323** Power wheelchair accessory, specialty joystick handle for hand control interface, prefabricated

✳ **E2324** Power wheelchair accessory, chin cup for chin control interface

✳ **E2325** Power wheelchair accessory, sip and puff interface, nonproportional, including all related electronics, mechanical stop switch, and manual swingaway mounting hardware

✳ **E2326** Power wheelchair accessory, breath tube kit for sip and puff interface

✳ **E2327** Power wheelchair accessory, head control interface, mechanical, proportional, including all related electronics, mechanical direction change switch, and fixed mounting hardware

✳ **E2328** Power wheelchair accessory, head control or extremity control interface, electronic, proportional, including all related electronics and fixed mounting hardware

✳ **E2329** Power wheelchair accessory, head control interface, contact switch mechanism, nonproportional, including all related electronics, mechanical stop switch, mechanical direction change switch, head array, and fixed mounting hardware

✳ **E2330** Power wheelchair accessory, head control interface, proximity switch mechanism, nonproportional, including all related electronics, mechanical stop switch, mechanical direction change switch, head array, and fixed mounting hardware

✳ **E2331** Power wheelchair accessory, attendant control, proportional, including all related electronics and fixed mounting hardware

✳ **E2340** Power wheelchair accessory, nonstandard seat frame width, 20-23 inches

✳ **E2341** Power wheelchair accessory, nonstandard seat frame width, 24-27 inches

✳ **E2342** Power wheelchair accessory, nonstandard seat frame depth, 20 or 21 inches

✳ **E2343** Power wheelchair accessory, nonstandard seat frame depth, 22-25 inches

✳ **E2351** Power wheelchair accessory, electronic interface to operate speech generating device using power wheelchair control interface

✳ **E2358** Power wheelchair accessory, Group 34 non-sealed lead acid battery, each

---

▶ New   → Revised   ✔ Reinstated   ~~deleted~~ Deleted
✪ Special coverage instructions   ◆ Not covered or valid by Medicare   ✳ Carrier discretion

* **E2359** Power wheelchair accessory, Group 34 sealed lead acid battery, each (e.g., gel cell, absorbed glassmat)

* **E2360** Power wheelchair accessory, 22 NF non-sealed lead acid battery, each

* **E2361** Power wheelchair accessory, 22NF sealed lead acid battery, each, (e.g. gel cell, absorbed glassmat)

* **E2362** Power wheelchair accessory, group 24 non-sealed lead acid battery, each

* **E2363** Power wheelchair accessory, group 24 sealed lead acid battery, each (e.g. gel cell, absorbed glassmat)

* **E2364** Power wheelchair accessory, U-1 non-sealed lead acid battery, each

* **E2365** Power wheelchair accessory, U-1 sealed lead acid battery, each (e.g. gel cell, absorbed glassmat)

* **E2366** Power wheelchair accessory, battery charger, single mode, for use with only one battery type, sealed or non-sealed, each

* **E2367** Power wheelchair accessory, battery charger, dual mode, for use with either battery type, sealed or non-sealed, each

→ * **E2368** Power wheelchair component, drive wheel motor, replacement only

→ * **E2369** Power wheelchair component, drive wheel gear box, replacement only

→ * **E2370** Power wheelchair component, integrated drive wheel motor and gear box combination, replacement only

* **E2371** Power wheelchair accessory, group 27 sealed lead acid battery, (e.g. gel cell, absorbed glass mat), each

* **E2372** Power wheelchair accessory, group 27 non-sealed lead acid battery, each

* **E2373** Power wheelchair accessory, hand or chin control interface, compact remote joystick, proportional, including fixed mounting hardware

⊙ **E2374** Power wheelchair accessory, hand or chin control interface, standard remote joystick (not including controller), proportional, including all related electronics and fixed mounting hardware, replacement only

⊙ **E2375** Power wheelchair accessory, non-expandable controller, including all related electronics and mounting hardware, replacement only

⊙ **E2376** Power wheelchair accessory, expandable controller, including all related electronics and mounting hardware, replacement only

⊙ **E2377** Power wheelchair accessory, expandable controller, including all related electronics and mounting hardware, upgrade provided at initial issue

▶ * **E2378** Power wheelchair component, actuator, replacement only

⊙ **E2381** Power wheelchair accessory, pneumatic drive wheel tire, any size, replacement only, each

⊙ **E2382** Power wheelchair accessory, tube for pneumatic drive wheel tire, any size, replacement only, each

⊙ **E2383** Power wheelchair accessory, insert for pneumatic drive wheel tire (removable), any type, any size, replacement only, each

⊙ **E2384** Power wheelchair accessory, pneumatic caster tire, any size, replacement only, each

⊙ **E2385** Power wheelchair accessory, tube for pneumatic caster tire, any size, replacement only, each

⊙ **E2386** Power wheelchair accessory, foam filled drive wheel tire, any size, replacement only, each

⊙ **E2387** Power wheelchair accessory, foam filled caster tire, any size, replacement only, each

⊙ **E2388** Power wheelchair accessory, foam drive wheel tire, any size, replacement only, each

⊙ **E2389** Power wheelchair accessory, foam caster tire, any size, replacement only, each

⊙ **E2390** Power wheelchair accessory, solid (rubber/plastic) drive wheel tire, any size, replacement only, each

⊙ **E2391** Power wheelchair accessory, solid (rubber/plastic) caster tire (removable), any size, replacement only, each

⊙ **E2392** Power wheelchair accessory, solid (rubber/plastic) caster tire with integrated wheel, any size, replacement only, each

⊙ **E2394** Power wheelchair accessory, drive wheel excludes tire, any size, replacement only, each

⊙ **E2395** Power wheelchair accessory, caster wheel excludes tire, any size, replacement only, each

---

▶ New   → Revised   ✔ Reinstated   ~~deleted~~ Deleted
⊙ Special coverage instructions   ◆ Not covered or valid by Medicare   * Carrier discretion

⊛ **E2396** Power wheelchair accessory, caster fork, any size, replacement only, each

✳ **E2397** Power wheelchair accessory, lithium-based battery, each

Negative Pressure

✳ **E2402** Negative pressure wound therapy electrical pump, stationary or portable

Bill DME/MAC

Document at least every 30 calendar days the quantitative wound characteristics, including wound surface area (length, width and depth)

Medicare coverage up to a maximum of 15 dressing kits (A6550) per wound per month unless documentation states that the wound size requires more than one dressing kit for each dressing change.

Speech Device

E2500-E2599: Bill DME/MAC

⊛ **E2500** Speech generating device, digitized speech, using pre-recorded messages, less than or equal to 8 minutes recording time

IOM: 100-03, 1, 50.1

⊛ **E2502** Speech generating device, digitized speech, using pre-recorded messages, greater than 8 minutes but less than or equal to 20 minutes recording time

IOM: 100-03, 1, 50.1

⊛ **E2504** Speech generating device, digitized speech, using pre-recorded messages, greater than 20 minutes but less than or equal to 40 minutes recording time

IOM: 100-03, 1, 50.1

⊛ **E2506** Speech generating device, digitized speech, using pre-recorded messages, greater than 40 minutes recording time

IOM: 100-03, 1, 50.1

⊛ **E2508** Speech generating device, synthesized speech, requiring message formulation by spelling and access by physical contact with the device

IOM: 100-03, 1, 50.1

⊛ **E2510** Speech generating device, synthesized speech, permitting multiple methods of message formulation and multiple methods of device access

IOM: 100-03, 1, 50.1

⊛ **E2511** Speech generating software program, for personal computer or personal digital assistant

IOM: 100-03, 1, 50.1

⊛ **E2512** Accessory for speech generating device, mounting system

IOM: 100-03, 1, 50.1

⊛ **E2599** Accessory for speech generating device, not otherwise classified

IOM: 100-03, 1, 50.1

Wheelchair, Cushion and Protection

E2601-E2621: Bill DME/MAC

✳ **E2601** General use wheelchair seat cushion, width less than 22 inches, any depth

✳ **E2602** General use wheelchair seat cushion, width 22 inches or greater, any depth

✳ **E2603** Skin protection wheelchair seat cushion, width less than 22 inches, any depth

✳ **E2604** Skin protection wheelchair seat cushion, width 22 inches or greater, any depth

✳ **E2605** Positioning wheelchair seat cushion, width less than 22 inches, any depth

✳ **E2606** Positioning wheelchair seat cushion, width 22 inches or greater, any depth

✳ **E2607** Skin protection and positioning wheelchair seat cushion, width less than 22 inches, any depth

✳ **E2608** Skin protection and positioning wheelchair seat cushion, width 22 inches or greater, any depth

✳ **E2609** Custom fabricated wheelchair seat cushion, any size

✳ **E2610** Wheelchair seat cushion, powered

✳ **E2611** General use wheelchair back cushion, width less than 22 inches, any height, including any type mounting hardware

✳ **E2612** General use wheelchair back cushion, width 22 inches or greater, any height, including any type mounting hardware

✳ **E2613** Positioning wheelchair back cushion, posterior, width less than 22 inches, any height, including any type mounting hardware

✳ **E2614** Positioning wheelchair back cushion, posterior, width 22 inches or greater, any height, including any type mounting hardware

---

▶ New → Revised ✔ Reinstated ~~deleted~~ Deleted

⊛ Special coverage instructions ◆ Not covered or valid by Medicare ✳ Carrier discretion

* **E2615**   Positioning wheelchair back cushion, posterior-lateral, width less than 22 inches, any height, including any type mounting hardware

* **E2616**   Positioning wheelchair back cushion, posterior-lateral, width 22 inches or greater, any height, including any type mounting hardware

* **E2617**   Custom fabricated wheelchair back cushion, any size, including any type mounting hardware

* **E2619**   Replacement cover for wheelchair seat cushion or back cushion, each

* **E2620**   Positioning wheelchair back cushion, planar back with lateral supports, width less than 22 inches, any height, including any type mounting hardware

* **E2621**   Positioning wheelchair back cushion, planar back with lateral supports, width 22 inches or greater, any height, including any type mounting hardware

SKIN PROTECTION, WHEELCHAIR (E2622-E2625)

* **E2622**   Skin protection wheelchair seat cushion, adjustable, width less than 22 inches, any depth

* **E2623**   Skin protection wheelchair seat cushion, adjustable, width 22 inches or greater, any depth

* **E2624**   Skin protection and positioning wheelchair seat cushion, adjustable, width less than 22 inches, any depth

* **E2625**   Skin protection and positioning wheelchair seat cushion, adjustable, width 22 inches or greater, any depth

ARM SUPPORT (E2626-E2633)

* **E2626**   Wheelchair accessory, shoulder elbow, mobile arm support attached to wheelchair, balanced, adjustable

* **E2627**   Wheelchair accessory, shoulder elbow, mobile arm support attached to wheelchair, balanced, adjustable rancho type

* **E2628**   Wheelchair accessory, shoulder elbow, mobile arm support attached to wheelchair, balanced, reclining

* **E2629**   Wheelchair accessory, shoulder elbow, mobile arm support attached to wheelchair, balanced, friction arm support (friction dampening to proximal and distal joints)

* **E2630**   Wheelchair accessory, shoulder elbow, mobile arm support, monosuspension arm and hand support, overhead elbow forearm hand sling support, yoke type suspension support

* **E2631**   Wheelchair accessory, addition to mobile arm support, elevating proximal arm

* **E2632**   Wheelchair accessory, addition to mobile arm support, offset or lateral rocker arm with elastic balance control

* **E2633**   Wheelchair accessory, addition to mobile arm support, supinator

Gait Trainer

E8000-E8002:   Bill DME/MAC

◆ **E8000**   Gait trainer, pediatric size, posterior support, includes all accessories and components

◆ **E8001**   Gait trainer, pediatric size, upright support, includes all accessories and components

◆ **E8002**   Gait trainer, pediatric size, anterior support, includes all accessories and components

---

▶ New   → Revised   ✔ Reinstated   ~~deleted~~ Deleted
☺ Special coverage instructions   ◆ Not covered or valid by Medicare   * Carrier discretion

TEMPORARY PROCEDURES/PROFESSIONAL SERVICES (G0000-G9999)

NOTE: This section contains national codes assigned by CMS on a temporary basis to identify procedures/professional services.

Administration, Vaccine

G0008-G0010:   Bill local carrier

✳ **G0008**   Administration of influenza virus vaccine

Coinsurance and deductible do not apply. If provided, report significant, separately identifiable E/M for medically necessary services (V04.81)

✳ **G0009**   Administration of pneumococcal vaccine

Reported once in a lifetime based on risk; Medicare covers cost of vaccine and administration (V03.82)

Copayment, coinsurance, and deductible waived. (https://www.cms.gov/MLNProducts/downloads/MPS_QuickReferenceChart_1.pdf)

✳ **G0010**   Administration of hepatitis B vaccine

Report for other than OPPs. Coinsurance and deductible apply; Medicare covers both cost of vaccine and administration (V05.3)

Copayment/coinsurance and deductible are waived. (https://www.cms.gov/MLNProducts/downloads/MPS_QuickReferenceChart_1.pdf)

Semen Analysis

✳ **G0027**   Semen analysis; presence and/or motility of sperm excluding Huhner

Bill local carrier

Laboratory Certification: Hematology

Screening, Cervical

☺ **G0101**   Cervical or vaginal cancer screening; pelvic and clinical breast examination

Bill local carrier

Covered once every two years and annually if high risk for cervical/vaginal cancer, or if childbearing age patient has had an abnormal Pap smear in preceding three years. High risk diagnosis, V15.89

Screening, Prostate

G0102-G0103:   Bill local carrier

☺ **G0102**   Prostate cancer screening; digital rectal examination

Covered annually by Medicare (V76.44). Not separately payable with an E/M code (99201-99499).

IOM: 100-02, 6, 10; 100-04, 4, 240

IOM: 100-04, 18, 50.1

☺ **G0103**   Prostate cancer screening; prostate specific antigen test (PSA)

Covered annually by Medicare (V76.44)

IOM: 100-02, 6, 10; 100-04, 4, 240

IOM: 100-04, 18, 50

Laboratory Certification: Routine chemistry

Screening, Colorectal

G0104-G0106:   Bill local carrier

☺ **G0104**   Colorectal cancer screening; flexible sigmoidoscopy

Covered once every 48 months for beneficiaries age 50+

Co-insurance waived under Section 4104.

☺ **G0105**   Colorectal cancer screening; colonoscopy on individual at high risk

Screening colonoscopy covered once every 24 months for high risk for developing colorectal cancer. May use modifier -53 if appropriate (physician fee schedule)

Co-insurance waived under Section 4104.

☺ **G0106**   Colorectal cancer screening; alternative to G0104, screening sigmoidoscopy, barium enema

Barium enema (not high risk) (alternative to G0104). Covered once every 4 years for beneficiaries age 50+. Use modifier -26 for professional component only.

▶ **New**   → **Revised**   ✔ **Reinstated**   ~~deleted~~ **Deleted**

☺ **Special coverage instructions**   ◆ **Not covered or valid by Medicare**   ✳ **Carrier discretion**

Training Services, Diabetes

G0108-G0109:   Bill local carrier

* ✳ **G0108**   Diabetes outpatient self-management training services, individual, per 30 minutes

    Report for beneficiaries diagnosed with diabetes

* ✳ **G0109**   Diabetes outpatient self-management training services, group session (2 or more) per 30 minutes

    Report for beneficiaries diagnosed with diabetes

Screening, Glaucoma

G0117-G0118:   Bill local carrier

* ✳ **G0117**   Glaucoma screening for high risk patients furnished by an optometrist or ophthalmologist

    Covered once per year (full 11 months between screenings). Bundled with all other ophthalmic services provided on same day. Diagnosis code V80.1

* ✳ **G0118**   Glaucoma screening for high risk patient furnished under the direct supervision of an optometrist or ophthalmologist

    Covered once per year (full 11 months between screenings). Diagnosis code V80.1

Screening, Colorectal, Other

G0120-G0122:   Bill local carrier

* ☼ **G0120**   Colorectal cancer screening; alternative to G0105, screening colonoscopy, barium enema

    Barium enema for patients with a high risk of developing colorectal. Covered once every 2 years. Used as an alternative to G0105. Use modifier 26 for professional component only

* ☼ **G0121**   Colorectal cancer screening; colonoscopy on individual not meeting criteria for high risk

    Screening colonoscopy for patients that are not high risk. Covered once every 10 years, but not within 48 months of a G0104. For non-Medicare patients report 45378.

    Co-insurance waived under Section 4104.

* ◆ **G0122**   Colorectal cancer screening; barium enema

    Medicare: this service is denied as noncovered, because it fails to meet the requirements of the benefit. The beneficiary is liable for payment.

Screening, Cytopathology

G0123-G0124:   Bill local carrier

* ☼ **G0123**   Screening cytopathology, cervical or vaginal (any reporting system), collected in preservative fluid, automated thin layer preparation, screening by cytotechnologist under physician supervision

    Use G0123 or G0143 or G0144 or G0145 or G0147 or G0148 or P3000 for Pap smears NOT requiring physician interpretation (technical component)

    IOM: 100-03, 3, 190.2; 100-04, 18, 30

    Laboratory Certification: Cytology

* ☼ **G0124**   Screening cytopathology, cervical or vaginal (any reporting system), collected in preservative fluid, automated thin layer preparation, requiring interpretation by physician

    Report professional component for Pap smears requiring physician interpretation

    IOM: 100-03, 3, 190.2; 100-04, 18, 30

    Laboratory Certification: Cytology

Trimming, Nail

* ☼ **G0127**   Trimming of dystrophic nails, any number

    Bill local carrier

    Must be used with a modifier (Q7, Q8, or Q9) to show that the foot care service is needed because the beneficiary has a systemic disease. Limit 1 unit of service

    IOM: 100-02, 15, 290

▶ New   → Revised   ✔ Reinstated   ~~deleted~~ Deleted
☼ Special coverage instructions   ◆ Not covered or valid by Medicare   ✳ Carrier discretion

Service, Nursing and OT

G0128-G0129: Bill local carrier

✿ **G0128** Direct (face-to-face with patient) skilled nursing services of a registered nurse provided in a comprehensive outpatient rehabilitation facility, each 10 minutes beyond the first 5 minutes

A separate nursing service that is clearly identifiable in the Plan of Treatment and not part of other services. Documentation must support this service. Examples include: Insertion of a urinary catheter, intramuscular injections, bowel disimpaction, nursing assessment, and education. Restricted coverage by Medicare.

Medicare Statute 1833(a)

✳ **G0129** Occupational therapy services requiring the skills of a qualified occupational therapist, furnished as a component of a partial hospitalization treatment program, per session (45 minutes or more)

Study, SEXA

✿ **G0130** Single energy x-ray absorptiometry (SEXA) bone density study, one or more sites; appendicular skeleton (peripheral) (eg, radius, wrist, heel)

Bill local carrier

Covered every 24 months (more frequently if medically necessary). Use modifier 26 for professional component only

Preventive service; no deductible

IOM: 100-03, 2, 150.3; 100-04, 13, 140.1

Screening, Cytopathology, Other

G0141-G0148: Bill local carrier

✳ **G0141** Screening cytopathology smears, cervical or vaginal, performed by automated system, with manual rescreening, requiring interpretation by physician

Co-insurance, copay, and deductible waived

Report professional component for Pap smears requiring physician interpretation. Refer to diagnosis of V15.89, V76.2, V76.47, or V76.49 to report appropriate risk level

Laboratory Certification: Cytology

✳ **G0143** Screening cytopathology, cervical or vaginal (any reporting system), collected in preservative fluid, automated thin layer preparation, with manual screening and rescreening by cytotechnologist under physician supervision

Co-insurance, copay, and deductible waived

Laboratory Certification: Cytology

✳ **G0144** Screening cytopathology, cervical or vaginal (any reporting system), collected in preservative fluid, automated thin layer preparation, with screening by automated system, under physician supervision

Co-insurance, copay, and deductible waived

Laboratory Certification: Cytology

✳ **G0145** Screening cytopathology, cervical or vaginal (any reporting system), collected in preservative fluid, automated thin layer preparation, with screening by automated system and manual rescreening under physician supervision

Co-insurance, copay, and deductible waived

Laboratory Certification: Cytology

✳ **G0147** Screening cytopathology smears, cervical or vaginal; performed by automated system under physician supervision

Co-insurance, copay, and deductible waived

Laboratory Certification: Cytology

✳ **G0148** Screening cytopathology smears, cervical or vaginal; performed by automated system with manual rescreening

Co-insurance, copay, and deductible waived

Laboratory Certification: Cytology

Services, Allied Health

G0151-G0166: Bill local carrier

✳ **G0151** Services performed by a qualified physical therapist in the home health or hospice setting, each 15 minutes

✳ **G0152** Services performed by a qualified occupational therapist in the home health or hospice setting, each 15 minutes

▶ New → Revised ✔ Reinstated deleted Deleted
✿ Special coverage instructions ◆ Not covered or valid by Medicare ✳ Carrier discretion

* **G0153** Services performed by a qualified speech-language pathologist in the home health or hospice setting, each 15 minutes

* **G0154** Direct skilled nursing services of a licensed nurse (LPN or RN) in the home health or hospice setting, each 15 minutes

* **G0155** Services of clinical social worker in home health or hospice settings, each 15 minutes

* **G0156** Services of home health/health aide in home health or hospice settings, each 15 minutes

* **G0157** Services performed by a qualified physical therapist assistant in the home health or hospice setting, each 15 minutes

* **G0158** Services performed by a qualified occupational therapist assistant in the home health or hospice setting, each 15 minutes

* **G0159** Services performed by a qualified physical therapist, in the home health setting, in the establishment or delivery of a safe and effective physical therapy maintenance program, each 15 minutes

* **G0160** Services performed by a qualified occupational therapist, in the home health setting, in the establishment or delivery of a safe and effective occupational therapy maintenance program, each 15 minutes

* **G0161** Services performed by a qualified speech-language pathologist, in the home health setting, in the establishment or delivery of a safe and effective speech-language pathology maintenance program, each 15 minutes

* **G0162** Skilled services by a registered nurse (RN) for management and evaluation of the plan of care; each 15 minutes (the patient's underlying condition or complication requires an RN to ensure that essential non-skilled care achieves its purpose in the home health or hospice setting)

   Transmittal No. 824 (CR7182)

* **G0163** Skilled services of a licensed nurse (LPN or RN) for the observation and assessment of the patient's condition, each 15 minutes (the of change in the patient's condition requires skilled nursing personnel to identify and evaluate the patient's need for possible modification of treatment in the home health or hospice setting)

   Transmittal No. 824 (CR7182)

* **G0164** Skilled services of a licensed nurse (LPN or RN), in the training and/or education of a patient or family member, in the home health or hospice setting, each 15 minutes

   Transmittal No. 824 (CR7182)

☼ **G0166** External counterpulsation, per treatment session

   IOM: 100-03, 1, 20.20

Wound Closure

* **G0168** Wound closure utilizing tissue adhesive(s) only

   Bill local carrier

   Report for wound closure with only tissue adhesive. If a practitioner utilizes tissue adhesive in addition to staples or sutures to close a wound, HCPCS code G0168 is not separately reportable, but is included in the tissue repair.

   The only closure material used for a simple repair, coverage based on payer.

Stereotactic Radiosurgery

☼ **G0173** Linear accelerator based stereotactic radiosurgery, complete course of therapy in one session

   Bill local carrier

   Do not bill with 77421

Team Conference

* **G0175** Scheduled interdisciplinary team conference (minimum of three exclusive of patient care nursing staff) with patient present

   Bill local carrier

▶ New   → Revised   ✔ Reinstated   deleted Deleted
☼ Special coverage instructions   ◆ Not covered or valid by Medicare   * Carrier discretion

Therapy, Activity

G0176-G0177:   Bill local carrier

OPPS not separately payable

⊛ **G0176**   Activity therapy, such as music, dance, art or play therapies not for recreation, related to the care and treatment of patient's disabling mental health problems, per session (45 minutes or more)

Paid in partial hospitalization

⊛ **G0177**   Training and educational services related to the care and treatment of patient's disabling mental health problems per session (45 minutes or more)

Paid in partial hospitalization

Physician Services

G0179-G0182:   Bill local carrier

✳ **G0179**   Physician re-certification for Medicare-covered home health services under a home health plan of care (patient not present), including contacts with home health agency and review of reports of patient status required by physicians to affirm the initial implementation of the plan of care that meets patient's needs, per re-certification period

The recertification code is used after a patient has received services for at least 60 days (or one certification period) when the physician signs the certification after the initial certification period.

✳ **G0180**   Physician certification for Medicare-covered home health services under a home health plan of care (patient not present), including contacts with home health agency and review of reports of patient status required by physicians to affirm the initial implementation of the plan of care that meets patient's needs, per certification period

This code can be billed only when the patient has not received Medicare covered home health services for at least 60 days.

✳ **G0181**   Physician supervision of a patient receiving Medicare-covered services provided by a participating home health agency (patient not present) requiring complex and multidisciplinary care modalities involving regular physician development and/or revision of care plans, review of subsequent reports of patient status, review of laboratory and other studies, communication (including telephone calls) with other health care professionals involved in the patient's care, integration of new information into the medical treatment plan and/or adjustment of medical therapy, within a calendar month, 30 minutes or more

✳ **G0182**   Physician supervision of a patient under a Medicare-approved hospice (patient not present) requiring complex and multidisciplinary care modalities involving regular physician development and/or revision of care plans, review of subsequent reports of patient status, review of laboratory and other studies, communication (including telephone calls) with other health care professionals involved in the patient's care, integration of new information into the medical treatment plan and/or adjustment of medical therapy, within a calendar month, 30 minutes or more

Destruction

✳ **G0186**   Destruction of localized lesion of choroid (for example, choroidal neovascularization); photocoagulation, feeder vessel technique (one or more sessions)

Bill local carrier

Mammography

G0202-G0206:   Bill local carrier

✳ **G0202**   Screening mammography, producing direct digital image, bilateral, all views

Screening mammogram reported based on technique, such as 76082, 76083, 76092, or G0202. Requires coinsurance, but no deductible. Diagnosis codes, V76.11 (high risk) or V76.12 (low risk). Use modifier 26 for professional component only

---

▶ New   → Revised   ✔ Reinstated   ̶d̶e̶l̶e̶t̶e̶d̶ Deleted

⊛ Special coverage instructions   ◆ Not covered or valid by Medicare   ✳ Carrier discretion

✳ **G0204**   Diagnostic mammography, producing direct digital image, bilateral, all views

Use modifier 26 for professional component only

✳ **G0206**   Diagnostic mammography, producing direct digital image, unilateral, all views

Use modifier 26 for professional component only

Imaging, PET

G0219-G0235:   Bill local carrier

◆ **G0219**   PET imaging whole body; melanoma for non-covered indications

Example: Assessing regional lymph nodes in melanoma. Medicare non-covered.

IOM: 100-03, 4, 220.6

◆ **G0235**   PET imaging, any site, not otherwise specified

Example: Prostate cancer diagnosis and initial staging. Medicare non-covered.

IOM: 100-03, 4, 220.6

Therapeutic Procedures

G0237-G0239:   Bill local carrier

✳ **G0237**   Therapeutic procedures to increase strength or endurance of respiratory muscles, face to face, one on one, each 15 minutes (includes monitoring)

✳ **G0238**   Therapeutic procedures to improve respiratory function, other than described by G0237, one on one, face to face, per 15 minutes (includes monitoring)

✳ **G0239**   Therapeutic procedures to improve respiratory function or increase strength or endurance of respiratory muscles, two or more individuals (includes monitoring)

Physician Service, Diabetic

G0245-G0246:   Bill local carrier

☺ **G0245**   Initial physician evaluation and management of a diabetic patient with diabetic sensory neuropathy resulting in a loss of protective sensation (LOPS) which must include (1) the diagnosis of LOPS, (2) a patient history, (3) a physical examination that consist of at least the following elements: (A) visual inspection of the forefoot, hindfoot and toe web spaces, (B) evaluation of a protective sensation, (C) evaluation of foot structure and biomechanics, (D) evaluation of vascular status and skin integrity, and (E) evaluation and recommendation of footwear, and (4) patient education

Report one of the following diagnosis codes in conjunction with this code: 250.60, 250.61, 250.62, 250.63, or 357.2

IOM: 100-03, 1, 70.2.1

☺ **G0246**   Follow-up physician evaluation and management of a diabetic patient with diabetic sensory neuropathy resulting in a loss of protective sensation (LOPS) to include at least the following: (1) a patient history, (2) a physical examination that includes: (A) visual inspection of the forefoot, hindfoot and toe web spaces, (B) evaluation of protective sensation, (C) evaluation of foot structure and biomechanics, (D) evaluation of vascular status and skin integrity, and (E) evaluation and recommendation of footwear, and (3) patient education

IOM: 100-03, 1, 70.2.1; 100-02, 15, 290

Foot Care

☺ **G0247**   Routine foot care by a physician of a diabetic patient with diabetic sensory neuropathy resulting in a loss of protective sensation (LOPS) to include, the local care of superficial wounds (i.e. superficial to muscle and fascia) and at least the following if present: (1) local care of superficial wounds, (2) debridement of corns and calluses, and (3) trimming and debridement of nails

Bill local carrier

IOM: 100-03, 1, 70.2.1

▶ New   → Revised   ✔ Reinstated   ~~deleted~~ Deleted

☺ Special coverage instructions   ◆ Not covered or valid by Medicare   ✳ Carrier discretion

Demonstration, INR

G0248-G0250:   Bill local carrier

⊛ **G0248**   Demonstration, prior to initiation, of home INR monitoring for patient with either mechanical heart valve(s), chronic atrial fibrillation, or venous thromboembolism who meets Medicare coverage criteria, under the direction of a physician; includes: face-to-face demonstration of use and care of the INR monitor, obtaining at least one blood sample, provision of instructions for reporting home INR test results, and documentation of patient's ability to perform testing and report results

⊛ **G0249**   Provision of test materials and equipment for home INR monitoring of patient with either mechanical heart valve(s), chronic atrial fibrillation, or venous thromboembolism who meets Medicare coverage criteria; includes provision of materials for use in the home and reporting of test results to physician; testing not occurring more frequently than once a week; testing materials, billing units of service include 4 tests

⊛ **G0250**   Physician review, interpretation, and patient management of home INR testing for patient with either mechanical heart valve(s), chronic atrial fibrillation, or venous thromboembolism who meets Medicare coverage criteria; testing not occurring more frequently than once a week; billing units of service include 4 tests

Stereotactic Radiosurgery

⊛ **G0251**   Linear accelerator based stereotactic radiosurgery, delivery including collimator changes and custom plugging, fractionated treatment, all lesions, per session, maximum five sessions per course of treatment

Bill local carrier

Cannot bill with 77421. The indicator is "0" and the edit cannot be bypassed with a modifier. (https://www.cms.gov/ NationalCorrectCodInitEd/NCCITrans/ list.asp)

Imaging, PET

◆ **G0252**   PET imaging, full and partial-ring PET scanners only, for initial diagnosis of breast cancer and/or surgical planning for breast cancer (e.g. initial staging of axillary lymph nodes)

Bill local carrier

IOM: 100-03, 4, 220.6

SNCT

◆ **G0255**   Current perception threshold/sensory nerve conduction test (SNCT), per limb, any nerve

Bill local carrier

IOM: 100-03, 2, 160.23

Dialysis, Emergency

⊛ **G0257**   Unscheduled or emergency dialysis treatment for an ESRD patient in a hospital outpatient department that is not certified as an ESRD facility

Bill local carrier

Injection, Arthrography

G0259-G0260:   Bill local carrier

⊛ **G0259**   Injection procedure for sacroiliac joint; arthrography

Replaces 27096 for reporting injections for Medicare beneficiaries

Used by Part A only (facility), not priced by Part B Medicare.

⊛ **G0260**   Injection procedure for sacroiliac joint; provision of anesthetic, steroid and/or other therapeutic agent, with or without arthrography

ASCs report when a therapeutic sacroiliac joint injection is administered in ASC

▶ New   → Revised   ✔ Reinstated   ~~deleted~~ Deleted
⊛ Special coverage instructions   ◆ Not covered or valid by Medicare   ✳ Carrier discretion

Removal, Cerumen

* **G0268** Removal of impacted cerumen (one or both ears) by physician on same date of service as audiologic function testing

  Bill local carrier

  Report only when a physician, not an audiologist, performs the procedure.

  Use with DX 380.4 when performed by physician.

Placement, Occlusive Device

☼ **G0269** Placement of occlusive device into either a venous or arterial access site, post surgical or interventional procedure (e.g. angioseal plug, vascular plug)

  Bill local carrier

  Report for replacement of vasoseal. Hospitals may report the closure device as a supply with C1760. Bundled status on Physician Fee Schedule.

Therapy, Nutrition

G0270-G0271: Bill local carrier

* **G0270** Medical nutrition therapy; reassessment and subsequent intervention(s) following second referral in same year for change in diagnosis, medical condition or treatment regimen (including additional hours needed for renal disease), individual, face to face with the patient, each 15 minutes

  Requires physician referral for beneficiaries with diabetes or renal disease. Services must be provided by dietitian/nutritionist. Co-insurance and deductible waived.

* **G0271** Medical nutrition therapy, reassessment and subsequent intervention(s) following second referral in same year for change in diagnosis, medical condition, or treatment regimen (including additional hours needed for renal disease), group (2 or more individuals), each 30 minutes

  Requires physician referral for beneficiaries with diabetes or renal disease. Services must be provided by dietitian/nutritionist. Co-insurance and deductible waived.

Angiography

G0275-G0278: Bill local carrier

* **G0275** Renal angiography, non-selective, one or both kidneys, performed at the same time as cardiac catheterization and/or coronary angiography, includes positioning or placement of any catheter in the abdominal aorta at or near the origins (OSTIA) of the renal arteries, injection of dye, flush aortogram, production of permanent images, and radiologic supervision and interpretation (list separately in addition to primary procedure)

  Routine "drive-by angiography" at time of cardiac catheterization performed in the absence of accepted clinical indications that support medical necessity will be denied by Medicare

* **G0278** Iliac and/or femoral artery angiography, non-selective, bilateral or ipsilateral to catheter insertion, performed at the same time as cardiac catheterization and/or coronary angiography, includes positioning or placement of the catheter in the distal aorta or ipsilateral femoral or iliac artery, injection of dye, production of permanent images, and radiologic supervision and interpretation (list separately in addition to primary procedure)

  Medicare specific code not reported for iliac injection used as a guiding shot for a closure device

Stimulation, Electrical

G0281-G0283: Bill local carrier

* **G0281** Electrical stimulation, (unattended), to one or more areas, for chronic stage III and stage IV pressure ulcers, arterial ulcers, diabetic ulcers, and venous stasis ulcers not demonstrating measurable signs of healing after 30 days of conventional care, as part of a therapy plan of care

  Reported by encounter/areas and not by site. Therapists report G0281 and G0283 rather than 97014

◆ **G0282** Electrical stimulation, (unattended), to one or more areas, for wound care other than described in G0281

  IOM: 100-03, 4, 270.1

▶ New → Revised ✔ Reinstated deleted Deleted
☼ Special coverage instructions ◆ Not covered or valid by Medicare ✱ Carrier discretion

✳ **G0283** Electrical stimulation (unattended), to one or more areas for indication(s) other than wound care, as part of a therapy plan of care

Reported by encounter/areas and not by site. Therapists report G0281 and G0283 rather than 97014

Angiography, Arthroscopy

G0288-G0289: Bill local carrier

✳ **G0288** Reconstruction, computed tomographic angiography of aorta for surgical planning for vascular surgery

✳ **G0289** Arthroscopy, knee, surgical, for removal of loose body, foreign body, debridement/shaving of articular cartilage (chondroplasty) at the time of other surgical knee arthroscopy in a different compartment of the same knee

Add-on code reported with knee arthroscopy code for major procedure performed—reported once per extra compartment

"The code may be reported twice (or with a unit of two) if the physician performs these procedures in two compartments, in addition to the compartment where the main procedure was performed." (http://www.ama-assn.org/resources/doc/cpt/orthopaedics.pdf)

Placement, Transcatheter

G0290-G0291: Bill local carrier

Includes angiography of same vessel.

~~G0290~~ ~~Transcatheter placement of a drug eluting intracoronary stent(s), percutaneous, with or without other therapeutic intervention, any method; single vessel~~ ✖

Cross Reference: CPT C9600, C9601, C9602, C9603, C9604

~~G0291~~ ~~Transcatheter placement of a drug eluting intracoronary stent(s), percutaneous, with or without other therapeutic intervention, any method; each additional vessel~~ ✖

Cross Reference: CPT C9605, C9606, C9607, C9608

Procedure, Non-Covered

G0293-G0294: Bill local carrier

☺ **G0293** Noncovered surgical procedure(s) using conscious sedation, regional, general or spinal anesthesia in a Medicare qualifying clinical trial, per day

☺ **G0294** Noncovered procedure(s) using either no anesthesia or local anesthesia only, in a Medicare qualifying clinical trial, per day

Therapy, Electromagnetic

◆ **G0295** Electromagnetic therapy, to one or more areas, for wound care other than described in G0329 or for other uses

Bill local carrier

IOM: 100-03, 4, 270.1

Services, Pulmonary Surgery

G0302-G0305: Bill local carrier

✳ **G0302** Pre-operative pulmonary surgery services for preparation for LVRS, complete course of services, to include a minimum of 16 days of services

✳ **G0303** Pre-operative pulmonary surgery services for preparation for LVRS, 10 to 15 days of services

✳ **G0304** Pre-operative pulmonary surgery services for preparation for LVRS, 1 to 9 days of services

✳ **G0305** Post-discharge pulmonary surgery services after LVRS, minimum of 6 days of services

Laboratory

G0306-G0328: Bill local carrier

✳ **G0306** Complete CBC, automated (HgB, HCT, RBC, WBC, without platelet count) and automated WBC differential count

Laboratory Certification: Hematology

✳ **G0307** Complete CBC, automated (HgB, HCT, RBC, WBC; without platelet count)

Laboratory Certification: Hematology

⊙ **G0328**   Colorectal cancer screening; fecal occult blood test, immunoassay, 1-3 simultaneous

Co-insurance and deductible waived

Reported for Medicare patients 50+; one FOBT per year, with either G0107 (guaiac-based) or G0328 (immunoassay-based)

Laboratory Certification: Routine Chemistry, Hematology

Therapy, Electromagnetic

✳ **G0329**   Electromagnetic therapy, to one or more areas for chronic stage III and stage IV pressure ulcers, arterial ulcers, and diabetic ulcers and venous stasis ulcers not demonstrating measurable signs of healing after 30 days of conventional care as part of a therapy plan of care

Bill local carrier

Fee, Pharmacy

⊙ **G0333**   Pharmacy dispensing fee for inhalation drug(s); initial 30-day supply as a beneficiary

Bill DME/MAC

Medicare will reimburse an initial dispensing fee to a pharmacy for initial 30-day period of inhalation drugs furnished through DME

Hospice

✳ **G0337**   Hospice evaluation and counseling services, pre-election

Bill local carrier

Radiosurgery, Robotic

G0339-G0340:   Bill local carrier

✳ **G0339**   Image-guided robotic linear accelerator-based stereotactic radiosurgery, complete course of therapy in one session or first session of fractionated treatment

Do not report with 77421

✳ **G0340**   Image-guided robotic linear accelerator-based stereotactic radiosurgery, delivery including collimator changes and custom plugging, fractionated treatment, all lesions, per session, second through fifth sessions, maximum five sessions per course of treatment

Do not report with 77421

Islet Cell

G0341-G0343:   Bill local carrier

⊙ **G0341**   Percutaneous islet cell transplant, includes portal vein catheterization and infusion

IOM: 100-03, 4, 260.3; 100-04, 32, 70

⊙ **G0342**   Laparoscopy for islet cell transplant, includes portal vein catheterization and infusion

IOM: 100-03, 4, 260.3

⊙ **G0343**   Laparotomy for islet cell transplant, includes portal vein catheterization and infusion

IOM: 100-03, 4, 260.3

Aspiration, Bone Marrow

✳ **G0364**   Bone marrow aspiration performed with bone marrow biopsy through the same incision on the same date of service

Bill local carrier

For Medicare patients, reported rather than 38220

Mapping, Vessel

G0365-G0372:   Bill local carrier

✳ **G0365**   Vessel mapping of vessels for hemodialysis access (services for preoperative vessel mapping prior to creation of hemodialysis access using an autogenous hemodialysis conduit, including arterial inflow and venous outflow)

Includes evaluation of the relevant arterial and venous vessels. Use modifier -26 for professional component only

⊙ **G0372**   Physician service required to establish and document the need for a power mobility device

Providers should bill the E/M code and G0372 on the same claim.

▶ New   → Revised   ✔ Reinstated   ~~deleted~~ Deleted
⊙ Special coverage instructions   ◆ Not covered or valid by Medicare   ✳ Carrier discretion

Services, Observation and ED

G0378-G0384: Bill local carrier

⊙ **G0378** Hospital observation service, per hour

Report all related services in addition to G0378. Report units of hours spent in observation (rounded to the nearest hour). Hospitals report the ED or clinic visit with a CPT code or, if applicable, G0379 (direct admit to observation) and G0378 (hospital observation services, per hour)

⊙ **G0379** Direct admission of patient for hospital observation care

Report all related services in addition to G0379. Report units of hours spent in observation (rounded to the nearest hour). Hospitals report the ED or clinic visit with a CPT code or, if applicable, G0379 (direct admit to observation) and G0378 (hospital observation services, per hour)

✳ **G0380** Level 1 hospital emergency department visit provided in a type B emergency department; (the ED must meet at least one of the following requirements: (1) it is licensed by the state in which it is located under applicable state law as an emergency room or emergency department; (2) it is held out to the public (by name, posted signs, advertising, or other means) as a place that provides care for emergency medical conditions on an urgent basis without requiring a previously scheduled appointment; or (3) during the calendar year immediately preceding the calendar year in which a determination under 42 CFR 489.24 is being made, based on a representative sample of patient visits that occurred during that calendar year, it provides at least one-third of all of its outpatient visits for the treatment of emergency medical conditions on an urgent basis without requiring a previously scheduled appointment)

✳ **G0381** Level 2 hospital emergency department visit provided in a type B emergency department; (the ED must meet at least one of the following requirements: (1) it is licensed by the state in which it is located under applicable state law as an emergency room or emergency department; (2) it is held out to the public (by name, posted signs, advertising, or other means) as a place that provides care for emergency medical conditions on an urgent basis without requiring a previously scheduled appointment; or (3) during the calendar year immediately preceding the calendar year in which a determination under 42 CFR 489.24 is being made, based on a representative sample of patient visits that occurred during that calendar year, it provides at least one-third of all of its outpatient visits for the treatment of emergency medical conditions on an urgent basis without requiring a previously scheduled appointment)

✳ **G0382** Level 3 hospital emergency department visit provided in a type B emergency department; (the ED must meet at least one of the following requirements: (1) it is licensed by the state in which it is located under applicable state law as an emergency room or emergency department; (2) it is held out to the public (by name, posted signs, advertising, or other means) as a place that provides care for emergency medical conditions on an urgent basis without requiring a previously scheduled appointment; or (3) during the calendar year immediately preceding the calendar year in which a determination under 42 CFR 489.24 is being made, based on a representative sample of patient visits that occurred during that calendar year, it provides at least one-third of all of its outpatient visits for the treatment of emergency medical conditions on an urgent basis without requiring a previously scheduled appointment)

▶ New → Revised ✔ Reinstated ~~deleted~~ Deleted

⊙ Special coverage instructions ◆ Not covered or valid by Medicare ✳ Carrier discretion

✳ **G0383** Level 4 hospital emergency department visit provided in a type B emergency department; (the ED must meet at least one of the following requirements: (1) it is licensed by the state in which it is located under applicable state law as an emergency room or emergency department; (2) it is held out to the public (by name, posted signs, advertising, or other means) as a place that provides care for emergency medical conditions on an urgent basis without requiring a previously scheduled appointment; or (3) during the calendar year immediately preceding the calendar year in which a determination under 42 CFR 489.24 is being made, based on a representative sample of patient visits that occurred during that calendar year, it provides at least one-third of all of its outpatient visits for the treatment of emergency medical conditions on an urgent basis without requiring a previously scheduled appointment)

✳ **G0384** Level 5 hospital emergency department visit provided in a type B emergency department; (the ED must meet at least one of the following requirements: (1) it is licensed by the state in which it is located under applicable state law as an emergency room or emergency department; (2) it is held out to the public (by name, posted signs, advertising, or other means) as a place that provides care for emergency medical conditions on an urgent basis without requiring a previously scheduled appointment; or (3) during the calendar year immediately preceding the calendar year in which a determination under 42 CFR § 489.24 is being made, based on a representative sample of patient visits that occurred during that calendar year, it provides at least one-third of all of its outpatient visits for the treatment of emergency medical conditions on an urgent basis without requiring a previously scheduled appointment)

Ultrasound, AAA

☼ **G0389** Ultrasound B-scan and/or real time with image documentation; for abdominal aortic aneurysm (AAA) screening

Bill local carrier

Use modifier -26 for professional component only

Eligible beneficiaries must receive a referral for an AAA ultrasound screening as a result of an IPPE (initial preventative physical examination). This is a once in a lifetime benefit per eligible beneficiary. (http://www.cms.gov/MLNProducts/downloads/MPS_QuickReferenceChart_1.pdf)

Team, Trauma Response

☼ **G0390** Trauma response team associated with hospital critical care service

Bill local carrier

Assessment/Intervention

G0396-G0397: Bill local carrier

✳ **G0396** Alcohol and/or substance (other than tobacco) abuse structured assessment (e.g., AUDIT, DAST), and brief intervention 15 to 30 minutes

Bill instead of 99408 and 99409

✳ **G0397** Alcohol and/or substance (other than tobacco) abuse structured assessment (e.g., AUDIT, DAST), and intervention, greater than 30 minutes

Bill instead of 99408 and 99409

Home Sleep Study Test

✳ **G0398** Home sleep study test (HST) with type II portable monitor, unattended; minimum of 7 channels: EEG, EOG, EMG, ECG/heart rate, airflow, respiratory effort and oxygen saturation

Bill local carrier

✳ **G0399** Home sleep test (HST) with type III portable monitor, unattended; minimum of 4 channels: 2 respiratory movement/airflow, 1 ECG/heart rate and 1 oxygen saturation

▶ New   → Revised   ✔ Reinstated   ~~deleted~~ Deleted
☼ Special coverage instructions   ◆ Not covered or valid by Medicare   ✳ Carrier discretion

✳ **G0400** Home sleep test (HST) with type IV portable monitor, unattended; minimum of 3 channels

Examination, Initial Medicare

✳ **G0402** Initial preventive physical examination; face-to-face visit, services limited to new beneficiary during the first 12 months of Medicare enrollment

Depending on circumstances, 99201-99215 may be assigned with modifier -25 to report an E/M service as a significant, separately identifiable service in addition to the Initial Preventive Physical Examination (IPPE), G0402.

Copayment and coinsurance waived, deductible waived.

Electrocardiogram

G0403-G0405: Bill local carrier

✳ **G0403** Electrocardiogram, routine ECG with 12 leads; performed as a screening for the initial preventive physical examination with interpretation and report

Optional service may be ordered or performed at discretion of physician. Once in a life-time screening, stemming from a referral from Initial Preventive Physical Examination (IPPE). Both deductible and co-payment apply.

✳ **G0404** Electrocardiogram, routine ECG with 12 leads; tracing only, without interpretation and report, performed as a screening for the initial preventive physical examination

✳ **G0405** Electrocardiogram, routine ECG with 12 leads; interpretation and report only, performed as a screening for the initial preventive physical examination

Telehealth

G0406-G0408: Bill local carrier

✳ **G0406** Follow-up inpatient consultation, limited, physicians typically spend 15 minutes communicating with the patient via telehealth

These telehealth modifers are required when billing for telehealth services with codes G0406-G0408 and G0425-G0427:
- GT, via interactive audio and video telecommunications system
- GQ, via asynchronous telecommunications system

✳ **G0407** Follow-up inpatient consultation, intermediate, physicians typically spend 25 minutes communicating with the patient via telehealth

✳ **G0408** Follow-up inpatient consultation, complex, physicians typically spend 35 minutes communicating with the patient via telehealth

Services, Social, Psychological

G0409-G0411: Bill local carrier

✳ **G0409** Social work and psychological services, directly relating to and/or furthering the patient's rehabilitation goals, each 15 minutes, face-to-face; individual (services provided by a CORF-qualified social worker or psychologist in a CORF)

✳ **G0410** Group psychotherapy other than of a multiple-family group, in a partial hospitalization setting, approximately 45 to 50 minutes

✳ **G0411** Interactive group psychotherapy, in a partial hospitalization setting, approximately 45 to 50 minutes

Treatment, Bone

G0412-G0415: Bill local carrier

✳ **G0412** Open treatment of iliac spine(s), tuberosity avulsion, or iliac wing fracture(s), unilateral or bilateral for pelvic bone fracture patterns which do not disrupt the pelvic ring includes internal fixation, when performed

▶ New　→ Revised　✔ Reinstated　deleted Deleted

☺ Special coverage instructions　◆ Not covered or valid by Medicare　✳ Carrier discretion

TEMPORARY PROCEDURES/PROFESSIONAL SERVICES　G0400 – G0412

* **G0413** Percutaneous skeletal fixation of posterior pelvic bone fracture and/or dislocation, for fracture patterns which disrupt the pelvic ring, unilateral or bilateral, (includes ilium, sacroiliac joint and/or sacrum)

* **G0414** Open treatment of anterior pelvic bone fracture and/or dislocation for fracture patterns which disrupt the pelvic ring, unilateral or bilateral, includes internal fixation when performed (includes pubic symphysis and/or superior/inferior rami)

* **G0415** Open treatment of posterior pelvic bone fracture and/or dislocation, for fracture patterns which disrupt the pelvic ring, unilateral or bilateral, includes internal fixation, when performed (includes ilium, sacroiliac joint and/or sacrum)

Pathology, Surgical

G0416-G0419: Bill local carrier

→ * **G0416** Surgical pathology, gross and microscopic examinations for prostate needle saturation biopsy sampling, 10-20 specimens

This testing requires a facility to have either a CLIA certificate of registration (certificate type code 9), a CLIA certificate of compliance (certificate type code 1), or a CLIA certificate of accreditation (certificate type code 3). A facility without a valid, current, CLIA certificate, with a current CLIA certificate of waiver (certificate type code 2) or with a current CLIA certificate for provider-performed microscopy procedures (certificate type code 4), must not be permitted to be paid for these tests. This code has a -TC, -26 (physician), or gobal component.

Laboratory Certification: Histopathology

* **G0417** Surgical pathology, gross and microscopic examination for prostate needle saturation biopsy sampling, 21-40 specimens

Laboratory Certification: Histopathology

* **G0418** Surgical pathology, gross and microscopic examination for prostate needle saturation biopsy sampling, 41-60 specimens

Use modifier 26 for professional component only

Laboratory Certification: Histopathology

* **G0419** Surgical pathology, gross and microscopic examination for prostate needle saturation biopsy sampling, greater than 60 specimens

Use modifier 26 for professional component only

Laboratory Certification: Histopathology

Educational Services, Rehabilitation, Telehealth, and Miscellaneous

G0420-G0441: Bill local carrier

* **G0420** Face-to-face educational services related to the care of chronic kidney disease; individual, per session, per one hour

CKD is kidney damage of 3 months or longer, regardless of the cause of kidney damage. Sessions billed in increments of one hour (if session is less than 1 hour, it must last at least 31 minutes to be billable. Sessions less than one hour and longer than 31 minutes is billable as one session. No more than 6 sessions of KDE services in a beneficiary's lifetime

* **G0421** Face-to-face educational services related to the care of chronic kidney disease; group, per session, per one hour

Group setting: 2 to 20, report codes G0420 and G0421 with diagnosis code 585.4.

* **G0422** Intensive cardiac rehabilitation; with or without continuous ECG monitoring with exercise, per session

Includes the same service as 93798 but at a greater frequency; may be reported with as many as six hourly sessions on a single date of service. Includes medical nutrition services to reduce cardiac disease risk factors.

▶ New   → Revised   ✔ Reinstated   ~~deleted~~ Deleted   ☺ Special coverage instructions   ◆ Not covered or valid by Medicare   * Carrier discretion

✳ **G0423** Intensive cardiac rehabilitation; with or without continuous ECG monitoring; without exercise, per session

Includes the same service as 93797 but at a greater frequency; may be reported with as many as six hourly sessions on a single date of service. Includes medical nutrition services to reduce cardiac disease risk factors.

✳ **G0424** Pulmonary rehabilitation, including exercise (includes monitoring), one hour, per session, up to two sessions per day

Includes therapeutic services and all related monitoring services to inprove respiratory function. Do not report with G0237, G0238, or G0239.

✳ **G0425** Telehealth consultation, emergency department or initial inpatient, typically 30 minutes communicating with the patient via telehealth

Problem Focused: Problem focused history and examination, with straightforward medical decision making complexity. Typically 30 minutes communicating with patient via telehealth

✳ **G0426** Initial inpatient telehealth consultation, emergency department or initial inpatient, typically 50 minutes communicating with the patient via telehealth

Detailed: Detailed history and examination, with moderate medical decision making complexity. Typically 50 minutes communicating with patient via telehealth

✳ **G0427** Initial inpatient telehealth consultation, emergency department or initial inpatient, typically 70 minutes or more communicating with the patient via telehealth

Comprehensive: Comprehensive history and examination, with high medical decision making complexity. Typically 70 minutes or more communicating with patient via telehealth.

◆ **G0428** Collagen meniscus implant procedure for filling meniscal defects (e.g., CMI, collagen scaffold, menaflex)

✳ **G0429** Dermal filler injection(s) for the treatment of facial lipodystrophy syndrome (LDS) (e.g., as a result of highly active antiretroviral therapy)

Designated for dermal fillers Sculptra® and Radiesse (Medicare). (https://www.cms.gov/ContractorLearningResources/downloads/JA6953.pdf)

✳ **G0431** Drug screen, qualitative; multiple drug classes by high complexity test method (e.g., immunoassay, enzyme assay), per patient encounter

http://www.cms.hhs.gov/mlnmattersarticles/downloads/se1001.pdf.

Laboratory Certification: Toxicology

✳ **G0432** Infectious agent antibody detection by enzyme immunoassay (EIA) technique, HIV-1 and/or HIV-2, screening

Laboratory Certification: Virology, General immunology

→ ✳ **G0433** Infectious agent antibody detection by enzyme-linked immunosorbent assay (ELISA) technique, HIV-1 and/or HIV-2, screening

Laboratory Certification: Virology, General immunology

→ ✳ **G0434** Drug screen, other than chromatographic; any number of drug classes, by CLIA waived test or moderate complexity test, per patient encounter

Laboratory Certification: Toxicology

✳ **G0435** Infectious agent antibody detection by rapid antibody test, HIV-1 and/or HIV-2, screening

✳ **G0436** Smoking and tobacco cessation counseling visit for the asymptomatic patient; intermediate, greater than 3 minutes, up to 10 minutes

✳ **G0437** Smoking and tobacco cessation counseling visit for the asymptomatic patient; intensive, greater than 10 minutes

✳ **G0438** Annual wellness visit; includes a personalized prevention plan of service (PPS), initial visit

✳ **G0439** Annual wellness visit, includes a personalized prevention plan of service (PPS), subsequent visit

✳ **G0442** Annual alcohol misuse screening, 15 minutes

✳ **G0443** Brief face-to-face behavioral counseling for alcohol misuse, 15 minutes

▶ New   → Revised   ✔ Reinstated   ~~deleted~~ Deleted
☉ Special coverage instructions   ◆ Not covered or valid by Medicare   ✳ Carrier discretion

❋ **G0444** Annual depression screening,
15 minutes

❋ **G0445** High intensity behavioral counseling to
prevent sexually transmitted infection;
face-to-face, individual, includes:
education, skills training and guidance
on how to change sexual behavior;
performed semi-annually, 30 minutes

→ ❋ **G0446** Annual, face-to-face intensive behavioral
therapy for cardiovascular disease,
individual, bi-annual, 15 minutes

❋ **G0447** Face-to-face behavioral counseling for
obesity, 15 minutes

❋ **G0448** Insertion or replacement of a
permanent pacing cardioverter-
defibrillator system with transvenous
lead(s), single or dual chamber with
insertion of pacing electrode, cardiac
venous system, for left ventricular
pacing

❋ **G0451** Development testing, with
interpretation and report, per
standardized instrument form

▶ ❋ **G0452** Molecular pathology procedure;
physician interpretation and report

▶ ❋ **G0453** Continuous intraoperative
neurophysiology monitoring, from
outside the operating room (remote or
nearby), per patient, (attention directed
exclusively to one patient) each 15
minutes (list in addition to primary
procedure)

▶ ❋ **G0454** Physician documentation of face-to-
face visit for durable medical
equipment determination performed by
nurse practitioner, physician assistant
or clinical nurse specialist

▶ ❋ **G0455** Preparation with instillation of fecal
microbiota by any method, including
assessment of donor specimen

▶ ❋ **G0456** Negative pressure wound therapy, (e. g.,
vacuum assisted drainage collection)
using a mechanically-powered device,
not durable medical equipment,
including provision of cartridge and
dressing(s), topical application(s),
wound assessment, and instructions for
ongoing care, per session; total
wounds(s) surface area less than or
equal to 50 square centimeters

▶ ❋ **G0457** Negative pressure wound therapy, (e. g.,
vacuum assisted drainage collection)
using a mechanically-powered device,
not durable medical equipment,
including provision of cartridge and
dressing(s), topical application(s),
wound assessment, and instructions for
ongoing care, per session; total
wounds(s) surface area greater than 50
square centimeters

▶ ❋ **G0458** Low dose rate (LDR) prostate
brachytherapy services, composite rate

❋ **G0908** Most recent hemoglobin (HGB) level
>12.0 g/dl

→ ❋ **G0909** Hemoglobin level measurement not
documented, reason not given

❋ **G0910** Most recent hemoglobin level
<= 12.0 g/dl

~~G0911~~   ~~Assessed level of activity and~~
~~symptoms~~   ✖

~~G0912~~   ~~Level of activity and symptoms~~
~~not assessed~~   ✖

❋ **G0913** Improvement in visual function
achieved within 90 days following
cataract surgery

❋ **G0914** Patient care survey was not completed
by patient

❋ **G0915** Improvement in visual function not
achieved within 90 days following
cataract surgery

❋ **G0916** Satisfaction with care achieved
within 90 days following cataract
surgery

❋ **G0917** Patient satisfaction survey was not
completed by patient

❋ **G0918** Satisfaction with care not achieved
within 90 days following cataract
surgery

❋ **G0919** Influenza immunization ordered or
recommended (to be given at alternate
location or alternate provider); vaccine
not available at time of visit

❋ **G0920** Type, anatomic location, and activity
all documented

→ ❋ **G0921** Documentation of patient reason(s) for
not being able to assess (e.g., patient
refuses endoscopic and/or radiologic
assessment)

→ ❋ **G0922** No documentation of disease type,
anatomic location, and activity, reason
not given

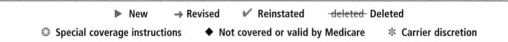

▶ New   → Revised   ✔ Reinstated   ~~deleted~~ Deleted

⊙ Special coverage instructions   ◆ Not covered or valid by Medicare   ❋ Carrier discretion

Tositumomab

✳ **G3001** Administration and supply of tositumomab, 450 mg

Bill local carrier

The therapeutic regimen consists of a dosimetric step of tositumomab infusion followed 7–14 days later by a therapeutic step of iodine I-131 tositumomab infusion.

Documentation

G8126-G9140: Bill local carrier

✳ **G8126** Patient documented as being treated with antidepressant medication during the entire 12 week acute treatment phase

✳ **G8127** Patient not documented as being treated with antidepressant medication during the entire 12 weeks acute treatment phase

✳ **G8128** Clinician documented that patient was not an eligible candidate for antidepressant medication during the entire 12 week acute treatment phase measure

✳ **G8395** Left ventricular ejection fraction (LVEF) > = 40% or documentation as normal or mildly depressed left ventricular systolic function

✳ **G8396** Left ventricular ejection fraction (LVEF) not performed or documented

✳ **G8397** Dilated macular or fundus exam performed, including documentation of the presence or absence of macular edema and level of severity of retinopathy

✳ **G8398** Dilated macular or fundus exam not performed

✳ **G8399** Patient with central dual-energy x-ray absorptiometry (DXA) results documented or ordered or pharmacologic therapy (other than minerals/vitamins) for osteoporosis prescribed)

→ ✳ **G8400** Patient with central dual-energy x-ray absorptiometry (DXA) results not documented or not ordered or pharmacologic therapy (other than minerals/vitamins) for osteoporosis not prescribed, reason not given

✳ **G8401** Clinician documented that patient was not an eligible candidate for screening or therapy for osteoporosis for women measure

✳ **G8404** Lower extremity neurological exam performed and documented

✳ **G8405** Lower extremity neurological exam not performed

✳ **G8406** Clinician documented that patient was not an eligible candidate for lower extremity neurological exam measure

✳ **G8410** Footwear evaluation performed and documented

✳ **G8415** Footwear evaluation was not performed

✳ **G8416** Clinician documented that patient was not an eligible candidate for footwear evaluation measure

→ ✳ **G8417** Calculated BMI above normal parameters and a follow-up plan was documented

→ ✳ **G8418** Calculated BMI below normal parameters and a follow-up plan was documented

→ ✳ **G8419** Calculated BMI outside normal parameters, no follow-up plan documented

✳ **G8420** Calculated BMI within normal parameters and documented

✳ **G8421** BMI not calculated

✳ **G8422** Patient not eligible for BMI calculation

→ ✳ **G8427** Eligible professional attests to documenting the patient's current medications to the best of his/her knowledge and ability

→ ✳ **G8428** Current medications not documented by the eligible professional, reason not given

→ ✳ **G8430** Eligible professional attests the patient is not eligible for medication documentation

→ ✳ **G8431** Positive screen for clinical depression with a documented follow-up plan

→ ✳ **G8432** Clinical depression screening not documented, reason not given

→ ✳ **G8433** Screening for clinical depression not documented; patient not eligible/appropriate

✳ **G8442** Documentation that patient is not eligible for pain assessment

~~G8447 Patient encounter was documented using an EHR system that has been certified by an authorized testing and certification body (ATCB)~~ ✖

~~G8448 Patient encounter was documented using a PQRI qualified EHR or other acceptable systems~~ ✖

▶ New → Revised ✔ Reinstated ~~deleted~~ Deleted
☼ Special coverage instructions ◆ Not covered or valid by Medicare ✳ Carrier discretion

➜ ✳ **G8450** Beta-blocker therapy prescribed

✳ **G8451** Clinician documented patient with left ventricular ejection fraction (LVEF) <40% or documentation as moderately or severely depressed left ventricular systolic function was not eligible candidate for beta-blocker therapy

➜ ✳ **G8452** Beta-blocker therapy not prescribed

✳ **G8458** Clinician documented that patient is not an eligible candidate for genotype testing; patient not receiving antiviral treatment for hepatitis C

✳ **G8459** Clinician documented that patient is receiving antiviral treatment for hepatitis C

✳ **G8460** Clinician documented that patient is not an eligible candidate for quantitative RNA testing at week 12; patient not receiving antiviral treatment for hepatitis C

✳ **G8461** Patient receiving antiviral treatment for hepatitis C

✳ **G8462** Clinician documented that patient is not an eligible candidate for counseling regarding contraception prior to antiviral treatment; patient not receiving antiviral treatment for hepatitis C

✳ **G8463** Patient receiving antiviral treatment for hepatitis C documented

✳ **G8464** Clinician documented that prostate cancer patient is not an eligible candidate for adjuvant hormonal therapy; low or intermediate risk of recurrence or risk of recurrence not determined

✳ **G8465** High risk of recurrence of prostate cancer

~~G8468~~ ~~Angiotensin converting enzyme (ACE) inhibitor or angiotensin receptor blocker (ARB) therapy prescribed for patients with a left ventricular ejection fraction (LVEF) <40% or documentation of moderately or severely depressed left ventricular systolic function~~ ✖

~~G8469~~ ~~Clinician documented that patient with a left ventricular ejection fraction (LVEF) <40% or documentation of moderately or severely depressed left ventricular systolic function was not an eligible candidate for angiotensin converting enzyme (ACE) inhibitor or angiotensin receptor blocker (ARB) therapy~~ ✖

~~G8470~~ ~~Patient with left ventricular ejection fraction (LVEF) > =40% or documentation as normal or mildly depressed left ventricular systolic function~~ ✖

~~G8471~~ ~~Left ventricular ejection fraction (LVEF) was not performed or documented~~ ✖

~~G8472~~ ~~Angiotensin converting enzyme (ACE) inhibitor or angiotensin receptor blocker (ARB) therapy not prescribed for patients with a left ventricular ejection fraction (LVEF) <40% or documentation of moderately or severely depressed left ventricular systolic function, reason not specified~~ ✖

✳ **G8473** Angiotensin converting enzyme (ACE) inhibitor or angiotensin receptor blocker (ARB) therapy prescribed

✳ **G8474** Angiotensin converting enzyme (ACE) inhibitor or angiotensin receptor blocker (ARB) therapy not prescribed for reasons documented by the clinician

➜ ✳ **G8475** Angiotensin converting enzyme (ACE) inhibitor or angiotensin receptor blocker (ARB) therapy not prescribed, reason not given

✳ **G8476** Most recent blood pressure has a systolic measurement of <130 mm/Hg and a diastolic measurement of <80 mm/Hg

✳ **G8477** Most recent blood pressure has a systolic measurement of > =130 mm/Hg and/or a diastolic measurement of > =80 mm/Hg

➜ ✳ **G8478** Blood pressure measurement not performed or documented, reason not given

✳ **G8482** Influenza immunization administered or previously received

➜ ✳ **G8483** Influenza immunization was not ordered or administered for reasons documented by clinician (e.g., patient allergy or other medical reason, patient declined or other patient reasons, or other system reasons)

➜ ✳ **G8484** Influenza immunization was not ordered or administered, reason not given

➜ ✳ **G8485** I intend to report the diabetes mellitus (DM) measures group

✳ **G8486** I intend to report the preventive care measures group

---

▶ New ➜ Revised ✔ Reinstated ~~deleted~~ Deleted

🌑 Special coverage instructions ◆ Not covered or valid by Medicare ✳ Carrier discretion

✳ **G8487** I intend to report the chronic kidney disease (CKD) measures group

✳ **G8489** I intend to report the coronary artery disease (CAD) measures group

→ ✳ **G8490** I intend to report the rheumatoid arthritis (RA) measures group

✳ **G8491** I intend to report the HIV/AIDS measures group

✳ **G8492** I intend to report the perioperative care measures group

✳ **G8493** I intend to report the back pain measures group

→ ✳ **G8494** All quality actions for the applicable measures in the diabetes mellitus (DM) measures group have been performed for this patient

Composite code, do not report with G8485

→ ✳ **G8495** All quality actions for the applicable measures in the chronic kidney disease (CKD) measures group have been performed for this patient

Composite code, do not report with G8487

✳ **G8496** All quality actions for the applicable measures in the Preventive Care measures group have been performed for this patient

Composite code, do not report with G8486

✳ **G8497** All quality actions for the applicable measures in the Coronary Artery Bypass Graft (CABG) measures group have been performed for this patient

Composite code.

✳ **G8498** All quality actions for the applicable measures in the Coronary Artery Disease (CAD) measures group have been performed for this patient

Composite code.

→ ✳ **G8499** All quality actions for the applicable measures in the rheumatoid arthritis (RA) measures group have been performed for this patient

Composite code, do not report with G8490

✳ **G8500** All quality actions for the applicable measures in the HIV/AIDS measures group have been performed for this patient

Composite code.

✳ **G8501** All quality actions for the applicable measures in the Perioperative Care measures group have been performed for this patient

Composite code, do not report with G8492

✳ **G8502** All quality actions for the applicable measures in the Back Pain measures group have been performed for this patient

Composite code, do not report with G8493

✳ **G8506** Patient receiving angiotensin converting enzyme (ACE) inhibitor or angiotensin receptor blocker (ARB) therapy

→ ✳ **G8509** Documentation of positive pain assessment; no documentation of a follow-up plan, reason not given

→ ✳ **G8510** Negative screen for clinical depression, follow-up not required

→ ✳ **G8511** Positive screen for clinical depression documented, follow up plan not documented, reason not given

~~G8524~~ ~~Patch closure used for patient undergoing conventional CEA~~   ✖

~~G8525~~ ~~Clinician documented that patient did not receive conventional CEA~~   ✖

~~G8526~~ ~~Patch closure not used for patient undergoing conventional CEA, reason not specified~~   ✖

✳ **G8530** Autogenous AV fistula received

✳ **G8531** Clinician documented that patient was not an eligible candidate for autogenous AV fistula

→ ✳ **G8532** Clinician documented that patient received vascular access other than autogenous AV fistula, reason not given

✳ **G8535** No documentation of an elder maltreatment screen, patient not eligible

→ ✳ **G8536** No documentation of an elder maltreatment screen, reason not given

→ ✳ **G8539** Documentation of a functional outcome assessment using a standardized tool and documentation of a care plan based on identified deficiencies on the date of the functional outcome assessment

✳ **G8540** Documentation that the patient is not eligible for a functional outcome assessment using a standardized tool

→ ✳ **G8541** Functional outcome assessment using a standardized tool not documented, reason not given

---

▶ **New**   → **Revised**   ✔ **Reinstated**   ~~deleted~~ **Deleted**

⊙ **Special coverage instructions**   ◆ **Not covered or valid by Medicare**   ✳ **Carrier discretion**

→ ✳ **G8542** Documentation of a functional outcome assessment using a standardized tool; no functional deficiencies identified, care plan not required

→ ✳ **G8543** Documentation of a functional outcome assessment using a standardized tool; care plan not documented, reason not given

✳ **G8544** I intend to report the coronary artery bypass graft (CABG) measures group

✳ **G8545** I intend to report the Hepatitis C measures group

~~G8546~~ ~~I intend to report the Community Acquired Pneumonia (CAP) measures group~~ ✖

✳ **G8547** I intend to report the Ischemic Vascular Disease (IVD) measures group

✳ **G8548** I intend to report the Heart Failure (HF) measures group

✳ **G8549** All quality actions for the applicable measures in the Hepatitis C measures group have been performed for this patient

Composite code, do not report with G8545

~~G8550~~ ~~All quality actions for the applicable measures in the Community Acquired Pneumonia (CAP) measures group have been performed for this patient~~ ✖

✳ **G8551** All quality actions for the applicable measures in the Heart Failure (HF) measures group have been performed for this patient

Composite code.

✳ **G8552** All quality actions for the applicable measures in the Ischemic Vascular Disease (IVD) measures group have been performed for this patient

Composite code, do not report with G8547

→ ✳ **G8553** Prescription(s) generated and transmitted via a qualified ERX system

✳ **G8556** Referred to a physician (preferably a physician with training in disorders of the ear) for an otologic evaluation

✳ **G8557** Patient is not eligible for the referral for otologic evaluation measure

→ ✳ **G8558** Not referred to a physician (preferably a physician with training in disorders of the ear) for an otologic evaluation, reason not given

✳ **G8559** Patient referred to a physician (preferably a physician with training in disorders of the ear) for an otologic evaluation

✳ **G8560** Patient has a history of active drainage from the ear within the previous 90 days

✳ **G8561** Patient is not eligible for the referral for otologic evaluation for patients with a history of active drainage measure

✳ **G8562** Patient does not have a history of active drainage from the ear within the previous 90 days

→ ✳ **G8563** Patient not referred to a physician (preferably a physician with training in disorders of the ear) for an otologic evaluation, reason not given

✳ **G8564** Patient was referred to a physician (preferably a physician with training in disorders of the ear) for an otologic evaluation, reason not specified)

✳ **G8565** Verification and documentation of sudden or rapidly progressive hearing loss

✳ **G8566** Patient is not eligible for the "referral for otologic evaluation for sudden or rapidly progressive hearing loss" measure

✳ **G8567** Patient does not have verification and documentation of sudden or rapidly progressive hearing loss

→ ✳ **G8568** Patient was not referred to a physician (preferably a physician with training in disorders of the ear) for an otologic evaluation, reason not given

✳ **G8569** Prolonged intubation (>24 hrs) required

✳ **G8570** Prolonged intubation (>24 hrs) not required

✳ **G8571** Development of deep sternal wound infection within 30 days postoperatively

✳ **G8572** No deep sternal wound infection

✳ **G8573** Stroke following isolated CABG surgery

✳ **G8574** No stroke following isolated CABG surgery

✳ **G8575** Developed postoperative renal failure or required dialysis

✳ **G8576** No postoperative renal failure/ dialysis not required

→ ✳ **G8577** Re-exploration required due to mediastinal bleeding with or without tamponade, graft occlusion, valve disfunction, or other cardiac reason

→ ✳ **G8578** Re-exploration not required due to mediastinal bleeding with or without tamponade, graft occlusion, valve dysfunction, or other cardiac reason

---

▶ **New**   → **Revised**   ✔ **Reinstated**   ~~deleted~~ **Deleted**

◎ **Special coverage instructions**   ◆ **Not covered or valid by Medicare**   ✳ **Carrier discretion**

✳ **G8579** Antiplatelet medication at discharge

✳ **G8580** Antiplatelet medication contraindicated

✳ **G8581** No antiplatelet medication at discharge

✳ **G8582** Beta-blocker at discharge

✳ **G8583** Beta-blocker contraindicated

✳ **G8584** No beta-blocker at discharge

✳ **G8585** Anti-lipid treatment at discharge

✳ **G8586** Anti-lipid treatment contraindicated

✳ **G8587** No anti-lipid treatment at discharge

✳ **G8588** Most recent systolic blood pressure < 140 mmhg

✳ **G8589** Most recent systolic blood pressure >= 140 mmhg

✳ **G8590** Most recent diastolic blood pressure < 90 mmhg

✳ **G8591** Most recent diastolic blood pressure >= 90 mmhg

→ ✳ **G8592** No documentation of blood pressure measurement, reason not given

✳ **G8593** Lipid profile results documented and reviewed (must include total cholesterol, HDL-C, triglycerides and calculated LDL-C)

→ ✳ **G8594** Lipid profile not performed, reason not given

✳ **G8595** Most recent LDL-C < 100 mg/dl

✳ **G8596** LDL-C was not performed

✳ **G8597** Most recent LDL-C >= 100 mg/dl

✳ **G8598** Aspirin or another antithrombotic therapy used

→ ✳ **G8599** Aspirin or another antithrombotic therapy not used, reason not given

✳ **G8600** IV T-PA initiated within three hours (<= 180 minutes) of time last known well

✳ **G8601** IV T-PA not initiated within three hours (<= 180 minutes) of time last known well for reasons documented by clinician

→ ✳ **G8602** IV T-PA not initiated within three hours (<= 180 minutes) of time last known well, reason not given

✳ **G8603** Score on the spoken language comprehension functional communication measure at discharge was higher than at admission

→ ✳ **G8604** Score on the spoken language comprehension functional communication measure at discharge was not higher than at admission, reason not given

✳ **G8605** Patient treated for spoken languge comprehension but not scored on the spoken language comprehension functional communication measure either at admission or at discharge

✳ **G8606** Score on the attention functional communication measure at discharge was higher than at admission

→ ✳ **G8607** Score on the attention functional communication measure at discharge was not higher than at admission, reason not given

✳ **G8608** Patient treated for attention but not scored on the attention functional communication measure either at admission or at discharge

✳ **G8609** Score on the memory functional communication measure at discharge was higher than at admission

→ ✳ **G8610** Score on the memory functional communication measure at discharge was not higher than at admission, reason not given

✳ **G8611** Patient treated for memory but not scored on the memory functional communication measure either at admission or at discharge

✳ **G8612** Score on the motor speech functional communication measure at discharge was higher than at admission

→ ✳ **G8613** Score on the motor speech functional communication measure at discharge was not higher than at admission, reason not given

✳ **G8614** Patient treated for motor speech but not scored on the motor speech comprehension functional communication measure either at admission or at discharge

✳ **G8615** Score on the reading functional communication measure at discharge was higher than at admission

→ ✳ **G8616** Score on the reading functional communication measure at discharge was not higher than at admission, reason not given

✳ **G8617** Patient treated for reading but not scored on the reading functional communication measure either at admission or at discharge

✳ **G8618** Score on the spoken language expression functional communication measure at discharge was higher than at admission

---

▶ New   → Revised   ✔ Reinstated   ~~deleted~~ Deleted

⊗ Special coverage instructions   ◆ Not covered or valid by Medicare   ✳ Carrier discretion

→ ✳ **G8619** Score on the spoken language expression functional communication measure at discharge was not higher than at admission, reason not given

✳ **G8620** Patient treated for spoken language expression but not scored on the spoken language expression functional communication measure either at admission or at discharge

✳ **G8621** Score on the writing functional communication measure at discharge was higher than at admission

→ ✳ **G8622** Score on the writing functional communication measure at discharge was not higher than at admission, reason not given

✳ **G8623** Patient treated for writing but not scored on the writing functional communication measure either at admission or at discharge

✳ **G8624** Score on the swallowing functional communication measure at discharge was higher than at admission

→ ✳ **G8625** Score on the swallowing functional communication measure at discharge was not higher than at admission, reason not given

✳ **G8626** Patient treated for swallowing but not scored on the swallowing functional communication measure at admission or at discharge

✳ **G8627** Surgical procedure performed within 30 days following cataract surgery for major complications (e.g. retained nuclear fragments, endophthalmitis, dislocated or wrong power IOL, retinal detachment, or wound dehiscence)

✳ **G8628** Surgical procedure not performed within 30 days following cataract surgery for major complications (e.g. retained nuclear fragments, endophthalmitis, dislocated or wrong power IOL, retinal detachment, or wound dehiscence)

✳ **G8629** Documentation of order for prophylactic parenteral antibiotic to be given within one hour (if fluoroquinolone or vancomycin, two hours) prior to surgical incision (or start of procedure when no incision is required)

✳ **G8630** Documentation that administration of prophylactic parenteral antibiotics was initiated within one hour (if fluoroquinolone or vancomycin, two hours) prior to surgical incision (or start of procedure when no incision is required), as ordered

✳ **G8631** Clinician documented that patient was not an eligible candidate for ordering prophylactic parenteral antibiotics to be given within one hour (if fluoroquinolone or vancomycin, two hours) prior to surgical incision (or start of procedure when no incision is required)

→ ✳ **G8632** Prophylactic parenteral antibiotics were not ordered to be given or given within one hour (if fluoroquinolone or vancomycin, two hours) prior to the surgical incision (or start of procedure when no incision is required), reason not given

✳ **G8633** Pharmacologic therapy (other than minierals/vitamins) for osteoporosis prescribed

✳ **G8634** Clinician documented patient not an eligible candidate to receive pharmacologic therapy for osteoporosis

→ ✳ **G8635** Pharmacologic therapy for osteoporosis was not prescribed, reason not given

✳ **G8642** The eligible professional practices in a rural area without sufficient high speed internet access and requests a hardship exemption from the application of the payment adjustment under Section 1848(a)(5)(a) of the Social Security Act

✳ **G8643** The eligible professional practices in an area without sufficient available pharmacies for electronic prescribing and requests a hardship exemption for the application of the payment adjustment under Section 1848(a)(5)(a) of the Social Security Act

✳ **G8644** Eligible professional does not have prescribing privileges

✳ **G8645** I intend to report the asthma measures group

✳ **G8646** All quality actions for the applicable measures in the asthma measures group have been performed for this patient

✳ **G8647** Risk-adjusted functional status change residual score for the knee successfully calculated and the score was equal to zero (0) or greater than zero (>0)

✳ **G8648** Risk-adjusted functional status change residual score for the knee successfully calculated and the score was less than zero (<0)

▶ New   → Revised   ✔ Reinstated   ~~deleted~~ Deleted
⊙ Special coverage instructions   ◆ Not covered or valid by Medicare   ✳ Carrier discretion

G8619 – G8648   TEMPORARY PROCEDURES/PROFESSIONAL SERVICES

✳ **G8649** Risk-adjusted functional status change residual scores for the knee not measured because the patient did not complete FOTO'S functional intake on admission and/or follow up status survey near discharge, patient not eligible/not appropriate

→ ✳ **G8650** Risk-adjusted functional status change residual scores for the knee not measured because the patient did not complete FOTO'S functional intake on admission and/or follow up status survey near discharge, reason not given

✳ **G8651** Risk-adjusted functional status change residual score for the hip successfully calculated and the score was equal to zero (0) or greater than zero (>0)

✳ **G8652** Risk-adjusted functional status change residual score for the hip successfully calculated and the score was less than zero (<0)

✳ **G8653** Risk-adjusted functional status change residual scores for the hip not measured because the patient did not complete FOTO'S functional intake on admission and/or follow up status survey near discharge, patient not eligible/not appropriate

→ ✳ **G8654** Risk-adjusted functional status change residual scores for the hip not measured because the patient did not complete FOTO'S functional intake on admission and/or follow up status survey near discharge, reason not given

✳ **G8655** Risk-adjusted functional status change residual score for the lower leg, foot or ankle successfully calculated and the score was equal to zero (0) or greater than zero (>0)

✳ **G8656** Risk-adjusted functional status change residual score for the lower leg, foot or ankle successfully calculated and the score was less than zero (<0)

✳ **G8657** Risk-adjusted functional status change residual scores for the lower leg, foot or ankle not measured because the patient did not complete FOTO'S functional intake on admission and/or follow up status survey near discharge, patient not eligible/not appropriate

→ ✳ **G8658** Risk-adjusted functional status change residual scores for the lower leg, foot or ankle not measured because the patient did not complete FOTO'S functional intake on admission and/or follow up status survey near discharge, reason not given

✳ **G8659** Risk-adjusted functional status change residual score for the lumbar spine successfully calculated and the score was equal to zero (0) or greater than zero (>0)

✳ **G8660** Risk-adjusted functional status change residual score for the lumbar spine successfully calculated and the score was less than zero (<0)

✳ **G8661** Risk-adjusted functional status change residual scores for the lumbar spine not measured because the patient did not complete FOTO'S functional intake on admission and/or follow up status survey near discharge, patient not eligible/not appropriate

→ ✳ **G8662** Risk-adjusted functional status change residual scores for the lumbar spine not measured because the patient did not complete FOTO'S functional intake on admission and/or follow up status survey near discharge, reason not given

✳ **G8663** Risk-adjusted functional status change residual score for the shoulder successfully calculated and the score was equal to zero (0) or greater than zero (>0)

✳ **G8664** Risk-adjusted functional status change residual score for the shoulder successfully calculated and the score was less than zero (<0)

✳ **G8665** Risk-adjusted functional status change residual scores for the shoulder not measured because the patient did not complete FOTO'S functional intake on admission and/or follow up status survey near discharge, patient not eligible/not appropriate

→ ✳ **G8666** Risk-adjusted functional status change residual scores for the shoulder not measured because the patient did not complete FOTO'S functional intake on admission and/or follow up status survey near discharge, reason not given

✳ **G8667** Risk-adjusted functional status change residual score for the elbow, wrist or hand successfully calculated and the score was equal to zero (0) or greater than zero (>0)

✳ **G8668** Risk-adjusted functional status change residual score for the elbow, wrist or hand successfully calculated and the score was less than zero (<0)

▶ New   → Revised   ✔ Reinstated   ~~deleted~~ Deleted
⊘ Special coverage instructions   ◆ Not covered or valid by Medicare   ✳ Carrier discretion

✳ **G8669** Risk-adjusted functional status change residual scores for the elbow, wrist or hand not measured because the patient did not complete FOTO'S functional intake on admission and/or follow up status survey near discharge, patient not eligible/not appropriate

→ ✳ **G8670** Risk-adjusted functional status change residual scores for the elbow, wrist or hand not measured because the patient did not complete FOTO'S functional intake on admission and/or follow up status survey near discharge, reason not given

✳ **G8671** Risk-adjusted functional status change residual score for the neck, cranium, mandible, thoracic spine, ribs, or other general orthopedic impairment successfully calculated and the score was equal to zero (0) or greater than zero (>0)

✳ **G8672** Risk-adjusted functional status change residual score for the neck, cranium, mandible, thoracic spine, ribs, or other general orthopedic impairment successfully calculated and the score was less than zero (<0)

✳ **G8673** Risk-adjusted functional status change residual scores for the neck, cranium, mandible, thoracic spine, ribs, or other general orthopedic impairment not measured because the patient did not complete FOTO'S functional intake on admission and/or follow up status survey near discharge, patient not eligible/not appropriate

→ ✳ **G8674** Risk-adjusted functional status change residual scores for the neck, cranium, mandible, thoracic spine, ribs, or other general orthopedic impairment not measured because the patient did not complete FOTO'S functional intake on admission and/or follow up status survey near discharge, reason not given

→ ✳ **G8682** LVF testing performed during the measurement period

→ ✳ **G8683** LVF testing not performed, patient not eligible

→ ✳ **G8685** LVF testing not performed, reason not given

✳ **G8694** Left ventriucular ejection fraction (LVEF) <40%

~~G8695~~ ~~Left ventricular ejection fraction (LVEF) >= 40% or documentation as mildly depressed left ventricular systolic function or normal~~ ✖

✳ **G8696** Antithrombotic therapy prescribed at discharge

→ ✳ **G8697** Antithrombotic therapy not prescribed for documented reasons (e.g., patients admitted for performance of elective carotid intervention, patient had stroke during hospital stay, patient expired during inpatient stay, other medical reason(s)); (e.g., patient left against medical advice, other patient reason(s))

→ ✳ **G8698** Antithrombotic therapy was not prescribed at discharge, reason not given

✳ **G8699** Rehabilitation services (occupational, physical or speech) ordered at or prior to discharge

✳ **G8700** Rehabilitation services (occupational, physical or speech) not indicated at or prior to discharge

✳ **G8701** Rehabilitation services were not ordered, reason not otherwise specified

✳ **G8702** Documentation that prophylactic antibiotics were given within 4 hours prior to surgical incision or intraoperatively

✳ **G8703** Documentation that prophylactic antibiotics were neither given within 4 hours prior to surgical incision nor intraoperatively

✳ **G8704** 12-lead electrocardiogram (ECG) performed

✳ **G8705** Documentation of medical reason(s) for not performing a 12-lead electrocardiogram (ECG)

✳ **G8706** Documentation of patient reason(s) for not performing a 12-lead electrocardiogram (ECG)

→ ✳ **G8707** 12-lead electrocardiogram (ECG) not performed, reason not given

✳ **G8708** Patient not prescribed or dispensed antibiotic

✳ **G8709** Patient prescribed or dispensed antibiotic for documented medical reason(s)

✳ **G8710** Patient prescribed or dispensed antibiotic

✳ **G8711** Prescribed or dispensed antibiotic

✳ **G8712** Antibiotic not prescribed or dispensed

✳ **G8713** SPKT/V greater than or equal to 1.2 (single-pool clearance of urea [KT] / volume [V])

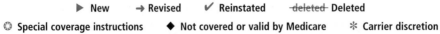

▶ New   → Revised   ✔ Reinstated   ~~deleted~~ Deleted
☉ Special coverage instructions   ◆ Not covered or valid by Medicare   ✳ Carrier discretion

→ ✳ **G8714** Hemodialysis treatment performed exactly three times per week for >90 days

~~**G8715** Hemodialysis treatment performed less than three times per week or greater than three times per week~~ ✘

~~**G8716** Documentation of reason(s) for patient not having greater than or equal to 1.2 (single-pool clearance of urea [KT] / volume [V])~~ ✘

→ ✳ **G8717** SPKT/V less than 1.2 (single-pool clearance of urea [KT] / volume [V]), reason not given

✳ **G8718** Total KT/V greater than or equal to 1.7 per week (total clearance of urea [KT] / volume [V])

→ ✳ **G8720** Total KT/V less than 1.7 per week (total clearance of urea [KT] / volume [V]), reason not given

✳ **G8721** PT category (primary tumor), PN category (regional lymph nodes), and histologic grade were documented in pathology report

→ ✳ **G8722** Medical reason(s) documented for not including PT category, PN category and histologic grade in the pathology report (e.g., anal canal)

✳ **G8723** Specimen site is other than anatomic location of primary tumor

→ ✳ **G8724** PT category, PN category and histologic grade were not documented in the pathology report, reason not given

✳ **G8725** Fasting lipid profile performed (triglycerides, LDL-C, HDL-C and total cholesterol)

→ ✳ **G8726** Clinician has documented reason for not performing fasting lipid profile (e.g., patient declined, other patient reasons)

~~**G8727** Patient receiving hemodialysis, peritoneal dialysis or kidney transplantation~~ ✘

→ ✳ **G8728** Fasting lipid profile not performed, reason not given

✳ **G8730** Pain assessment documented as positive utilizing a standardized tool and a follow-up plan is documented

✳ **G8731** Pain assessment documented as negative, no follow-up plan is required

→ ✳ **G8732** No documentation of pain assessment, reason not given

→ ✳ **G8733** Documentation of a positive elder maltreatment screen and documented follow-up plan at the time of the positive screen

✳ **G8734** Elder maltreatment screen documented as negative, no follow-up required

→ ✳ **G8735** Elder maltreatment screen documented as positive, follow-up plan not documented, reason not given

✳ **G8736** Most current LDL-C <100 mg/dl

✳ **G8737** Most current LDL-C >=100 mg/dl

✳ **G8738** Left ventricular ejection fraction (LVEF) <40% or documentation of severely or moderately depressed left ventricular systolic function

✳ **G8739** Left ventricular ejection fraction (LVEF) >= 40% or documentation as normal or mildly depressed left ventricular systolic function

→ ✳ **G8740** Left ventricular ejection fraction (LVEF) not performed or assessed, reason not given

✳ **G8741** Patient not treated for spoken language comprehension disorder

✳ **G8742** Patient not treated for attention disorder

✳ **G8743** Patient not treated for memory disorder

✳ **G8744** Patient not treated for motor speech disorder

✳ **G8745** Patient not treated for reading disorder

✳ **G8746** Patient not treated for spoken language expression disorder

✳ **G8747** Patient not treated for writing disorder

✳ **G8748** Patient not treated for swallowing disorder

✳ **G8749** Absence of signs of melanoma (cough, dyspnea, tenderness, localized neurologic signs such as weakness, jaundice or any other sign suggesting systemic spread) or absence of symptoms of melanoma (pain, paresthesia, or any other symptom suggesting the possibility of systemic spread of melanoma)

~~**G8750** Presence of signs of melanoma (cough, dyspnea, tenderness, localized neurologic signs such as weakness, jaundice or any other sign suggesting systemic spread) or presence of symptoms of melanoma (pain, paresthesia, or any other symptom suggesting the possibility of systemic spread of melanoma)~~ ✘

▶ **New** → **Revised** ✔ **Reinstated** ~~deleted~~ **Deleted**
⊘ **Special coverage instructions** ◆ **Not covered or valid by Medicare** ✳ **Carrier discretion**

* **G8751** Smoking status and exposure to second-hand smoke in the home not assessed, reason not given

* **G8752** Most recent systolic blood pressure <140 mm hg

* **G8753** Most recent systolic blood pressure >= 140 mm hg

* **G8754** Most recent diastolic blood pressure <90 mm hg

* **G8755** Most recent diastolic blood pressure >= 90 mm hg

→ * **G8756** No documentation of blood pressure measurement, reason not given

→ * **G8757** All quality actions for the applicable measures in the chronic obstructive pulmonary disease (COPD) measures group have been performed for this patient

→ * **G8758** All quality actions for the applicable measures in the inflammatory bowel disease (IBD) measures group have been performed for this patient

→ * **G8759** All quality actions for the applicable measures in the sleep apnea measures group have been performed for this patient

~~G8760~~ ~~All quality actions for the applicable measures in the epilepsy measures group have been performed for this patient~~ ✖

* **G8761** All quality actions for the applicable measures in the dementia measures group have been performed for this patient

* **G8762** All quality actions for the applicable measures in the Parkinson's disease measures group have been performed for this patient

→ * **G8763** All quality actions for the applicable measures in the hypertension (HTN) measures group have been performed for this patient

* **G8764** All quality actions for the applicable measures in the cardiovascular prevention measures group have been performed for this patient

* **G8765** All quality actions for the applicable measures in the cataract measures group have been performed for this patient

* **G8767** Lipid panel results documented and reviewed (must include total cholesterol, HDL-C, triglycerides and calculated LDL-C)

* **G8768** Documentation of medical reason(s) for not performing lipid profile (e.g., patients who have a terminal illness or for whom treatment of hypertension with standard treatment goals is not clinically appropriate)

→ * **G8769** Lipid profile not performed, reason not given

* **G8770** Urine protein test result documented and reviewed

* **G8771** Documentation of diagnosis of chronic kidney disease

* **G8772** Documentation of medical reason(s) for not performing urine protein test (e.g., patients who have a terminal illness or for whom treatment of hypertension with standard treatment goals is not clinically appropriate)

→ * **G8773** Urine protein test was not performed, reason not given

* **G8774** Serum creatinine test result documented and reviewed

* **G8775** Documentation of medical reason(s) for not performing serum creatinine test (e.g., patients who have a terminal illness or for whom treatment of hypertension with standard treatment goals is not clinically appropriate)

→ * **G8776** Serum creatinine test not performed, reason not given

* **G8777** Diabetes screening test performed

* **G8778** Documentation of medical reason(s) for not performing diabetes screening test (e.g., patients who have a terminal illness or for whom treatment of hypertension with standard treatment goals is not clinically appropriate, or patients with a diagnosis of diabetes)

→ * **G8779** Diabetes screening test not performed, reason not given

* **G8780** Counseling for diet and physical activity performed

* **G8781** Documentation of medical reason(s) for patient not receiving counseling for diet and physical activity (e.g., patients who have a terminal illness or for whom treatment of hypertension with standard treatment goals is not clinically appropriate)

→ * **G8782** Counseling for diet and physical activity not performed, reason not given

→ * **G8783** Normal blood pressure reading documented, follow-up not required

▶ New   → Revised   ✔ Reinstated   ~~deleted~~ Deleted

⊚ Special coverage instructions   ◆ Not covered or valid by Medicare   * Carrier discretion

→ ✳ **G8784** Blood pressure reading not documented, patient not eligible/not appropriate

→ ✳ **G8785** Blood pressure reading not documented, reason not given

~~G8786~~ ~~Severity of angina assessed according to level of activity~~ ✖

~~G8787~~ ~~Angina assessed as present~~ ✖

~~G8788~~ ~~Angina assessed as absent~~ ✖

~~G8789~~ ~~Severity of angina not assessed according to level of activity~~ ✖

✳ **G8790** Most recent office visit systolic blood pressure <130 mm hg

✳ **G8791** Most recent office visit systolic blood pressure, 130-139 mm hg

✳ **G8792** Most recent office visit systolic blood pressure >=140 mm hg

✳ **G8793** Most recent office visit diastolic blood pressure, <80 mm hg

✳ **G8794** Most recent office visit diastolic blood pressure, 80-89 mm hg

✳ **G8795** Most recent office visit diastolic blood pressure >=90 mm hg

→ ✳ **G8796** Blood pressure measurement not documented, reason not given

✳ **G8797** Specimen site other than anatomic location of esophagus

✳ **G8798** Specimen site other than anatomic location of prostate

✳ **G8799** Anticoagulation ordered

✳ **G8800** Anticoagulation not ordered for reasons documented by clinician

→ ✳ **G8801** Anticoagulation was not ordered, reason not given

~~G8802~~ ~~Pregnancy test (urine or serum) ordered~~ ✖

~~G8803~~ ~~Pregnancy test (urine or serum) not ordered for reasons documented by clinician~~ ✖

~~G8805~~ ~~Pregnancy test (urine or serum) was not ordered, reason not specified~~ ✖

✳ **G8806** Performance of trans-abdominal or trans-vaginal ultrasound

→ ✳ **G8807** Trans-abdominal or trans-vaginal ultrasound not performed for reasons documented by clinician (e.g., patient has visited the ED multiple times within 72 hours, patient has a documented intrauterine pregnancy [IUP])

→ ✳ **G8808** Performance of trans-abdominal or trans-vaginal ultrasound not ordered, reason not given

✳ **G8809** Rh-immunoglobulin (RhoGAM) ordered

→ ✳ **G8810** Rh-immunoglobulin (RhoGAM) not ordered for reasons documented by clinician (e.g., patient had prior documented report of rhogam within 12 weeks)

→ ✳ **G8811** Documentation RH-immunoglobulin (RhoGAM) was not ordered, reason not given

→ ✳ **G8812** Patient is not eligible for follow-up CTA, duplex, or MRA (e.g., patient death, failure to return for scheduled follow-up exam, planned follow-up study which will meet numerator criteria has not yet occurred at the time of reporting)

✳ **G8813** Follow-up CTA, duplex, or MRA of the abdomen and pelvis performed

✳ **G8814** Follow-up CTA, duplex, or MRA of the abdomen and pelvis not performed

→ ✳ **G8815** Statin therapy not prescribed for documented reasons (e.g., medical intolerance to statin, death of patient prior to discharge, transfer of care to another acute care or federal hospital, hospice admission, left against medical advice)

✳ **G8816** Statin medication prescribed at discharge

→ ✳ **G8817** Statin therapy not prescribed at discharge, reason not given

✳ **G8818** Patient discharge to home no later than post-operative day #7

~~G8819~~ ~~Aneurysm minor diameter <= 5.5 cm~~ ✖

~~G8820~~ ~~Aneurysm minor diameter 5.6-6.0 cm~~ ✖

~~G8821~~ ~~Abdominal aortic aneurysm is not infarenal~~ ✖

~~G8822~~ ~~Male patients with aneurysms minor diameter >6 cm~~ ✖

~~G8823~~ ~~Female patients with aneurysm minor diameter >6 cm~~ ✖

~~G8824~~ ~~Female patients with aneurysm minor diameter 5.6-6.0 cm~~ ✖

✳ **G8825** Patient not discharged to home by post-operative day #7

✳ **G8826** Patient discharge to home no later than post-operative day #2 following EVAR

▶ New   → Revised   ✔ Reinstated   ~~deleted~~ Deleted
☼ Special coverage instructions   ◆ Not covered or valid by Medicare   ✳ Carrier discretion

* **G8827** Aneurysm minor diameter <= 5.5 cm for women

~~G8828~~ ~~Aneurysm minor diameter~~ ~~<= 5.5 cm for men~~ ✖

~~G8829~~ ~~Aneurysm minor diameter~~ ~~5.6-6.0 cm for men~~ ✖

~~G8830~~ ~~Aneurysm minor diameter~~ ~~>6 cm for men~~ ✖

~~G8831~~ ~~Aneurysm minor diameter~~ ~~>6 cm for women~~ ✖

~~G8832~~ ~~Aneurysm minor diameter~~ ~~5.6-6.0 cm for women~~ ✖

→ * **G8833** Patient not discharged to home by post-operative day #2 following EVAR

* **G8834** Patient discharged to home no later than post-operative day #2 following CEA

* **G8835** Asymptomatic patient with no history of any transient ischemic attack or stroke in any carotid or vertebrobasilar territory

~~G8836~~ ~~Symptomatic patient with~~ ~~ipsilateral stroke or TIA within 120~~ ~~days prior to CEA~~ ✖

~~G8837~~ ~~Other symptomatic patient with~~ ~~ipsilateral carotid territory TIA or~~ ~~stroke >120 days prior to CEA, or~~ ~~contralateral carotid territory TIA or~~ ~~stroke or vertebrobasilar TIA or stroke~~ ✖

→ * **G8838** Patient not discharged to home by post-operative day #2 following CEA

* **G8839** Sleep apnea symptoms assessed, including presence or absence of snoring and daytime sleepiness

* **G8840** Documentation of reason(s) for not performing an assessment of sleep symptoms (e.g., patient didn't have initial daytime sleepiness, patient visits between initial testing and initiation of therapy)

→ * **G8841** Sleep apnea symptoms not assessed, reason not given

* **G8842** Apnea Hypopnea Index (AHI) or Respiratory Disturbance Index (RDI) measured at the time of initial diagnosis

→ * **G8843** Documentation of reason(s) for not measuring an Apnea Hypopnea Index (AHI) or a Respiratory Disturbance Index (RDI) at the time of initial diagnosis (e.g., abnormal anatomy, patient declined, financial, insurance coverage)

→ * **G8844** Apnea Hypopnea Index (AHI) or Respiratory Disturbance Index (RDI) not measured at the time of initial diagnosis, reason not given

* **G8845** Positive airway pressure therapy prescribed

* **G8846** Moderate or severe obstructive sleep apnea (Apnea Hypopnea Index (AHI) or Respiratory Disturbance Index (RDI) of 15 or greater)

~~G8847~~ ~~Positive airway pressure therapy~~ ~~not prescribed~~ ✖

* **G8848** Mild obstructive sleep apnea (Apnea Hypopnea Index (AHI) or Respiratory Disturbance Index (RDI) of less than 15)

→ * **G8849** Documentation of reason(s) for not prescribing positive airway pressure therapy (e.g., patient unable to tolerate, alternative therapies use, patient declined, financial, insurance coverage)

→ * **G8850** Positive airway pressure therapy not prescribed, reason not given

* **G8851** Objective measurement of adherence to positive airway pressure therapy, documented

* **G8852** Positive airway pressure therapy prescribed

* **G8853** Positive airway pressure therapy not prescribed

→ * **G8854** Documentation of reason(s) for not objectively measuring adherence to positive airway pressure therapy (e.g., patient didn't bring data from continuous positive airway pressure [CPAP], therapy was not yet initiated, not available on machine)

→ * **G8855** Objective measurement of adherence to positive airway pressure therapy not performed, reason not given

* **G8856** Referral to a physician for an otologic evaluation performed

* **G8857** Patient is not eligible for the referral for otologic evaluation measure (e.g., patients who are already under the care of a physician for acute or chronic dizziness)

▶ New   → Revised   ✔ Reinstated   ~~deleted~~ Deleted

⊙ Special coverage instructions   ◆ Not covered or valid by Medicare   ✳ Carrier discretion

→ ✳ **G8858** Referral to a physician for an otologic evaluation not performed, reason not given

✳ **G8859** Patient receiving corticosteroids greater than or equal to 10 mg/day for 60 or greater consecutive days

✳ **G8860** Patients who have received dose of corticosteroids greater than or equal to 10 mg/day for 60 or greater consecutive days

✳ **G8861** Central dual-energy x-ray absorptiometry (DXA) ordered or documented, review of systems and medication history or pharmacologic therapy (other than minerals/vitamins) for osteoporosis prescribed

✳ **G8862** Patients not receiving corticosteroids greater than or equal to 10 mg/day for 60 or greater consecutive days

→ ✳ **G8863** Patients not assessed for risk of bone loss, reason not given

✳ **G8864** Pneumococcal vaccine administered or previously received

✳ **G8865** Documentation of medical reason(s) for not administering or previously receiving pneumococcal vaccine (e.g., patient allergic reaction, potential adverse drug reaction)

✳ **G8866** Documentation of patient reason(s) for not administering or previously receiving pneumococcal vaccine (e.g., patient refusal)

→ ✳ **G8867** Pneumococcal vaccine not administered or previously received, reason not given

✳ **G8868** Patients receiving a first course of anti-TNF therapy

✳ **G8869** Patient has documented immunity to hepatitis B and is receiving a first course of anti-TNF therapy

✳ **G8870** Hepatitis B vaccine injection administered or previously received and is receiving a first course of anti-TNF therapy

✳ **G8871** Patient not receiving a first course of anti-TNF therapy

✳ **G8872** Excised tissue evaluated by imaging intraoperatively to confirm successful inclusion of targeted lesion

→ ✳ **G8873** Patients with needle localization specimens which are not amenable to intraoperative imaging such as MRI needle wire localization, or targets which are tentatively identified on mammogram or ultrasound which do not contain a biopsy marker but which can be verified on intraoperative inspection or pathology (e.g., needle biopsy site where the biopsy marker is remote from the actual biopsy site)

✳ **G8874** Excised tissue not evaluated by imaging intraoperatively to confirm successful inclusion of targeted lesion

✳ **G8875** Clinician diagnosed breast cancer preoperatively by a minimally invasive biopsy method

→ ✳ **G8876** Documentation of reason(s) for not performing minimally invasive biopsy to diagnose breast cancer properatively (e.g., clinical and imaging findings consistent with a benign lesion, lesion too close to skin, implant, chest wall, etc., lesion could not be adequately visualized for needle biopsy, patient condition prevents needle biopsy [weight, breast thickness, etc.], duct excision without imaging abnormality, prophylactic mastectomy, reduction mammoplasty, excisional biopsy performed by another physician)

→ ✳ **G8877** Clinician did not attempt to achieve the diagnosis of breast cancer preoperatively by a minimally invasive biopsy method, reason not given

✳ **G8878** Sentinel lymph node biopsy procedure performed

✳ **G8879** Clinically node negative (T1N0M0 or T2N0M0) invasive breast cancer

→ ✳ **G8880** Documentation of reason(s) sentinel lymph node biopsy not performed (e.g., cancer diagnosed at prophylactic mastectomy, non-invasive cancer, incidental discovery of breast cancer on prophylactic mastectomy, incidental discovery of breast cancer on reduction mammoplasty, biopsy proven lymph node (LN) metastases [e.g., pre-op FNA or core biopsy, inflammatory carcinoma, recurrent invasive breast cancer], patient refusal after informed consent)

✳ **G8881** Stage of breast cancer is greater than T1N0M0 or T2N0M0

✳ **G8882** Sentinel lymph node biopsy procedure not performed

---

▶ New   → Revised   ✔ Reinstated   ~~deleted~~ Deleted
☺ Special coverage instructions   ◆ Not covered or valid by Medicare   ✳ Carrier discretion

* **G8883** Biopsy results reviewed, communicated, tracked and documented

* **G8884** Clinician documented reason that patient's biopsy results were not reviewed

* **G8885** Biopsy results not reviewed, communicated, tracked or documented

* **G8886** Most recent blood pressure under control

→ * **G8887** Documentation of medical reason(s) for most recent blood pressure not being under control (e.g., patients who had a terminal illness or for whom treatment of hypertension with standard treatment goals is not clinically appropriate)

* **G8888** Most recent blood pressure not under control, results documented and reviewed

→ * **G8889** No documentation of blood pressure measurement, reason not given

* **G8890** Most recent LDL-C under control, results documented and reviewed

* **G8891** Documentation of medical reason(s) for most recent LSL-C not under control (e.g., patients who had a terminal illness or for whom treatment of hypertension with standard treatment goals is not clinically appropriate)

* **G8892** Documentation of medical reason(s) for not performing LDL-C test (e.g., patients who had a terminal illness or for whom treatment of hypertension with standard treatment goals is not clinically appropriate)

* **G8893** Most recent LDL-C not under control, results documented and reviewed

→ * **G8894** LDL-C not performed, reason not given

→ * **G8895** Oral aspirin or other antithrombotic therapy prescribed

→ * **G8896** Documentation of medical reason(s) for not prescribing oral aspirin or other antithrombotic therapy (e.g., patient documented to be low risk or patient with terminal illness or treatment of hypertension with standard treatment goals is not clinically appropriate or for whom risk of aspirin or other antithrombotic therapy exceeds potential benefits such as for individuals whose blood pressure is poorly controlled)

→ * **G8897** Oral aspirin or other antithrombotic therapy was not prescribed, reason not given

→ * **G8898** I intend to report the chronic obstructive pulmonary disease (COPD) measures group

→ * **G8899** I intend to report the inflammatory bowel disease (IBD) measures group

→ * **G8900** I intend to report the sleep apnea measures group

~~G8901~~ ~~I intend to report the epilepsy measures group~~ ✖

* **G8902** I intend to report the dementia measures group

* **G8903** I intend to report the Parkinson's disease measures group

→ * **G8904** I intend to report the hypertension (HTN) measures group

* **G8905** I intend to report the cardiovascular prevention measures group

* **G8906** I intend to report the cataract measures group

▶ * **G8907** Patient documented not to have experienced any of the following events: a burn prior to discharge; a fall within the facility; wrong site/side/patient/procedure/implant event; or a hospital transfer or hospital admission upon discharge from the facility

▶ * **G8908** Patient documented to have received a burn prior to discharge

▶ * **G8909** Patient documented not to have received a burn prior to discharge

▶ * **G8910** Patient documented to have experienced a fall within ASC

▶ * **G8911** Patient documented not to have experienced a fall within ambulatory surgical center

▶ * **G8912** Patient documented to have experienced a wrong site, wrong side, wrong patient, wrong procedure or wrong implant event

▶ * **G8913** Patient documented not to have experienced a wrong site, wrong side, wrong patient, wrong procedure or wrong implant event

▶ * **G8914** Patient documented to have experienced a hospital transfer or hospital admission upon discharge from ASC

▶ * **G8915** Patient documented not to have experienced a hospital transfer or hospital admission upon discharge from ASC

▶ New → Revised ✔ Reinstated ~~deleted~~ Deleted

☺ Special coverage instructions ◆ Not covered or valid by Medicare * Carrier discretion

▶ ✳ **G8916** Patient with preoperative order for IV antibiotic surgical site infection (SSI) prophylaxis, antibiotic initiated on time

▶ ✳ **G8917** Patient with preoperative order for IV antibiotic surgical site infection (SSI) prophylaxis, antibiotic not initiated on time

▶ ✳ **G8918** Patient without preoperative order for IV antibiotic surgical site infection(SSI) prophylaxis

▶ ✳ **G8919** Most recent systolic blood pressure <140 mmhg

▶ ✳ **G8920** Most recent systolic blood pressure >= 140 mmhg

▶ ✳ **G8921** Most recent diastolic blood pressure <90 mmhg

▶ ✳ **G8922** Most recent diastolic blood pressure >= 90 mmhg

▶ ✳ **G8923** Left ventricular ejection fraction (LVEF) <40% or documentation of moderately or severely depressed left ventricular systolic function

▶ ✳ **G8924** Spirometry test results demonstrate FEV1/FVC <60% with COPD symptoms (e.g., dyspnea, cough/sputum, wheezing)

▶ ✳ **G8925** Spirometry test results demonstrate FEV1/FVC >=60% or patient does not have COPD symptoms

▶ ✳ **G8926** Spirometry test not performed or documented, reason not given

▶ ✳ **G8927** Adjuvant chemotherapy referred, prescribed or previously received for AJCC stage III, colon cancer

▶ ✳ **G8928** Adjuvant chemotherapy not prescribed or previously received, reason given

▶ ✳ **G8929** Adjuvant chemotherapy not prescribed or previously received, reason not given

▶ ✳ **G8930** Assessment of depression severity not documented, reason not given

▶ ✳ **G8931** Assessment of depression severity not documented, reason not given

▶ ✳ **G8932** Suicide risk assessed at the initial evaluation

▶ ✳ **G8933** Suicide risk not assessed at the initial evaluation, reason not given

▶ ✳ **G8934** Left ventricular ejection fraction (LVEF) <40% or documentation of moderately or severely depressed left ventricular systolic function

▶ ✳ **G8935** Clinician prescribed angiotensin converting enzyme (ACE) inhibitor or angiotensin receptor blocker (ARB) therapy

▶ ✳ **G8936** Clinician documented that patient was not an eligible candidate for angiotensin converting enzyme (ACE) inhibitor or angiotensin receptor blocker (ARB) therapy

▶ ✳ **G8937** Clinician did not prescribe angiotensin converting enzyme (ACE) inhibitor or angiotensin receptor blocker (ARB) therapy, reason not given

▶ ✳ **G8938** BMI is calculated, but patient not eligible for follow-up plan

▶ ✳ **G8939** Pain assessment documented, follow-up plan not documented, patient not eligible/appropriate

▶ ✳ **G8940** Screening for clinical depression documented, follow-up plan not documented, patient not eligible/appropriate

▶ ✳ **G8941** Elder maltreatment screen documented, patient not eligible for follow-up

▶ ✳ **G8942** Documented functional outcomes assessment and care plan within the previous 30 days

▶ ✳ **G8943** LDL-C result not present or not within 12 months prior

▶ ✳ **G8944** AJCC melanoma cancer stage 0 through IIC melanoma

▶ ✳ **G8945** Aneurysm minor diameter <= 6 cm for men

▶ ✳ **G8946** Minimally invasive biopsy method attempted but not diagnostic of breast cancer(e.g., high risk lesion of breast such as atypical ductal hyperplasia, lobular neoplasia, atypical lobular carcinoma in situ, atypical columnar hyperplasica, flat epithelial atypia, radial scar, complex sclerosing lesion, papillary lesion, or any lesion with spindle cells)

▶ ✳ **G8947** One or more neuropsychiatric symptoms

▶ ✳ **G8948** No neuropsychiatric symptoms

▶ ✳ **G8949** Documentation of patient reason(s) for patient not receiving counseling for diet and physical activity (e.g., patient is not willing to discuss diet or exercise interventions to help control blood pressure, or the patient said he/she refused to make these changes)

▶ New → Revised ✔ Reinstated ~~deleted~~ Deleted

☺ Special coverage instructions ◆ Not covered or valid by Medicare ✳ Carrier discretion

▶ ✳ **G8950** Pre-hypertensive or hypertensive blood pressure reading documented, indicated follow-up documented

▶ ✳ **G8951** Pre-hypertensive or hypertensive blood pressure reading documented, indicated follow-up not documented, patient not eligible/not appropriate

▶ ✳ **G8952** Pre-hypertensive or hypertensive blood pressure reading documented, indicated follow-up not documented, reason not given

▶ ✳ **G8953** All quality actions for the applicable measures in the oncology measures group have been performed for this patient

▶ ✳ **G8954** Complete and appropriate patient data were reported to a qualified clinical database registry

▶ ✳ **G8955** Most recent assessment of adequacy of volume management

▶ ✳ **G8956** Patient receiving maintenance hemodialysis in an outpatient dialysis facility

▶ ✳ **G8957** Patient not receiving maintenance hemodialysis in an outpatient dialysis facility

▶ ✳ **G8958** Assessment of adequacy of volume management not documented, reason not given

▶ ✳ **G8959** Clinician treating major depressive disorder communicates to clinician treating comorbid condition

▶ ✳ **G8960** Clinician treating major depressive disorder did not communicate to clinician treating comorbid condition, reason not given

▶ ✳ **G8961** Cardiac stress imaging test primarily performed on low-risk surgery patient for preoperative evaluation within 30 days preceding this surgery

▶ ✳ **G8962** Cardiac stress imaging test performed on patient for any reason including those who did not have low risk surgery or test that was performed more than 30 days preceding low risk surgery

▶ ✳ **G8963** Cardiac stress imaging performed primarily for monitoring of asymptomatic patient who had PCI within 2 years

▶ ✳ **G8964** Cardiac stress imaging test performed primarily for any other reason than monitoring of asymptomatic patient who had PCI within 2 years (e.g., symptomatic patient, patient greater than 2 years since PCI, initial evaluation, etc.)

▶ ✳ **G8965** Cardiac stress imaging test primarily performed on low CHD risk patient for initial detection and risk assessment

▶ ✳ **G8966** Cardiac stress imaging test performed on symptomatic or higher than low CHD risk patient or for any reason other than initial detection and risk assessment

▶ ✳ **G8967** Warfarin or another oral anticoagulant that is FDA approved prescribed

▶ ✳ **G8968** Documentation of medical reason(s) for not prescribing warfarin or another oral anticoagulant that is FDA approved not prescribed (e.g., allergy, risk of bleeding, transient or reversible causes of atrial fibrillation, other medical reasons including, but not limited to pregnancy, mitral stenosis, prosthetic heart valve or patient is in the postoperative period)

▶ ✳ **G8969** Documentation of patient reason(s) for not prescribing warfarin or another oral anticoagulant that is FDA approved (e.g., economic, social, and/or religious impediments, noncompliance or patient refusal, other patient reasons)

▶ ✳ **G8970** No risk factors or one moderate risk factor for thromboembolism

▶ ✳ **G8971** Warfarin or another oral anticoagulant that is FDA approved not prescribed, reason not given

▶ ✳ **G8972** One or more high risk factors for thromboembolism or more than one moderate risk factor for thromboembolism

▶ ✳ **G8973** Most recent hemoglobin (Hgb) level <10 g/dl

▶ ✳ **G8974** Hemoglobin level measurement not documented, reason not given

---

▶ New   → Revised   ✔ Reinstated   ~~deleted~~ Deleted
⊙ Special coverage instructions   ◆ Not covered or valid by Medicare   ✳ Carrier discretion

▶ ✳ **G8975** Documentation of medical reason(s) for patient having a hemoglobin level <10 g/dl (e.g., patients who have non-renal etiologies of anemia [e.g., sickle cell anemia or other hemoglobinopathies, hypersplenism, primary bone marrow disease, anemia related to chemotherapy for diagnosis of malignancy, postoperative bleeding, active bloodstream or peritoneal infection], other medical reasons)

▶ ✳ **G8976** Most recent hemoglobin (Hgb) level >= 10 g/dl

▶ ✳ **G8977** I intend to report the oncology measures group

▶ ✳ **G8978** Mobility: walking & moving around functional limitation, current status, at therapy episode outset and at reporting intervals

▶ ✳ **G8979** Mobility: walking & moving around functional limitation, projected goal status, at therapy episode outset, at reporting intervals, and at discharge or to end reporting

▶ ✳ **G8980** Mobility: walking & moving around functional limitation, discharge status, at discharge from therapy or to end reporting

▶ ✳ **G8981** Changing & maintaining body position functional limitation, current status, at therapy episode outset and at reporting intervals

▶ ✳ **G8982** Changing & maintaining body position functional limitation, projected goal status, at therapy episode outset, at reporting intervals, and at discharge or to end reporting

▶ ✳ **G8983** Changing & maintaining body position functional limitation, discharge status, at discharge from therapy or to end reporting

▶ ✳ **G8984** Carrying, moving & handling objects functional limitation, current status, at therapy episode outset and at reporting intervals

▶ ✳ **G8985** Carrying, moving & handling objects functional limitation, current status, at therapy episode outset and at reporting intervals

▶ ✳ **G8986** Carrying, moving & handling objects functional limitation, discharge status, at discharge from therapy or to end reporting

▶ ✳ **G8987** Self-care functional limitation, current status, at therapy episode outset and at reporting intervals

▶ ✳ **G8988** Self-care functional limitation, projected goal status, at therapy episode outset, at reporting intervals, and at discharge or to end reporting

▶ ✳ **G8989** Self-care functional limitation, discharge status, at discharge from therapy or to end reporting

▶ ✳ **G8990** Other physical or occupational primary functional limitation, current status, at therapy episode outset and at reporting intervals

▶ ✳ **G8991** Other physical or occupational primary functional limitation, projected goal status, at therapy episode outset, at reporting intervals, and at discharge or to end reporting

▶ ✳ **G8992** Other physical or occupational primary functional limitation, discharge status, at discharge from therapy or to end reporting

▶ ✳ **G8993** Other physical or occupational subsequent functional limitation, current status, at therapy episode outset and at reporting intervals

▶ ✳ **G8994** Other physical or occupational subsequent functional limitation, projected goal status, at therapy episode outset, at reporting intervals, and at discharge or to end reporting

▶ ✳ **G8995** Other physical or occupational subsequent functional limitation, discharge status, at discharge from therapy or to end reporting

▶ ✳ **G8996** Swallowing functional limitation, current status at time of initial therapy treatment/episode outset and reporting intervals

▶ ✳ **G8997** Swallowing functional limitation, projected goal status, at initial therapy treatment/outset and at discharge from therapy

▶ ✳ **G8998** Swallowing functional limitation, discharge status, at discharge from therapy/end of reporting on limitation

▶ ✳ **G8999** Motor speech functional limitation, current status at time of initial therapy treatment/episode outset and reporting intervals

☺ **G9001** Coordinated care fee, initial rate

☺ **G9002** Coordinated care fee, maintenance rate

▶ New → Revised ✔ Reinstated ~~deleted~~ Deleted
☺ Special coverage instructions ◆ Not covered or valid by Medicare ✳ Carrier discretion

⊙ **G9003**   Coordinated care fee, risk adjusted high, initial

⊙ **G9004**   Coordinated care fee, risk adjusted low, initial

⊙ **G9005**   Coordinated care fee, risk adjusted maintenance

⊙ **G9006**   Coordinated care fee, home monitoring

⊙ **G9007**   Coordinated care fee, scheduled team conference

⊙ **G9008**   Coordinated care fee, physician coordinated care oversight services

⊙ **G9009**   Coordinated care fee, risk adjusted maintenance, level 3

⊙ **G9010**   Coordinated care fee, risk adjusted maintenance, level 4

⊙ **G9011**   Coordinated care fee, risk adjusted maintenance, level 5

⊙ **G9012**   Other specified case management services not elsewhere classified

◆ **G9013**   ESRD demo basic bundle Level I

Medicare non-covered.

◆ **G9014**   ESRD demo expanded bundle, including venous access and related services

Medicare non-covered.

◆ **G9016**   Smoking cessation counseling, individual, in the absence of or in addition to any other evaluation and management service, per session (6-10 minutes) [demo project code only]

Medicare non-covered.

✳ **G9017**   Amantadine hydrochloride, oral, per 100 mg (for use in a Medicare-approved demonstration project)

✳ **G9018**   Zanamivir, inhalation powder, administered through inhaler, per 10 mg (for use in a Medicare-approved demonstration project)

✳ **G9019**   Oseltamivir phosphate, oral, per 75 mg (for use in a Medicare-approved demonstration project)

✳ **G9020**   Rimantadine hydrochloride, oral, per 100 mg (for use in a Medicare-approved demonstration project)

✳ **G9033**   Amantadine hydrochloride, oral brand, per 100 mg (for use in a Medicare-approved demonstration project)

✳ **G9034**   Zanamivir, inhalation powder, administered through inhaler, brand, per 10 mg (for use in a Medicare-approved demonstration project)

✳ **G9035**   Oseltamivir phosphate, oral, brand, per 75 mg (for use in a Medicare-approved demonstration project)

✳ **G9036**   Rimantadine hydrochloride, oral, brand, per 100 mg (for use in a Medicare-approved demonstration project)

◆ **G9050**   Oncology; primary focus of visit; work-up, evaluation, or staging at the time of cancer diagnosis or recurrence (for use in a Medicare-approved demonstration project)

◆ **G9051**   Oncology; primary focus of visit; treatment decision-making after disease is staged or restaged, discussion of treatment options, supervising/ coordinating active cancer directed therapy or managing consequences of cancer directed therapy (for use in a Medicare-approved demonstration project)

◆ **G9052**   Oncology; primary focus of visit; surveillance for disease recurrence for patient who has completed definitive cancer-directed therapy and currently lacks evidence of recurrent disease; cancer directed therapy might be considered in the future (for use in a Medicare-approved demonstration project)

◆ **G9053**   Oncology; primary focus of visit; expectant management of patient with evidence of cancer for whom no cancer directed therapy is being administered or arranged at present; cancer directed therapy might be considered in the future (for use in a Medicare-approved demonstration project)

◆ **G9054**   Oncology; primary focus of visit; supervising, coordinating or managing care of patient with terminal cancer or for whom other medical illness prevents further cancer treatment; includes symptom management, end-of-life care planning, management of palliative therapies (for use in a Medicare-approved demonstration project)

◆ **G9055**   Oncology; primary focus of visit; other, unspecified service not otherwise listed (for use in a Medicare-approved demonstration project)

◆ **G9056**   Oncology; practice guidelines; management adheres to guidelines (for use in a Medicare-approved demonstration project)

▶ New   → Revised   ✔ Reinstated   ~~deleted~~ Deleted

⊙ Special coverage instructions   ◆ Not covered or valid by Medicare   ✳ Carrier discretion

◆ **G9057** Oncology; practice guidelines; management differs from guidelines as a result of patient enrollment in an institutional review board approved clinical trial (for use in a Medicare-approved demonstration project)

◆ **G9058** Oncology; practice guidelines; management differs from guidelines because the treating physician disagrees with guideline recommendations (for use in a Medicare-approved demonstration project)

◆ **G9059** Oncology; practice guidelines; management differs from guidelines because the patient, after being offered treatment consistent with guidelines, has opted for alternative treatment or management, including no treatment (for use in a Medicare-approved demonstration project)

◆ **G9060** Oncology; practice guidelines; management differs from guidelines for reason(s) associated with patient comorbid illness or performance status not factored into guidelines (for use in a Medicare-approved demonstration project)

◆ **G9061** Oncology; practice guidelines; patient's condition not addressed by available guidelines (for use in a Medicare-approved demonstration project)

◆ **G9062** Oncology; practice guidelines; management differs from guidelines for other reason(s) not listed (for use in a Medicare-approved demonstration project)

✳ **G9063** Oncology; disease status; limited to non-small cell lung cancer; extent of disease initially established as stage I (prior to neo-adjuvant therapy, if any) with no evidence of disease progression, recurrence, or metastases (for use in a Medicare-approved demonstration project)

✳ **G9064** Oncology; disease status; limited to non-small cell lung cancer; extent of disease initially established as stage II (prior to neo-adjuvant therapy, if any) with no evidence of disease progression, recurrence, or metastases (for use in a Medicare-approved demonstration project)

✳ **G9065** Oncology; disease status; limited to non-small cell lung cancer; extent of disease initially established as stage IIIA (prior to neo-adjuvant therapy, if any) with no evidence of disease progression, recurrence, or metastases (for use in a Medicare-approved demonstration project)

✳ **G9066** Oncology; disease status; limited to non-small cell lung cancer; stage IIIB-IV at diagnosis, metastatic, locally recurrent, or progressive (for use in a Medicare-approved demonstration project)

✳ **G9067** Oncology; disease status; limited to non-small cell lung cancer; extent of disease unknown, staging in progress, or not listed (for use in a Medicare-approved demonstration project)

✳ **G9068** Oncology; disease status; limited to small cell and combined small cell/non-small cell; extent of disease initially established as limited with no evidence of disease progression, recurrence, or metastases (for use in a Medicare-approved demonstration project)

✳ **G9069** Oncology; disease status; small cell lung cancer, limited to small cell and combined small cell/non-small cell; extensive stage at diagnosis, metastatic, locally recurrent, or progressive (for use in a Medicare-approved demonstration project)

✳ **G9070** Oncology; disease status; small cell lung cancer, limited to small cell and combined small cell/non-small cell; extent of disease unknown, staging in progress, or not listed (for use in a Medicare-approved demonstration project)

✳ **G9071** Oncology; disease status; invasive female breast cancer (does not include ductal carcinoma in situ); adenocarcinoma as predominant cell type; stage I or stage IIA-IIB; or T3, N1, M0; and ER and/or PR positive; with no evidence of disease progression, recurrence, or metastases (for use in a Medicare-approved demonstration project)

▶ New → Revised ✔ Reinstated deleted Deleted
○ Special coverage instructions ◆ Not covered or valid by Medicare ✳ Carrier discretion

* **G9072** Oncology; disease status; invasive female breast cancer (does not include ductal carcinoma in situ); adenocarcinoma as predominant cell type; stage I, or stage IIA-IIB; or T3, N1, M0; and ER and PR negative; with no evidence of disease progression, recurrence, or metastases (for use in a Medicare-approved demonstration project)

* **G9073** Oncology; disease status; invasive female breast cancer (does not include ductal carcinoma in situ); adenocarcinoma as predominant cell type; stage IIIA-IIIB; and not T3, N1, M0; and ER and/or PR positive; with no evidence of disease progression, recurrence, or metastases (for use in a Medicare-approved demonstration project)

* **G9074** Oncology; disease status; invasive female breast cancer (does not include ductal carcinoma in situ); adenocarcinoma as predominant cell type; stage IIIA-IIIB; and not T3, N1, M0; and ER and PR negative; with no evidence of disease progression, recurrence, or metastases (for use in a Medicare-approved demonstration project)

* **G9075** Oncology; disease status; invasive female breast cancer (does not include ductal carcinoma in situ); adenocarcinoma as predominant cell type; M1 at diagnosis, metastatic, locally recurrent, or progressive (for use in a Medicare-approved demonstration project)

* **G9077** Oncology; disease status; prostate cancer, limited to adenocarcinoma as predominant cell type; T1-T2c and Gleason 2-7 and PSA < or equal to 20 at diagnosis with no evidence of disease progression, recurrence, or metastases (for use in a Medicare-approved demonstration project)

* **G9078** Oncology; disease status; prostate cancer, limited to adenocarcinoma as predominant cell type; T2 or T3a Gleason 8-10 or PSA > 20 at diagnosis with no evidence of disease progression, recurrence, or metastases (for use in a Medicare-approved demonstration project)

* **G9079** Oncology; disease status; prostate cancer, limited to adenocarcinoma as predominant cell type; T3b-T4, any N; any T, N1 at diagnosis with no evidence of disease progression, recurrence, or metastases (for use in a Medicare-approved demonstration project)

* **G9080** Oncology; disease status; prostate cancer, limited to adenocarcinoma; after initial treatment with rising PSA or failure of PSA decline (for use in a Medicare-approved demonstration project)

* **G9083** Oncology; disease status; prostate cancer, limited to adenocarcinoma; extent of disease unknown, staging in progress, or not listed (for use in a Medicare-approved demonstration project)

* **G9084** Oncology; disease status; colon cancer, limited to invasive cancer, adenocarcinoma as predominant cell type; extent of disease initially established as T1-3, N0, M0 with no evidence of disease progression, recurrence, or metastases (for use in a Medicare-approved demonstration project)

* **G9085** Oncology; disease status; colon cancer, limited to invasive cancer, adenocarcinoma as predominant cell type; extent of disease initially established as T4, N0, M0 with no evidence of disease progression, recurrence, or metastases (for use in a Medicare-approved demonstration project)

* **G9086** Oncology; disease status; colon cancer, limited to invasive cancer, adenocarcinoma as predominant cell type; extent of disease initially established as T1-4, N1-2, M0 with no evidence of disease progression, recurrence, or metastases (for use in a Medicare-approved demonstration project)

* **G9087** Oncology; disease status; colon cancer, limited to invasive cancer, adenocarcinoma as predominant cell type; M1 at diagnosis, metastatic, locally recurrent, or progressive with current clinical, radiologic, or biochemical evidence of disease (for use in a Medicare-approved demonstration project)

▶ New   → Revised   ✔ Reinstated   ~~deleted~~ Deleted
○ Special coverage instructions   ◆ Not covered or valid by Medicare   * Carrier discretion

✳ **G9088** Oncology; disease status; colon cancer, limited to invasive cancer, adenocarcinoma as predominant cell type; M1 at diagnosis, metastatic, locally recurrent, or progressive without current clinical, radiologic, or biochemical evidence of disease (for use in a Medicare-approved demonstration project)

✳ **G9089** Oncology; disease status; colon cancer, limited to invasive cancer, adenocarcinoma as predominant cell type; extent of disease unknown, staging in progress, or not listed (for use in a Medicare-approved demonstration project)

✳ **G9090** Oncology; disease status; rectal cancer, limited to invasive cancer, adenocarcinoma as predominant cell type; extent of disease initially established as T1-2, N0, M0 (prior to neo-adjuvant therapy, if any) with no evidence of disease progression, recurrence, or metastases (for use in a Medicare-approved demonstration project)

✳ **G9091** Oncology; disease status; rectal cancer, limited to invasive cancer, adenocarcinoma as predominant cell type; extent of disease initially established as T3, N0, M0 (prior to neo-adjuvant therapy, if any) with no evidence of disease progression, recurrence, or metastases (for use in a Medicare-approved demonstration project)

✳ **G9092** Oncology; disease status; rectal cancer, limited to invasive cancer, adenocarcinoma as predominant cell type; extent of disease initially established as T1-3, N1-2, M0 (prior to neo-adjuvant therapy, if any) with no evidence of disease progression, recurrence or metastases (for use in a Medicare-approved demonstration project)

✳ **G9093** Oncology; disease status; rectal cancer, limited to invasive cancer, adenocarcinoma as predominant cell type; extent of disease initially established as T4, any N, M0 (prior to neo-adjuvant therapy, if any) with no evidence of disease progression, recurrence, or metastases (for use in a Medicare-approved demonstration project)

✳ **G9094** Oncology; disease status; rectal cancer, limited to invasive cancer, adenocarcinoma as predominant cell type; M1 at diagnosis, metastatic, locally recurrent, or progressive (for use in a Medicare-approved demonstration project)

✳ **G9095** Oncology; disease status; rectal cancer, limited to invasive cancer, adenocarcinoma as predominant cell type; extent of disease unknown, staging in progress, or not listed (for use in a Medicare-approved demonstration project)

✳ **G9096** Oncology; disease status; esophageal cancer, limited to adenocarcinoma or squamous cell carcinoma as predominant cell type; extent of disease initially established as T1-T3, N0-N1 or NX (prior to neo-adjuvant therapy, if any) with no evidence of disease progression, recurrence, or metastases (for use in a Medicare-approved demonstration project)

✳ **G9097** Oncology; disease status; esophageal cancer, limited to adenocarcinoma or squamous cell carcinoma as predominant cell type; extent of disease initially established as T4, any N, M0 (prior to neo-adjuvant therapy, if any) with no evidence of disease progression, recurrence, or metastases (for use in a Medicare-approved demonstration project)

✳ **G9098** Oncology; disease status; esophageal cancer, limited to adenocarcinoma or squamous cell carcinoma as predominant cell type; M1 at diagnosis, meta-static, locally recurrent, or progressive (for use in a Medicare-approved demonstration project)

✳ **G9099** Oncology; disease status; esophageal cancer, limited to adenocarcinoma or squamous cell carcinoma as predominant cell type; extent of disease unknown, staging in progress, or not listed (for use in a Medicare-approved demonstration project)

✳ **G9100** Oncology; disease status; gastric cancer, limited to adenocarcinoma as predominant cell type; post R0 resection (with or without neoadjuvant therapy) with no evidence of disease recurrence, progression, or metastases (for use in a Medicare-approved demonstration project)

▶ New	→ Revised	✔ Reinstated	~~deleted~~ Deleted
☼ Special coverage instructions	◆ Not covered or valid by Medicare	✳ Carrier discretion	

✳ **G9101**   Oncology; disease status; gastric cancer, limited to adenocarcinoma as predominant cell type; post R1 or R2 resection (with or without neoadjuvant therapy) with no evidence of disease progression, or metastases (for use in a Medicare-approved demonstration project)

✳ **G9102**   Oncology; disease status; gastric cancer, limited to adenocarcinoma as predominant cell type; clinical or pathologic M0, unresectable with no evidence of disease progression, or metastases (for use in a Medicare-approved demonstration project)

✳ **G9103**   Oncology; disease status; gastric cancer, limited to adenocarcinoma as predominant cell type; clinical or pathologic M1 at diagnosis, metastatic, locally recurrent, or progressive (for use in a Medicare-approved demonstration project)

✳ **G9104**   Oncology; disease status; gastric cancer, limited to adenocarcinoma as predominant cell type; extent of disease unknown, staging in progress, or not listed (for use in a Medicare-approved demonstration project)

✳ **G9105**   Oncology; disease status; pancreatic cancer, limited to adenocarcinoma as predominant cell type; post R0 resection without evidence of disease progression, recurrence, or metastases (for use in a Medicare-approved demonstration project)

✳ **G9106**   Oncology; disease status; pancreatic cancer, limited to adenocarcinoma; post R1 or R2 resection with no evidence of disease progression or metastases (for use in a Medicare-approved demonstration project)

✳ **G9107**   Oncology; disease status; pancreatic cancer, limited to adenocarcinoma; unresectable at diagnosis, M1 at diagnosis, metastatic, locally recurrent, or progressive (for use in a Medicare-approved demonstration project)

✳ **G9108**   Oncology; disease status; pancreatic cancer, limited to adenocarcinoma; extent of disease unknown, staging in progress, or not listed (for use in a Medicare-approved demonstration project)

✳ **G9109**   Oncology; disease status; head and neck cancer, limited to cancers of oral cavity, pharynx and larynx with squamous cell as predominant cell type; extent of disease initially established as T1-T2 and N0, M0 (prior to neo-adjuvant therapy, if any) with no evidence of disease progression, recurrence, or metastases (for use in a Medicare-approved demonstration project)

✳ **G9110**   Oncology; disease status; head and neck cancer, limited to cancers of oral cavity, pharynx, and larynx with squamous cell as predominant cell type; extent of disease initially established as T3-4 and/ or N1-3, M0 (prior to neo-adjuvant therapy, if any) with no evidence of disease progression, recurrence, or metastases (for use in a Medicare-approved demonstration project)

✳ **G9111**   Oncology; disease status; head and neck cancer, limited to cancers of oral cavity, pharynx and larynx with squamous cell as predominant cell type; M1 at diagnosis, metastatic, locally recurrent, or progressive (for use in a Medicare-approved demonstration project)

✳ **G9112**   Oncology; disease status; head and neck cancer, limited to cancers of oral cavity, pharynx and larynx with squamous cell as predominant cell type; extent of disease unknown, staging in progress, or not listed (for use in a Medicare-approved demonstration project)

✳ **G9113**   Oncology; disease status; ovarian cancer, limited to epithelial cancer; pathologic stage IA-B (grade 1) without evidence of disease progression, recurrence, or metastases (for use in a Medicare-approved demonstration project)

✳ **G9114**   Oncology; disease status; ovarian cancer, limited to epithelial cancer; pathologic stage IA-B (grade 2-3); or stage IC (all grades); or stage II; without evidence of disease progression, recurrence, or metastases (for use in a Medicare-approved demonstration project)

✳ **G9115**   Oncology; disease status; ovarian cancer, limited to epithelial cancer; pathologic stage III-IV; without evidence of progression, recurrence, or metastases (for use in a Medicare-approved demonstration project)

▶ New   → Revised   ✔ Reinstated   ~~deleted~~ Deleted

⊘ Special coverage instructions   ◆ Not covered or valid by Medicare   ✳ Carrier discretion

✳ **G9116** Oncology; disease status; ovarian cancer, limited to epithelial cancer; evidence of disease progression, or recurrence and/or platinum resistance (for use in a Medicare-approved demonstration project)

✳ **G9117** Oncology; disease status; ovarian cancer, limited to epithelial cancer; extent of disease unknown, staging in progress, or not listed (for use in a Medicare-approved demonstration project)

✳ **G9123** Oncology; disease status; chronic myelogenous leukemia, limited to Philadelphia chromosome positive and/or BCR-ABL positive; chronic phase not in hematologic, cytogenetic, or molecular remission (for use in a Medicare-approved demonstration project)

✳ **G9124** Oncology; disease status; chronic myelogenous leukemia, limited to Philadelphia chromosome positive and/or BCR-ABL positive; accelerated phase not in hematologic cytogenetic, or molecular remission (for use in a Medicare-approved demonstration project)

✳ **G9125** Oncology; disease status; chronic myelogenous leukemia, limited to Philadelphia chromosome positive and/or BCR-ABL positive; blast phase not in hematologic, cytogenetic, or molecular remission (for use in a Medicare-approved demonstration project)

✳ **G9126** Oncology; disease status; chronic myelogenous leukemia, limited to Philadelphia chromosome positive and/or BCR-ABL positive; in hematologic, cytogenetic, or molecular remission (for use in a Medicare-approved demonstration project)

G9128 Oncology: disease status; limited to multiple myeloma, systemic disease; smouldering, stage I (for use in a Medicare-approved demonstration project)

✳ **G9129** Oncology; disease status; limited to multiple myeloma, systemic disease; stage II or higher (for use in a Medicare-approved demonstration project)

✳ **G9130** Oncology; disease status; limited to multiple myeloma, systemic disease; extent of disease unknown, staging in progress, or not listed (for use in a Medicare-approved demonstration project)

✳ **G9131** Oncology; disease status; invasive female breast cancer (does not include ductal carcinoma in situ); adenocarcinoma as predominant cell type; extent of disease unknown, staging in progress, or not listed (for use in a Medicare-approved demonstration project)

✳ **G9132** Oncology; disease status; prostate cancer, limited to adenocarcinoma; hormone-refractory/androgen-independent (e.g., rising PSA on anti-androgen therapy or post-orchiectomy); clinical metastases (for use in a Medicare-approved demonstration project)

✳ **G9133** Oncology; disease status; prostate cancer, limited to adenocarcinoma; hormone-responsive; clinical metastases or M1 at diagnosis (for use in a Medicare-approved demonstration project)

✳ **G9134** Oncology; disease status; non-Hodgkin's lymphoma, any cellular classification; stage I, II at diagnosis, not relapsed, not refractory (for use in a Medicare-approved demonstration project)

✳ **G9135** Oncology; disease status; non-Hodgkin's lymphoma, any cellular classification; stage III, IV, not relapsed, not refractory (for use in a Medicare-approved demonstration project)

✳ **G9136** Oncology; disease status; non-Hodgkin's lymphoma, transformed from original cellular diagnosis to a second cellular classification (for use in a Medicare-approved demonstration project)

✳ **G9137** Oncology; disease status; non-Hodgkin's lymphoma, any cellular classification; relapsed/refractory (for use in a Medicare-approved demonstration project)

✳ **G9138** Oncology; disease status; non-Hodgkin's lymphoma, any cellular classification; diagnostic evaluation, stage not determined, evaluation of possible relapse or non-response to therapy, or not listed (for use in a Medicare-approved demonstration project)

▶ New   → Revised   ✔ Reinstated   deleted Deleted

✪ Special coverage instructions   ◆ Not covered or valid by Medicare   ✳ Carrier discretion

✳ **G9139** Oncology; disease status; chronic myelogenous leukemia, limited to Philadelphia chromosome positive and/or BCR-ABL positive; extent of disease unknown, staging in progress, not listed (for use in a Medicare-approved demonstration project)

✳ **G9140** Frontier extended stay clinic demonstration; for a patient stay in a clinic approved for the CMS demonstration project; the following measures should be present: the stay must be equal to or greater than 4 hours; weather or other conditions must prevent transfer or the case falls into a category of monitoring and observation cases that are permitted by the rules of the demonstration; there is a maximum frontier extended stay clinic (FESC) visit of 48 hours, except in the case when weather or other conditions prevent transfer; payment is made on each period up to 4 hours, after the first 4 hours

Influenza A (H1N1) and Warfarin Responsiveness Testing

~~G9141~~ ~~Influenza A (H1N1) immunization administration (includes the physician counseling the patient/family)~~ ✖

~~G9142~~ ~~Influenza A (H1N1) vaccine, any route of administration~~ ✖

→ ✳ **G9143** Warfarin responsiveness testing by genetic technique using any method, any number of specimen(s)

This would be a once-in-a-lifetime test unless there is a reason to believe that the patient's personal genetic characteristics would change over time. (https://www.cms.gov/ContractorLearningResources/downloads/JA6715.pdf)

Laboratory Certification: General immunology, hematology

◆ **G9147** Outpatient intravenous insulin treatment (OIVIT) either pulsatile or continuous, by any means, guided by the results of measurements for: respiratory quotient; and/or, urine urea nitrogen (UUN); and/or, arterial, venous or capillary glucose; and/or potassium concentration

On December 23, 2009, CMS issued a national non-coverage decision on the use of OIVIT. CR 6775.

Not covered on Physician Fee Schedule

▶ ✳ **G9148** National committee for quality assurance - level 1 medical home

▶ ✳ **G9149** National committee for quality assurance - level 2 medical home

▶ ✳ **G9150** National committee for quality assurance - level 3 medical home

▶ ✳ **G9151** MAPCP demonstration - state provided services

▶ ✳ **G9152** MAPCP demonstration - community health teams

▶ ✳ **G9153** MAPCP demonstration - physician incentive pool

✳ **G9156** Evaluation for wheelchair requiring face to face visit with physician

▶ ✳ **G9157** Transesophageal doppler use for cardiac monitoring

▶ ✳ **G9158** Motor speech functional limitation, discharge status at discharge from therapy/end of reporting on limitation

▶ ✳ **G9159** Spoken language comprehension functional limitation, current status at time of initial therapy treatment/episode outset and reporting intervals

▶ ✳ **G9160** Spoken language comprehension functional limitation, projected goal status at initial therapy treatment/outset and at discharge from therapy

▶ ✳ **G9161** Spoken language comprehension functional limitation, discharge status at discharge from therapy/end of reporting on limitation

▶ ✳ **G9162** Spoken language expression functional limitation, current status at time of initial therapy treatment/episode outset and reporting intervals

▶ ✳ **G9163** Spoken language expression functional limitation, projected goal status at initial therapy treatment/outset and at discharge from therapy

▶ ✳ **G9164** Spoken language expression functional limitation, discharge status at discharge from therapy/end of reporting on limitation

▶ ✳ **G9165** Attention functional limitation, current status at time of initial therapy treatment/episode outset and reporting intervals

▶ ✳ **G9166** Attention functional limitation, projected goal status at initial therapy treatment/outset and at discharge from therapy

▶ ✳ **G9167** Attention functional limitation, discharge status at discharge from therapy/end of reporting on limitation

---

▶ New   → Revised   ✔ Reinstated   ~~deleted~~ Deleted

☺ Special coverage instructions   ◆ Not covered or valid by Medicare   ✳ Carrier discretion

▶ ✳ **G9168**   Memory functional limitation, current status at time of initial therapy treatment/episode outset and reporting intervals

▶ ✳ **G9169**   Memory functional limitation, projected goal status at initial therapy treatment/outset and at discharge from therapy

▶ ✳ **G9170**   Memory functional limitation, discharge status at discharge from therapy/end of reporting on limitation

▶ ✳ **G9171**   Voice functional limitation, current status at time of initial therapy treatment/episode outset and reporting intervals

▶ ✳ **G9172**   Voice functional limitation, projected goal status at initial therapy treatment/outset and at discharge from therapy

▶ ✳ **G9173**   Voice functional limitation, discharge status at discharge from therapy/end of reporting on limitation

▶ ✳ **G9174**   Other speech language pathology functional limitation, current status at time of initial therapy treatment/episode outset and reporting intervals

▶ ✳ **G9175**   Other speech language pathology functional limitation, projected goal status at initial therapy treatment/outset and at discharge from therapy

▶ ✳ **G9176**   Other speech language pathology functional limitation, discharge status at discharge from therapy/end of reporting on limitation

▶ ✳ **G9186**   Motor speech functional limitation, projected goal status at initial therapy treatment/outset and at discharge from therapy

BEHAVIORAL HEALTH AND/OR SUBSTANCE ABUSE TREATMENT SERVICES (H0001-H9999)

Used by Medicaid state agencies because no national code exists to meet the reporting needs of these agencies.

◆ **H0001**   Alcohol and/or drug assessment

◆ **H0002**   Behavioral health screening to determine eligibility for admission to treatment program

◆ **H0003**   Alcohol and/or drug screening; laboratory analysis of specimens for presence of alcohol and/or drugs

◆ **H0004**   Behavioral health counseling and therapy, per 15 minutes

◆ **H0005**   Alcohol and/or drug services; group counseling by a clinician

◆ **H0006**   Alcohol and/or drug services; case management

◆ **H0007**   Alcohol and/or drug services; crisis intervention (outpatient)

◆ **H0008**   Alcohol and/or drug services; sub-acute detoxification (hospital inpatient)

◆ **H0009**   Alcohol and/or drug services; acute detoxification (hospital inpatient)

◆ **H0010**   Alcohol and/or drug services; sub-acute detoxification (residential addiction program inpatient)

◆ **H0011**   Alcohol and/or drug services; acute detoxification (residential addiction program inpatient)

◆ **H0012**   Alcohol and/or drug services; sub-acute detoxification (residential addiction program outpatient)

◆ **H0013**   Alcohol and/or drug services; acute detoxification (residential addiction program outpatient)

◆ **H0014**   Alcohol and/or drug services; ambulatory detoxification

◆ **H0015**   Alcohol and/or drug services; intensive outpatient (treatment program that operates at least 3 hours/day and at least 3 days/week and is based on an individualized treatment plan), including assessment, counseling; crisis intervention, and activity therapies or education

◆ **H0016**   Alcohol and/or drug services; medical/somatic (medical intervention in ambulatory setting)

◆ **H0017**   Behavioral health; residential (hospital residential treatment program), without room and board, per diem

◆ **H0018**   Behavioral health; short-term residential (non-hospital residential treatment program), without room and board, per diem

◆ **H0019**   Behavioral health; long-term residential (non-medical, non-acute care in a residential treatment program where stay is typically longer than 30 days), without room and board, per diem

◆ **H0020**   Alcohol and/or drug services; methadone administration and/or service (provision of the drug by a licensed program)

◆ **H0021**   Alcohol and/or drug training service (for staff and personnel not employed by providers)

◆ **H0022**   Alcohol and/or drug intervention service (planned facilitation)

◆ **H0023**   Behavioral health outreach service (planned approach to reach a targeted population)

◆ **H0024**   Behavioral health prevention information dissemination service (one-way direct or non-direct contact with service audiences to affect knowledge and attitude)

◆ **H0025**   Behavioral health prevention education service (delivery of services with target population to affect knowledge, attitude and/or behavior)

◆ **H0026**   Alcohol and/or drug prevention process service, community-based (delivery of services to develop skills of impactors)

◆ **H0027**   Alcohol and/or drug prevention environmental service (broad range of external activities geared toward modifying systems in order to mainstream prevention through policy and law)

◆ **H0028**   Alcohol and/or drug prevention problem identification and referral service (e.g. student assistance and employee assistance programs), does not include assessment

◆ **H0029**   Alcohol and/or drug prevention alternatives service (services for populations that exclude alcohol and other drug use e.g. alcohol-free social events)

◆ **H0030**   Behavioral health hotline service

◆ **H0031**   Mental health assessment, by non-physician

◆ **H0032**   Mental health service plan development by non-physician

◆ **H0033**   Oral medication administration, direct observation

---

▶ New   → Revised   ✔ Reinstated   ~~deleted~~ Deleted

○ Special coverage instructions   ◆ Not covered or valid by Medicare   ✳ Carrier discretion

◆ **H0034** Medication training and support, per 15 minutes

◆ **H0035** Mental health partial hospitalization, treatment, less than 24 hours

◆ **H0036** Community psychiatric supportive treatment, face-to-face, per 15 minutes

◆ **H0037** Community psychiatric supportive treatment program, per diem

◆ **H0038** Self-help/peer services, per 15 minutes

◆ **H0039** Assertive community treatment, face-to-face, per 15 minutes

◆ **H0040** Assertive community treatment program, per diem

◆ **H0041** Foster care, child, non-therapeutic, per diem

◆ **H0042** Foster care, child, non-therapeutic, per month

◆ **H0043** Supported housing, per diem

◆ **H0044** Supported housing, per month

◆ **H0045** Respite care services, not in the home, per diem

◆ **H0046** Mental health services, not otherwise specified

◆ **H0047** Alcohol and/or other drug abuse services, not otherwise specified

◆ **H0048** Alcohol and/or other drug testing: collection and handling only, specimens other than blood

◆ **H0049** Alcohol and/or drug screening

◆ **H0050** Alcohol and/or drug services, brief intervention, per 15 minutes

◆ **H1000** Prenatal care, at-risk assessment

◆ **H1001** Prenatal care, at-risk enhanced service; antepartum management

◆ **H1002** Prenatal care, at-risk enhanced service; care coordination

◆ **H1003** Prenatal care, at-risk enhanced service; education

◆ **H1004** Prenatal care, at-risk enhanced service; follow-up home visit

◆ **H1005** Prenatal care, at-risk enhanced service package (includes H1001-H1004)

◆ **H1010** Non-medical family planning education, per session

◆ **H1011** Family assessment by licensed behavioral health professional for state defined purposes

◆ **H2000** Comprehensive multidisciplinary evaluation

◆ **H2001** Rehabilitation program, per 1/2 day

◆ **H2010** Comprehensive medication services, per 15 minutes

◆ **H2011** Crisis intervention service, per 15 minutes

◆ **H2012** Behavioral health day treatment, per hour

◆ **H2013** Psychiatric health facility service, per diem

◆ **H2014** Skills training and development, per 15 minutes

◆ **H2015** Comprehensive community support services, per 15 minutes

◆ **H2016** Comprehensive community support services, per diem

◆ **H2017** Psychosocial rehabilitation services, per 15 minutes

◆ **H2018** Psychosocial rehabilitation services, per diem

◆ **H2019** Therapeutic behavioral services, per 15 minutes

◆ **H2020** Therapeutic behavioral services, per diem

◆ **H2021** Community-based wrap-around services, per 15 minutes

◆ **H2022** Community-based wrap-around services, per diem

◆ **H2023** Supported employment, per 15 minutes

◆ **H2024** Supported employment, per diem

◆ **H2025** Ongoing support to maintain employment, per 15 minutes

◆ **H2026** Ongoing support to maintain employment, per diem

◆ **H2027** Psychoeducational service, per 15 minutes

◆ **H2028** Sexual offender treatment service, per 15 minutes

◆ **H2029** Sexual offender treatment service, per diem

◆ **H2030** Mental health clubhouse services, per 15 minutes

◆ **H2031** Mental health clubhouse services, per diem

◆ **H2032** Activity therapy, per 15 minutes

◆ **H2033** Multisystemic therapy for juveniles, per 15 minutes

◆ **H2034** Alcohol and/or drug abuse halfway house services, per diem

◆ **H2035** Alcohol and/or other drug treatment program, per hour

◆ **H2036** Alcohol and/or other drug treatment program, per diem

◆ **H2037** Developmental delay prevention activities, dependent child of client, per 15 minutes

---

▶ New   → Revised   ✔ Reinstated   ~~deleted~~ Deleted

☼ Special coverage instructions   ◆ Not covered or valid by Medicare   ✳ Carrier discretion

DRUGS OTHER THAN CHEMOTHERAPY (J0100-J9999)

J0120-J3570: Bill local carrier if incident to a physician's service or used in an implanted infusion pump. If other, bill DME/MAC.

⊛ **J0120** Injection, tetracycline, **up to 250 mg**

Other: Achromycin

IOM: 100-02, 15, 50

✻ **J0129** Injection, abatacept, **10 mg**

Other: Orencia

⊛ **J0130** Injection, abciximab, **10 mg** (Code may be used for Medicare when drug administered under the direct supervision of a physician; not for use when drug is self-administered)

NDC: ReoPro

IOM: 100-02, 15, 50

✻ **J0131** Injection, acetaminophen, **10 mg**

✻ **J0132** Injection, acetylcysteine, **100 mg**

NDC: Acetadote

✻ **J0133** Injection, acyclovir, **5 mg**

✻ **J0135** Injection, adalimumab, **20 mg**

NDC: Humira

IOM: 100-02, 15, 50

⊛ **J0150** Injection, adenosine, for therapeutic use, **6 mg** (not to be used to report any adenosine phosphate compounds, instead use A9270)

NDC: Adenocard

IOM: 100-02, 15, 50

✻ **J0152** Injection, adenosine, for diagnostic use, **30 mg** (not to be used to report any adenosine phosphate compounds; instead use A9270)

NDC: Adenoscan

⊛ **J0171** Injection, adrenalin, epinephrine, **0.1 mg**

IOM: 100-02, 15, 50

▶ ✻ **J0178** Injection, aflibercept, **1 mg**

✻ **J0180** Injection, agalsidase beta, **1 mg**

NDC: Fabrazyme

IOM: 100-02, 15, 50

⊛ **J0190** Injection, biperiden lactate, **per 5 mg**

Other: Akineton

IOM: 100-02, 15, 50

⊛ **J0200** Injection, alatrofloxacin mesylate, **100 mg**

Other: Trovan

IOM: 100-02, 15, 50

⊛ **J0205** Injection, alglucerase, **per 10 units**

NDC: Ceredase

IOM: 100-02, 15, 50

⊛ **J0207** Injection, amifostine, **500 mg**

NDC: Ethyol

IOM: 100-02, 15, 50

⊛ **J0210** Injection, methyldopate HCL, **up to 250 mg**

Other: Aldomet

IOM: 100-02, 15, 50

✻ **J0215** Injection, alefacept, **0.5 mg**

NDC: Amevive

✻ **J0220** Injection, alglucosidase alfa, not otherwise specified, **10 mg**

NDC: Myozyme

Other: Lumizyme

✻ **J0221** Injection, alglucosidase alfa, (lumizyme), **10 mg**

⊛ **J0256** Injection, alpha 1 - proteinase inhibitor (human), not otherwise specified, **10 mg**

NDC: Aralast, Aralast NP, Prolastin, Prolastin-C, Zemaira

IOM: 100-02, 15, 50

⊛ **J0257** Injection, alpha 1 proteinase inhibitor (human), (glassia), **10 mg**

IOM: 100-02, 15, 50

⊛ **J0270** Injection, alprostadil, **per 1.25 mcg** (Code may be used for Medicare when drug administered under the direct supervision of a physician, not for use when drug is self administered)

NDC: Caverject, Caverject Impulse, Edex, Prostin VR

Other: Prostaglandin E1

IOM: 100-02, 15, 50

⊛ **J0275** Alprostadil urethral suppository (Code may be used for Medicare when drug administered under the direct supervision of a physician, not for use when drug is self administered)

Other: Muse

IOM: 100-02, 15, 50

✻ **J0278** Injection, amikacin sulfate, **100 mg**

Other: Amikin

▶ New → Revised ✔ Reinstated ~~deleted~~ Deleted
⊛ Special coverage instructions ◆ Not covered or valid by Medicare ✻ Carrier discretion

⚙ **J0280** Injection, aminophylline, **up to 250 mg**
IOM: 100-02, 15, 50

⚙ **J0282** Injection, amiodarone hydrochloride, **30 mg**
Other: Cordarone
IOM: 100-02, 15, 50

⚙ **J0285** Injection, amphotericin B, **50 mg**
Other: ABLC, Amphocin, Fungizone
IOM: 100-02, 15, 50

⚙ **J0287** Injection, amphotericin B lipid complex, **10 mg**
NDC: Abelcet
IOM: 100-02, 15, 50

⚙ **J0288** Injection, amphotericin B cholesteryl sulfate complex, **10 mg**
NDC: Amphotec
IOM: 100-02, 15, 50

⚙ **J0289** Injection, amphotericin B liposome, **10 mg**
NDC: AmBisome
IOM: 100-02, 15, 50

⚙ **J0290** Injection, ampicillin sodium, **500 mg**
Other: Omnipen-N, Polycillin-N, Totacillin-N
IOM: 100-02, 15, 50

⚙ **J0295** Injection, ampicillin sodium/sulbactam sodium, **per 1.5 gm**
NDC: Unasyn
Other: Omnipen-N, Polycillin-N, Totacillin-N
IOM: 100-02, 15, 50

⚙ **J0300** Injection, amobarbital, **up to 125 mg**
Other: Amytal
IOM: 100-02, 15, 50

⚙ **J0330** Injection, succinylcholine chloride, **up to 20 mg**
Other: Anectine, Quelicin
IOM: 100-02, 15, 50

✳ **J0348** Injection, anidulafungin, **1 mg**
NDC: Eraxis

⚙ **J0350** Injection, anistreplase, **per 30 units**
Other: Eminase
IOM: 100-02, 15, 50

⚙ **J0360** Injection, hydralazine hydrochloride, **up to 20 mg**
Other: Apresoline
IOM: 100-02, 15, 50

✳ **J0364** Injection, apomorphine hydrochloride, **1 mg**
NDC: Apokyn

⚙ **J0365** Injection, aprotinin, **10,000 KIU**
NDC: Trasylol
IOM: 100-02, 15, 50

⚙ **J0380** Injection, metaraminol bitartrate, **per 10 mg**
Other: Aramine
IOM: 100-02, 15, 50

⚙ **J0390** Injection, chloroquine hydrochloride, **up to 250 mg**
Benefit only for diagnosed malaria or amebiasis
Other: Aralen
IOM: 100-02, 15, 50

⚙ **J0395** Injection, arbutamine HCL, **1 mg**
IOM: 100-02, 15, 50

✳ **J0400** Injection, aripiprazole, intramuscular, **0.25 mg**
Other: Abilify

⚙ **J0456** Injection, azithromycin, **500 mg**
NDC: Zithromax
IOM: 100-02, 15, 50

⚙ **J0461** Injection, atropine sulfate, **0.01 mg**
IOM: 100-02, 15, 50

⚙ **J0470** Injection, dimercaprol, per 100 mg
NDC: BAL In Oil
IOM: 100-02, 15, 50

⚙ **J0475** Injection, baclofen, **10 mg**
NDC: Gablofen, Lioresal
IOM: 100-02, 15, 50

⚙ **J0476** Injection, baclofen **50 mcg** for intrathecal trial
NDC: Gablofen, Lioresal
IOM: 100-02, 15, 50

⚙ **J0480** Injection, basiliximab, **20 mg**
NDC: Simulect
IOM: 100-02, 15, 50

▶ ✳ **J0485** Injection, belatacept, **1 mg**

✳ **J0490** Injection, belimumab, **10 mg**
NDC: Benlysta

▶ New → Revised ✔ Reinstated ~~deleted~~ Deleted

⚙ Special coverage instructions ◆ Not covered or valid by Medicare ✳ Carrier discretion

⊗ **J0500**   Injection, dicyclomine HCL, **up to 20 mg**

NDC: Bentyl

Other: Antispas, Dibent, Dicyclocot, Dilomine, Di-Spa, Neoquess, Or-Tyl, Spasmoject

IOM: 100-02, 15, 50

⊗ **J0515**   Injection, benztropine mesylate, **per 1 mg**

NDC: Cogentin

IOM: 100-02, 15, 50

⊗ **J0520**   Injection, bethanechol chloride, myotonachol or urecholine, **up to 5 mg**

IOM: 100-02, 15, 50

✳ **J0558**   Injection, penicillin G benzathine and penicillin G procaine, **100,000 units**

NDC: Bicillin C-R

⊗ **J0561**   Injection, penicillin G benzathine, **100,000 units**

NDC: Bicillin L-A

IOM: 100-02, 15, 50

✳ **J0583**   Injection, bivalirudin, **1 mg**

NDC: Angiomax

✳ **J0585**   Injection, onabotulinumtoxinaA, **1 unit**

NDC: Botox, Botox Cosmetic

Other: Oculinum

IOM: 100-02, 15, 50

✳ **J0586**   Injection, abobotulinumtoxinaA, **5 units**

NDC: Dysport

✳ **J0587**   Injection, rimabotulinumtoxinB, **100 units**

NDC: Myobloc

IOM: 100-02, 15, 50

✳ **J0588**   Injection, incobotulinumtoxin A, **1 unit**

NDC: Xeomin

⊗ **J0592**   Injection, buprenorphine hydrochloride, **0.1 mg**

IOM: 100-02, 15, 50

✳ **J0594**   Injection, busulfan, **1 mg**

✳ **J0595**   Injection, butorphanol tartrate, **1 mg**

NDC: Stadol

✳ **J0597**   Injection, C-1 esterase inhibitor (human), Berinet, **10 units**

✳ **J0598**   Injection, C1 esterase inhibitor (human), cinryze, **10 units**

⊗ **J0600**   Injection, edetate calcium disodium, **up to 1000 mg**

Other: Calcium Disodium Versenate

IOM: 100-02, 15, 50

⊗ **J0610**   Injection, calcium gluconate, **per 10 ml**

Other: Kaleinate

IOM: 100-02, 15, 50

⊗ **J0620**   Injection, calcium glycerophosphate and calcium lactate, **per 10 ml**

Other: Calphosan

MCM 2049

IOM: 100-02, 15, 50

⊗ **J0630**   Injection, calcitonin (salmon), **up to 400 units**

NDC: Miacalcin

Other: Calcimar, Calcitonin-salmon

IOM: 100-02, 15, 50

⊗ **J0636**   Injection, calcitriol, **0.1 mcg**

Non-dialysis use

NDC: Calcijex

Other: Calcitriol in almond oil

IOM: 100-02, 15, 50

✳ **J0637**   Injection, caspofungin acetate, **5 mg**

NDC: Cancidas

✳ **J0638**   Injection, canakinumab, **1 mg**

NDC: Ilaris

⊗ **J0640**   Injection, leucovorin calcium, **per 50 mg**

NDC: Calcium Folinate (Hungarian import)

Other: Wellcovorin

IOM: 100-02, 15, 50

⊗ **J0641**   Injection, levoleucovorin calcium, **0.5 mg**

Part of treatment regimen for osteosarcoma

⊗ **J0670**   Injection, mepivacaine HCL, **per 10 ml**

NDC: Polocaine, Polocaine-MPF

Other: Carbocaine, Isocaine HCl

IOM: 100-02, 15, 50

⊗ **J0690**   Injection, cefezolin sodium, **500 mg**

Other: Ancef, Kefzol

IOM: 100-02, 15, 50

✳ **J0692**   Injection, cefepime HCL, **500 mg**

NDC: Maxipime

▶ New   ➡ Revised   ✔ Reinstated   ~~deleted~~ Deleted

⊗ Special coverage instructions   ◆ Not covered or valid by Medicare   ✳ Carrier discretion

⚙ **J0694** Injection, cefoxitin sodium, **1 gm**

NDC: Mefoxin

IOM: 100-02, 15, 50,

Cross Reference Q0090

⚙ **J0696** Injection, ceftriaxone sodium, **per 250 mg**

NDC: Rocephin

IOM: 100-02, 15, 50

⚙ **J0697** Injection, sterile cefuroxime sodium, **per 750 mg**

NDC: Zinacef

Other: Kefurox

IOM: 100-02, 15, 50

⚙ **J0698** Injection, cefotaxime sodium, **per g**

NDC: Claforan

IOM: 100-02, 15, 50

⚙ **J0702** Injection, betamethasone acetate **3 mg** and betamethasone sodium phosphate **3 mg**

NDC: Celestone Soluspan

Other: Betameth

IOM: 100-02, 15, 50

✳ **J0706** Injection, caffeine citrate, **5 mg**

Other: Cafcit, Cipro IV, Ciprofloxacin

⚙ **J0710** Injection, cephapirin sodium, **up to 1 gm**

Other: Cefadyl

IOM: 100-02, 15, 50

✳ **J0712** Injection, ceftaroline fosamil, **10 mg**

NDC: Teflaro

⚙ **J0713** Injection, ceftazidime, **per 500 mg**

NDC: Fortaz, Tazicef

IOM: 100-02, 15, 50

⚙ **J0715** Injection, ceftizoxime sodium, **per 500 mg**

Other: Cefizox

IOM: 100-02, 15, 50

▶ ✳ **J0716** Injection, centruroides immune F(ab)2, up to 120 milligrams

✳ **J0718** Injection, certolizumab pegol, **1 mg**

NDC: Cimzia

⚙ **J0720** Injection, chloramphenicol sodium succinate, **up to 1 gm**

IOM: 100-02, 15, 50

⚙ **J0725** Injection, chorionic gonadotropin, **per 1,000 USP units**

NDC: Novarel

Other: A.P.L., Chorex-5, Chorex-10, Chorignon, Choron-10, Corgonject-5, Follutein, Glukor, Gonic, Pregnyl, Profasi HP

IOM: 100-02, 15, 50

⚙ **J0735** Injection, clonidine hydrochloride (HCL), **1 mg**

NDC: Duraclon

IOM: 100-02, 15, 50

⚙ **J0740** Injection, cidofovir, **375 mg**

NDC: Vistide

IOM: 100-02, 15, 50

⚙ **J0743** Injection, cilastatin sodium; imipenem, **per 250 mg**

NDC: Primaxin

IOM: 100-02, 15, 50

✳ **J0744** Injection, ciprofloxacin for intravenous infusion, **200 mg**

Other: Cipro IV

⚙ **J0745** Injection, codeine phosphate, **per 30 mg**

IOM: 100-02, 15, 50

⚙ **J0760** Injection, colchicine, **per 1 mg**

IOM: 100-02, 15, 50

⚙ **J0770** Injection, colistimethate sodium, **up to 150 mg**

NDC: Coly-Mycin M Parenteral

IOM: 100-02, 15, 50

✳ **J0775** Injection, collagenase, clostridium histolyticum, **0.01 mg**

NDC: Xiaflex

⚙ **J0780** Injection, prochlorperazine, **up to 10 mg**

Other: Compa-Z, Compazine, Cotranzine, Ultrazine-10

IOM: 100-02, 15, 50

⚙ **J0795** Injection, corticorelin ovine triflutate, **1 microgram**

NDC: Acthrel

IOM: 100-02, 15, 50

⚙ **J0800** Injection, corticotropin, **up to 40 units**

NDC: Acthar H.P.

Other: H.P. Acthar, ACTH

IOM: 100-02, 15, 50

▶ New → Revised ✔ Reinstated ~~deleted~~ Deleted

⚙ Special coverage instructions ◆ Not covered or valid by Medicare ✳ Carrier discretion

* **J0833** Injection, cosyntropin, not otherwise specified, **0.25 mg**

* **J0834** Injection, cosyntropin (Cortrosyn), **0.25 mg**

* **J0840** Injection, crotalidae polyvalent immune fab (ovine), **up to 1 gram**

NDC: Crofab Powder for Solution

☺ **J0850** Injection, cytomegalovirus immune globulin intravenous (human), **per vial**

Prophylaxis to prevent cytomegalovirus disease associated with transplantation of kidney, lung, liver, pancreas, and heart.

NDC: CytoGam

IOM: 100-02, 15, 50

* **J0878** Injection, daptomycin, **1 mg**

NDC: Cubicin

☺ **J0881** Injection, darbepoetin alfa, **1 microgram** (non-ESRD use)

NDC: Aranesp

☺ **J0882** Injection, darbepoetin alfa, **1 microgram** (for ESRD on dialysis)

NDC: Aranesp

IOM: 100-02, 6, 10; 100-04, 4, 240

☺ **J0885** Injection, epoetin alfa, (for non-ESRD use), **1000 units**

NDC: Epogen, Procrit

IOM: 100-02, 15, 50

☺ **J0886** Injection, epoetin alfa, **1000 units** (for ESRD on dialysis)

NDC: Epogen, Procrit

IOM: 100-02, 6, 10; 100-04, 4, 240

▶ * **J0890** Injection, peginesatide, 0.1 mg (for ESRD on dialysis)

* **J0894** Injection, decitabine, **1 mg**

Indicated for treatment of myelodysplastic syndromes (MDS)

☺ **J0895** Injection, deferoxamine mesylate, **500 mg**

NDC: Desferal

Other: Desferal mesylate

IOM: 100-02, 15, 50,

Cross Reference Q0087

* **J0897** Injection, denosumab, **1 mg**

NDC: Prolia, Xgeva

☺ **J0900** Injection, testosterone enanthate and estradiol valerate, **up to 1 cc**

Other: Andrest 90-4, Andro-Estro 90-4, Androgyn L.A., Deladumone, Deladumone OB, Delatest, Delatestadiol, Ditate-DS, Dua-Gen LA, Duoval PA, Estra-Testrin, TEEV, Testadiate, Testradiol 90/4, Valertest

IOM: 100-02, 15, 50

☺ **J0945** Injection, brompheniramine maleate, **per 10 mg**

Other: Codimal-A, Cophene-B, Dehist, Histaject, Nasahist B, ND Stat, Oraminic II, Sinusol-B

IOM: 100-02, 15, 50

☺ **J1000** Injection, depo-estradiol cypionate, **up to 5 mg**

Other: Depogen, DepGynogen, Dura-Estrin, Estra-D, Estro-Cyp, Estroject LA, Estronol-LA

IOM: 100-02, 15, 50

☺ **J1020** Injection, methylprednisolone acetate, **20 mg**

NDC: Depo-Medrol, Methylpred

Other: DepMedalone, Depoject, Depopred, D-Med 80, Duralone, Medralone, M-Prednisol, Rep-Pred

IOM: 100-02, 15, 50

☺ **J1030** Injection, methylprednisolone acetate, **40 mg**

NDC: Depo-Medrol

Other: DepMedalone, Depoject, Depropred, D-Med 80, Duralone, Medralone, M-Prednisol, Rep-Pred

IOM: 100-02, 15, 50

☺ **J1040** Injection, methylprednisolone acetate, **80 mg**

NDC: Depo-Medrol

Other: DepMedalone, Depoject, Depropred, D-Med 80, Duralone, Medralone, M-Prednisol, Rep-Pred

IOM: 100-02, 15, 50

▶ * **J1050** Injection, medroxyprogesterone acetate, 1 mg

~~J1051~~ ~~Injection, medroxyprogesterone~~ ✖
~~acetate, 50 mg~~

~~J1055~~ ~~Injection, medroxyprogesterone~~ ✖
~~acetate for contraceptive use, 150 mg~~

▶ New → Revised ✔ Reinstated ~~deleted~~ Deleted

☺ Special coverage instructions ◆ Not covered or valid by Medicare * Carrier discretion

~~J1056~~   ~~Injection, medroxyprogesterone~~
~~acetate/estradiol cypionate, 5 mg/25 mg~~   ✖

⊛ **J1060**   Injection, testosterone cypionate and
estradiol cypionate, **up to 1 ml**

*Other: Andro/Fem, De-Comberol,
DepAndrogyn, Depo-Testadiol,
Depotestogen, Duratestrin, Estradiol
cypionate, Test-Estro-C, Test-Estro
Cypionates, Valertest No. 1*

IOM: 100-02, 15, 50

⊛ **J1070**   Injection, testosterone cypionate, **up to
100 mg**

NDC: Depo-Testosterone

*Other: Andro-Cyp, Andronaq-LA,
Andronate, DepAndro, Depotest,
Duratest, Testa-C, Testadiate-Depo,
Testaject-LA, Testoject-LA,*

IOM: 100-02, 15, 50

⊛ **J1080**   Injection, testosterone cypionate, **1 cc,
200 mg**

NDC: Depo-Testosterone

*Other: Andro-Cyp, Andronaq-LA,
Andronate, DepAndro, Depotest,
Duratest, Testa-C, Testadiate-Depo,
Testaject-LA, Testoject-LA*

IOM: 100-02, 15, 50

⊛ **J1094**   Injection, dexamethasone acetate, **1 mg**

*Other: Cortastat LA, Dalalone LA,
Decadrone LA, Decaject LA,
Dexacen-LA-8, Dexamethasone
Micronized, Dexasone L.A., Dexone-LA*

IOM: 100-02, 15, 50

⊛ **J1100**   Injection, dexamethasone sodium
phosphate, **1 mg**

*Other: Cortastat 10, Dalalone, Decadron
Phosphate, Decaject, Dexacen-4, Dexone,
Hexadrol Phosphate, Solurex*

IOM: 100-02, 15, 50

⊛ **J1110**   Injection, dihydroergotamine mesylate,
per 1 mg

NDC: D.H.E. 45

IOM: 100-02, 15, 50

⊛ **J1120**   Injection, acetazolamide sodium, **up to
500 mg**

Other: Diamox

IOM: 100-02, 15, 50

⊛ **J1160**   Injection, digoxin, **up to 0.5 mg**

NDC: Lanoxin

IOM: 100-02, 15, 50

⊛ **J1162**   Injection, digoxin immune Fab (ovine),
per vial

NDC: Digibind, DigiFab

IOM: 100-02, 15, 50

⊛ **J1165**   Injection, phenytoin sodium, **per
50 mg**

Other: Dilantin

IOM: 100-02, 15, 50

⊛ **J1170**   Injection, hydromorphone, **up to 4 mg**

Other: Dilaudid

IOM: 100-02, 15, 50

⊛ **J1180**   Injection, dyphylline, **up to 500 mg**

Other: Dilor, Lufyllin

IOM: 100-02, 15, 50

⊛ **J1190**   Injection, dexrazoxane hydrochloride,
per 250 mg

NDC: Totect, Zinecard

IOM: 100-02, 15, 50

⊛ **J1200**   Injection, diphenhydramine HCL, **up to
50 mg**

NDC: Benadryl

Other: Bena-D, Truxadryl

IOM: 100-02, 15, 50

⊛ **J1205**   Injection, chlorothiazide sodium, **per
500 mg**

NDC: Diuril

IOM: 100-02, 15, 50

⊛ **J1212**   Injection, DMSO, dimethyl sulfoxide,
50%, **50 ml**

NDC: Rimso-50

IOM: 100-02, 15, 50; 100-03, 4, 230.12

⊛ **J1230**   Injection, methadone HCL,
up to 10 mg

MCM 2049

IOM: 100-02, 15, 50

⊛ **J1240**   Injection, dimenhydrinate,
up to 50 mg

*Other: Dinate, Dommanate, Dramamine,
Dramanate, Dramilin, Dramocen,
Dramoject, Dymenate, Hydrate,
Marmine, Wehamine*

IOM: 100-02, 15, 50

⊛ **J1245**   Injection, dipyridamole, **per 10 mg**

Other: Persantine

IOM: 100-04, 15, 50; 100-04, 12, 30.6

▶ New   → Revised   ✔ Reinstated   ~~deleted~~ Deleted
⊛ Special coverage instructions   ◆ Not covered or valid by Medicare   ✳ Carrier discretion

⊗ **J1250**   Injection, dobutamine HCL,
per 250 mg

Other: Dobutrex

IOM: 100-02, 15, 50

⊗ **J1260**   Injection, dolasetron mesylate, **10 mg**

NDC: Anzemet

IOM: 100-02, 15, 50

✳ **J1265**   Injection, dopamine HCL, **40 mg**

✳ **J1267**   Injection, doripenem, **10 mg**

NDC: Doribax

✳ **J1270**   Injection, doxercalciferol, **1 mcg**

NDC: Hectorol

✳ **J1290**   Injection, ecallantide, **1 mg**

NDC: Kalbitor

✳ **J1300**   Injection, eculizumab, **10 mg**

NDC: Soliris

⊗ **J1320**   Injection, amitriptyline HCL, **up to
20 mg**

Other: Elavil, Enovil

IOM: 100-02, 15, 50

✳ **J1324**   Injection, enfuvirtide, **1 mg**

Other: Fuzeon

⊗ **J1325**   Injection, epoprostenol, **0.5 mg**

NDC: Flolan

IOM: 100-02, 15, 50

⊗ **J1327**   Injection, eptifibatide, **5 mg**

NDC: Integrilin

IOM: 100-02, 15, 50

⊗ **J1330**   Injection, ergonovine maleate, **up to
0.2 mg**

Benefit limited to obstetrical diagnosis

IOM: 100-02, 15, 50

✳ **J1335**   Injection, ertapenem sodium, **500 mg**

NDC: Invanz

⊗ **J1364**   Injection, erythromycin lactobionate,
per 500 mg

IOM: 100-02, 15, 50

⊗ **J1380**   Injection, estradiol valerate, **up to
10 mg**

NDC: Delestrogen

*Other: Dioval, Duragen, Estra-L,
Gynogen L.A., L.A.E. 20, Valergen*

IOM: 100-02, 15, 50

⊗ **J1410**   Injection, estrogen conjugated,
per 25 mg

NDC: Premarin

IOM: 100-02, 15, 50

⊗ **J1430**   Injection, ethanolamine oleate, **100 mg**

Other: Ethamolin

IOM: 100-02, 15, 50

⊗ **J1435**   Injection, estrone, **per 1 mg**

*Other: Estragyn, Estronol, Kestrone 5,
Theelin Aqueous*

IOM: 100-02, 15, 50

⊗ **J1436**   Injection, etidronate disodium, **per
300 mg**

Other: Didronel

IOM: 100-02, 15, 50

⊗ **J1438**   Injection, etanercept, **25 mg** (Code may
be used for Medicare when drug
administered under the direct
supervision of a physician, not for use
when drug is self-administered.)

NDC: Enbrel

IOM: 100-02, 15, 50

⊗ **J1440**   Injection, filgrastim (G-CSF), **300 mcg**

NDC: Neupogen

IOM: 100-02, 15, 50

⊗ **J1441**   Injection, filgrastim (G-CSF), **480 mcg**

Other: Neupogen

IOM: 100-02, 15, 50

⊗ **J1450**   Injection, fluconazole, **200 mg**

NDC: Diflucan

IOM: 100-02, 15, 50

⊗ **J1451**   Injection, fomepizole, **15 mg**

NDC: Antizol

IOM: 100-02, 15, 50

⊗ **J1452**   Injection, fomivirsen sodium,
intraocular, **1.65 mg**

IOM: 100-02, 15, 50

✳ **J1453**   Injection, fosaprepitant, **1 mg**

Prevents chemotherapy-induced nausea
and vomiting

NDC: Emend

⊗ **J1455**   Injection, foscarnet sodium, **per
1000 mg**

NDC: Foscavir

IOM: 100-02, 15, 50

✳ **J1457**   Injection, gallium nitrate, **1 mg**

NDC: Ganite

✳ **J1458**   Injection, galsulfase, **1 mg**

NDC: Naglazyme

✳ **J1459**   Injection, immune globulin (Privigen),
intravenous, non-lyophilized (e.g.,
liquid), **500 mg**

▶ New   → Revised   ✔ Reinstated   ~~deleted~~ Deleted

⊗ Special coverage instructions   ◆ Not covered or valid by Medicare   ✳ Carrier discretion

✲ **J1460** Injection, gamma globulin, intramuscular, **1 cc**

NDC: GamaSTAN

Other: Gammar

IOM: 100-02, 15, 50

✳ **J1557** Injection, immune globulin, (gammaplex), intravenous, non-lyophilized (e.g., liquid), **500 mg**

✳ **J1559** Injection, immune globulin, (hizentra), **100 mg**

✲ **J1560** Injection, gamma globulin, intramuscular, **over 10 cc**

NDC: GamaSTAN, Immune Globin (Human)

Other: Gammar

IOM: 100-02, 15, 50

→ ✲ **J1561** Injection, immune globulin, (Gamunex-C/Gammaked), non-lyophilized (e.g. liquid), **500 mg**

NDC: Gamunex

IOM: 100-02, 15, 50

✳ **J1562** Injection, immune globulin (Vivaglobin), **100 mg**

✲ **J1566** Injection, immune globulin, intravenous, lyophilized (e.g., powder), not otherwise specified, **500 mg**

NDC: Carimune, Gammagard S/D

Other: Polygam

IOM: 100-02, 15, 50

✳ **J1568** Injection, immune globulin, (Octagam), intravenous, non-lyophilized (e.g., liquid), **500 mg**

→ ✲ **J1569** Injection, immune globulin, (Gammagard Liquid), non-lyophilized, (e.g. liquid), **500 mg**

IOM: 100-02, 15, 50

✲ **J1570** Injection, ganciclovir sodium, **500 mg**

NDC: Cytovene

IOM: 100-02, 15, 50

✲ **J1571** Injection, hepatitis B immune globulin (HepaGam B), intramuscular, **0.5 ml**

IOM: 100-02, 15, 50

✲ **J1572** Injection, immune globulin, (flebogamma/flebogamma DIF) intravenous, non-lyophilized (e.g. liquid), **500 mg**

IOM: 100-02, 15, 50

✳ **J1573** Injection, hepatitis B immune globulin (HepaGam B), intravenous, **0.5 ml**

✲ **J1580** Injection, Garamycin, gentamicin, **up to 80 mg**

NDC: Gentamicin Sulfate

Other: Jenamicin

IOM: 100-02, 15, 50

✳ **J1590** Injection, gatifloxacin, **10 mg**

Other: Tequin

✲ **J1595** Injection, glatiramer acetate, **20 mg**

Other: Copaxone

IOM: 100-02, 15, 50

✳ **J1599** Injection, immune globulin, intravenous, non-lyophilized (e.g., liquid), not otherwise specified, **500 mg**

✲ **J1600** Injection, gold sodium thiomalate, **up to 50 mg**

NDC: Myochrysine

IOM: 100-02, 15, 50

✲ **J1610** Injection, glucagon hydrochloride, **per 1 mg**

NDC: GlucaGen, Glucagon Emergency

IOM: 100-02, 15, 50

✲ **J1620** Injection, gonadorelin hydrochloride, **per 100 mcg**

Other: Factrel

IOM: 100-02, 15, 50

✲ **J1626** Injection, granisetron hydrochloride, **100 mcg**

NDC: Kytril

IOM: 100-02, 15, 50

✲ **J1630** Injection, haloperidol, **up to 5 mg**

NDC: Haldol, Haloperidol Lactate

IOM: 100-02, 15, 50

✲ **J1631** Injection, haloperidol decanoate, **per 50 mg**

IOM: 100-02, 15, 50

✲ **J1640** Injection, hemin, **1 mg**

NDC: Panhematin

IOM: 100-02, 15, 50

✲ **J1642** Injection, heparin sodium, (heparin lock flush), **per 10 units**

NDC: Heparin (Porcine) Lock Flush, Heparin Sodium Flush,

Other: Hep-Lock U/P

IOM: 100-02, 15, 50

▶ New   → Revised   ✔ Reinstated   ~~deleted~~ Deleted

✲ Special coverage instructions   ◆ Not covered or valid by Medicare   ✳ Carrier discretion

⚙ **J1644** Injection, heparin sodium, **per 1000 units**

NDC: Heparin (Porcine), Heparin Sodium (Porcine)

Other: Liquaemin Sodium

IOM: 100-02, 15, 50

⚙ **J1645** Injection, dalteparin sodium, **per 2500 IU**

NDC: Fragmin

IOM: 100-02, 15, 50

✳ **J1650** Injection, enoxaparin sodium, **10 mg**

NDC: Lovenox

⚙ **J1652** Injection, fondaparinux sodium, **0.5 mg**

NDC: Arixtra

IOM: 100-02, 15, 50

✳ **J1655** Injection, tinzaparin sodium, **1000 IU**

Other: Innohep

⚙ **J1670** Injection, tetanus immune globulin, human, **up to 250 units**

Indicated for transient protection against tetanus post-exposure to tetanus (V03.7).

NDC: Hypertet S/D

Other: Hyper-tet

IOM: 100-02, 15, 50

⚙ **J1675** Injection, histrelin acetate, **10 micrograms**

IOM: 100-02, 15, 50

~~J1680~~ ~~Injection, human fibrinogen concentrate, 100 mg~~ ✖

⚙ **J1700** Injection, hydrocortisone acetate, **up to 25 mg**

Other: Hydrocortone Acetate

IOM: 100-02, 15, 50

⚙ **J1710** Injection, hydrocortisone sodium phosphate, **up to 50 mg**

Other: A-hydroCort, Hydrocortone phosphate, Solu-Cortef

IOM: 100-02, 15, 50

⚙ **J1720** Injection, hydrocortisone sodium succinate, **up to 100 mg**

NDC: Solu-Cortef

Other: A-Hydrocourt

IOM: 100-02, 15, 50

✳ **J1725** Injection, hydroxyprogesterone caproate, **1 mg**

⚙ **J1730** Injection, diazoxide, **up to 300 mg**

Other: Hyperstat

IOM: 100-02, 15, 50

✳ **J1740** Injection, ibandronate sodium, **1 mg**

NDC: Boniva

▶ ✳ **J1741** Injection, ibuprofen, **100 mg**

⚙ **J1742** Injection, ibutilide fumarate, **1 mg**

NDC: Corvert

IOM: 100-02, 15, 50

✳ **J1743** Injection, idursulfase, **1 mg**

Other: Elaprase

▶ ✳ **J1744** Injection, icatibant, **1 mg**

⚙ **J1745** Injection, infliximab, **10 mg**

Report total number of 10 mg increments administered; medical record must document failed or incomplete control of arthritis with use of other antirheumatic modalities

NDC: Remicade

IOM: 100-02, 15, 50

⚙ **J1750** Injection, iron dextran, **50 mg**

IOM: 100-02, 15, 50

NDC: Dexferrum, Infed

✳ **J1756** Injection, iron sucrose, **1 mg**

NDC: Venofer

⚙ **J1786** Injection, imiglucerase, **10 units**

NDC: Cerezyme

IOM: 100-02, 15, 50

⚙ **J1790** Injection, droperidol, **up to 5 mg**

NDC: Inapsine

IOM: 100-02, 15, 50

⚙ **J1800** Injection, propranolol HCL, **up to 1 mg**

Other: Inderal

IOM: 100-02, 15, 50

⚙ **J1810** Injection, droperidol and fentanyl citrate, **up to 2 ml ampule**

Other: Innovar

IOM: 100-02, 15, 50

⚙ **J1815** Injection, insulin, **per 5 units**

NDC: Humalog, Humulin, Lantus, Novolin, Novolog

IOM: 100-02, 15, 50; 100-03, 4, 280.14

✳ **J1817** Insulin for administration through DME (i.e., insulin pump) **per 50 units**

NDC: Humalog, Humulin, Novolin, Novolog

Other: Apidra Solostar, Insulin Lispro

▶ New   → Revised   ✔ Reinstated   ~~deleted~~ Deleted

⚙ Special coverage instructions   ◆ Not covered or valid by Medicare   ✳ Carrier discretion

◆ **J1826** Injection, interferon beta-1a, **30 mcg**

✿ **J1830** Injection interferon beta-1b, **0.25 mg** (Code may be used for Medicare when drug administered under the direct supervision of a physician, not for use when drug is self administered)

Other: Betaseron

IOM: 100-02, 15, 50

✳ **J1835** Injection, itraconazole, **50 mg**

Other: Sporanox

✿ **J1840** Injection, kanamycin sulfate, **up to 500 mg**

Other: Kantrex, Klebcil

IOM: 100-02, 15, 50

✿ **J1850** Injection, kanamycin sulfate, **up to 75 mg**

Other: Kantrex, Klebcil

IOM: 100-02, 15, 50

✿ **J1885** Injection, ketorolac tromethamine, **per 15 mg**

Other: Toradol

IOM: 100-02, 15, 50

✿ **J1890** Injection, cephalothin sodium, **up to 1 gram**

Other: Keflin

IOM: 100-02, 15, 50

✳ **J1930** Injection, lanreotide, **1 mg**

Treats acromegaly and symptoms caused by neuroendocrine tumors

NDC: Somatuline Depot

✳ **J1931** Injection, laronidase, **0.1 mg**

NDC: Aldurazyme

✿ **J1940** Injection, furosemide, **up to 20 mg**

Other: Lasix

MCM 2049

IOM: 100-02, 15, 50

✿ **J1945** Injection, lepirudin, **50 mg**

NDC: Refludan

IOM: 100-02, 15, 50

✿ **J1950** Injection, leuprolide acetate (for depot suspension), **per 3.75 mg**

NDC: Lupron Depot, Lupron Depot-Ped

IOM: 100-02, 15, 50

✳ **J1953** Injection, levetiracetam, **10 mg**

✿ **J1955** Injection, levocarnitine, **per 1 gm**

NDC: Carnitor

Other: L-Carnitine

IOM: 100-02, 15, 50

✿ **J1956** Injection, levofloxacin, **250 mg**

NDC: Levaquin

IOM: 100-02, 15, 50

✿ **J1960** Injection, levorphanol tartrate, **up to 2 mg**

Other: Levo-Dromoran

MCM 2049

IOM: 100-02, 15, 50

✿ **J1980** Injection, hyoscyamine sulfate, **up to 0.25 mg**

NDC: Levsin

IOM: 100-02, 15, 50

✿ **J1990** Injection, chlordiazepoxide HCL, **up to 100 mg**

Other: Librium

IOM: 100-02, 15, 50

✿ **J2001** Injection, lidocaine HCL for intravenous infusion, **10 mg**

NDC: Lidocaine in D5W, Xylocaine (Cardiac)

Other: Anestacaine, Caine-1, Dilocaine, L-Caine, Lidoject, Nervocaine, Nulicaine, Xylocaine

IOM: 100-02, 15, 50

✿ **J2010** Injection, lincomycin HCL, **up to 300 mg**

NDC: Lincocin

IOM: 100-02, 15, 50

✳ **J2020** Injection, linezolid, **200 mg**

NDC: Zyvox

✿ **J2060** Injection, lorazepam, **2 mg**

NDC: Ativan

IOM: 100-02, 15, 50

✿ **J2150** Injection, mannitol, **25% in 50 ml**

MCM 2049

IOM: 100-02, 15, 50

✳ **J2170** Injection, mecasermin, **1 mg**

Other: Increlex

✿ **J2175** Injection, meperidine hydrochloride, **per 100 mg**

NDC: Demerol

IOM: 100-02, 15, 50

✿ **J2180** Injection, meperidine and promethazine HCL, **up to 50 mg**

Other: Mepergan

IOM: 100-02, 15, 50

▶ New　→ Revised　✔ Reinstated　~~deleted~~ Deleted

✿ Special coverage instructions　◆ Not covered or valid by Medicare　✳ Carrier discretion

* **J2185**   Injection, meropenem, **100 mg**

  NDC: Merrem

☼ **J2210**   Injection, methylergonovine maleate, **up to 0.2 mg**

  Benefit limited to obstetrical diagnoses for prevention and control of post-partum hemorrhage

  NDC: Methergine

  IOM: 100-02, 15, 50

▶ * **J2212**   Injection, methylnaltrexone, **0.1 mg**

* **J2248**   Injection, micafungin sodium, **1 mg**

  Other: Mycamine

☼ **J2250**   Injection, midazolam hydrochloride, **per 1 mg**

  Other: Versed

  IOM: 100-02, 15, 50

☼ **J2260**   Injection, milrinone lactate, **5 mg**

  Other: Primacor

  IOM: 100-02, 15, 50

* **J2265**   Injection, minocycline hydrochloride, **1 mg**

☼ **J2270**   Injection, morphine sulfate, **up to 10 mg**

  Other: Astromorph PF, Duramorph

  IOM: 100-02, 15, 50

☼ **J2271**   Injection, morphine sulfate, **100 mg**

  Other: Astramorph PF, Duramorph

  IOM: 100-02, 15, 50; 100-03, 4, 280.1

☼ **J2275**   Injection, morphine sulfate (preservative-free sterile solution), **per 10 mg**

  NDC: Astramorph, Duramorph, Infumorph

  IOM: 100-02, 15, 50; 100-03, 4, 280.1

☼ **J2278**   Injection, ziconotide, **1 microgram**

  NDC: Prialt

* **J2280**   Injection, moxifloxacin, **100 mg**

  NDC: Avelox

☼ **J2300**   Injection, nalbuphine hydrochloride, **per 10 mg**

  Other: Nubain

  IOM: 100-02, 15, 50

☼ **J2310**   Injection, naloxone hydrochloride, **per 1 mg**

  Other: Narcan

  IOM: 100-02, 15, 50

* **J2315**   Injection, naltrexone, depot form, **1 mg**

  NDC: Vivitrol

☼ **J2320**   Injection, nandrolone decanoate, **up to 50 mg**

  Other: Anabolin LA 100, Androlone, Deca-Durabolin, Decolone, Hybolin Decanoate, Nandrobolic LA, Neo-Durabolic

  IOM: 100-02, 15, 50

* **J2323**   Injection, natalizumab, **1 mg**

  Other: Tysabri

☼ **J2325**   Injection, nesiritide, **0.1 mg**

  NDC: Natrecor

  IOM: 100-02, 15, 50

* **J2353**   Injection, octreotide, depot form for intramuscular injection, **1 mg**

  NDC: Sandostatin LAR Depot

* **J2354**   Injection, octreotide, non-depot form for subcutaneous or intravenous injection, **25 mcg**

  Other: Sandostatin LAR Depot

☼ **J2355**   Injection, oprelvekin, **5 mg**

  NDC: Neumega

  IOM: 100-02, 15, 50

* **J2357**   Injection, omalizumab, **5 mg**

  NDC: Xolair

* **J2358**   Injection, olanzapine, long-acting, **1 mg**

  NDC: Zyprexa, Relprevv

☼ **J2360**   Injection, orphenadrine citrate, **up to 60 mg**

  NDC: Norflex

  Other: Antiflex, Banflex, Flexoject, Flexon, K-Flex, Mio-Rel, Neocyten, O-Flex, Orfro, Orphenate

  IOM: 100-02, 15, 50

☼ **J2370**   Injection, phenylephrine HCL, **up to 1 ml**

  Other: Neo-Synephrine

  IOM: 100-02, 15, 50

☼ **J2400**   Injection, chloroprocaine hydrochloride, **per 30 ml**

  NDC: Nesacaine, Nesacaine-MPF

  IOM: 100-02, 15, 50

☼ **J2405**   Injection, ondansetron hydrochloride, **per 1 mg**

  NDC: Zofran

  IOM: 100-02, 15, 50

☼ **J2410**   Injection, oxymorphone HCL, **up to 1 mg**

  NDC: Opana

  Other: Numorphan

  IOM: 100-02, 15, 50

▶ New   → Revised   ✔ Reinstated   ~~deleted~~ Deleted

☼ Special coverage instructions   ◆ Not covered or valid by Medicare   * Carrier discretion

✳ **J2425** Injection, palifermin, **50 micrograms**

NDC: Kepivance

✳ **J2426** Injection, paliperidone palmitate extended release, **1 mg**

NDC: Invega Sustenna

☺ **J2430** Injection, pamidronate disodium, **per 30 mg**

NDC: Aredia

IOM: 100-02, 15, 50

☺ **J2440** Injection, papaverine HCL, **up to 60 mg**

IOM: 100-02, 15, 50

☺ **J2460** Injection, oxytetracycline HCL, **up to 50 mg**

Other: Terramycin IM

IOM: 100-02, 15, 50

✳ **J2469** Injection, palonosetron HCL, **25 mcg**

Example: 0.25 mgm dose = 10 units. Example of use is acute, delayed, nausea and vomiting due to chemotherapy

NDC: Aloxi

☺ **J2501** Injection, paricalcitol, **1 mcg**

NDC: Zemplar

IOM: 100-02, 15, 50

✳ **J2503** Injection, pegaptanib sodium, **0.3 mg**

NDC: Macugen

☺ **J2504** Injection, pegademase bovine, **25 IU**

NDC: Adagen

IOM: 100-02, 15, 50

✳ **J2505** Injection, pegfilgrastim, **6 mg**

Report 1 unit per 6 mg.

NDC: Neulasta

✳ **J2507** Injection, pegloticase, **1 mg**

NDC: Krystexxa

☺ **J2510** Injection, penicillin G procaine, aqueous, **up to 600,000 units**

NDC: Wycillin

Other: Crysticillin, Duracillin AS, Pfizerpen AS

IOM: 100-02, 15, 50

☺ **J2513** Injection, pentastarch, 10% solution, **100 ml**

IOM: 100-02, 15, 50

☺ **J2515** Injection, pentobarbital sodium, **per 50 mg**

NDC: Nembutal

IOM: 100-02, 15, 50

☺ **J2540** Injection, penicillin G potassium, **up to 600,000 units**

NDC: Pfizerpen-G

IOM: 100-02, 15, 50

☺ **J2543** Injection, piperacillin sodium/ tazobactam sodium, **1 gram/ 0.125 grams (1.125 grams)**

NDC: Zosyn

IOM: 100-02, 15, 50

☺ **J2545** Pentamidine isethionate, inhalation solution, FDA-approved final product, non-compounded, administered through DME, unit dose form, **per 300 mg**

NDC: Nebupent

☺ **J2550** Injection, promethazine HCL, **up to 50 mg**

Administration of phenergan suppository considered part of E/M encounter

NDC: Phenergan

Other: Anergan, Phenazine, Prorex, Prothazine

IOM: 100-02, 15, 50

☺ **J2560** Injection, phenobarbital sodium, **up to 120 mg**

IOM: 100-02, 15, 50

✳ **J2562** Injection, plerixafor, **1 mg**

FDA approved for non-Hodgkin lymphoma and multiple myeloma in 2008.

NDC: Mozobil

☺ **J2590** Injection, oxytocin, **up to 10 units**

NDC: Pitocin

Other: Syntocinon

IOM: 100-02, 15, 50

☺ **J2597** Injection, desmopressin acetate, **per 1 mcg**

NDC: DDAVP

IOM: 100-02, 15, 50

☺ **J2650** Injection, prednisolone acetate, **up to 1 ml**

Other: Cotolone, Key-Pred, Predalone, Predcor, Predicort

IOM: 100-02, 15, 50

☺ **J2670** Injection, tolazoline HCL, **up to 25 mg**

Other: Priscoline Hydrochloride

IOM: 100-02, 15, 50

▶ New   → Revised   ✔ Reinstated   ~~deleted~~ Deleted

☺ Special coverage instructions   ◆ Not covered or valid by Medicare   ✳ Carrier discretion

⚙ **J2675** Injection, progesterone, **per 50 mg**

Other: Gesterol 50, Progestaject

IOM: 100-02, 15, 50

⚙ **J2680** Injection, fluphenazine decanoate, **up to 25 mg**

Other: Prolixin Decanoate

MCM 2049

IOM: 100-02, 15, 50

⚙ **J2690** Injection, procainamide HCL, **up to 1 gm**

Benefit limited to obstetrical diagnoses

Other: Pronestyl, Prostaphlin

IOM: 100-02, 15, 50

⚙ **J2700** Injection, oxacillin sodium, **up to 250 mg**

NDC: Bactocill

IOM: 100-02, 15, 50

⚙ **J2710** Injection, neostigmine methylsulfate, **up to 0.5 mg**

Other: Prostigmin

IOM: 100-02, 15, 50

⚙ **J2720** Injection, protamine sulfate, **per 10 mg**

IOM: 100-02, 15, 50

✳ **J2724** Injection, protein C concentrate, intravenous, human, **10 IU**

NDC: Ceprotin

⚙ **J2725** Injection, protirelin, **per 250 mcg**

Other: Relefact TRH, Thypinone

IOM: 100-02, 15, 50

⚙ **J2730** Injection, pralidoxime chloride, **up to 1 gm**

NDC: Protopam Chloride

IOM: 100-02, 15, 50

⚙ **J2760** Injection, phentolamine mesylate, **up to 5 mg**

Other: Regitine

IOM: 100-02, 15, 50

⚙ **J2765** Injection, metoclopramide HCL, **up to 10 mg**

NDC: Reglan

IOM: 100-02, 15, 50

⚙ **J2770** Injection, quinupristin/dalfopristin, **500 mg (150/350)**

NDC: Synercid

IOM: 100-02, 15, 50

✳ **J2778** Injection, ranibizumab, **0.1 mg**

May be reported for exudative senile macular degeneration (wet AMD) with 67028 (RT or LT)

Other: Lucentis

⚙ **J2780** Injection, ranitidine hydrochloride, **25 mg**

NDC: Zantac

IOM: 100-02, 15, 50

✳ **J2783** Injection, rasburicase, **0.5 mg**

NDC: Elitek

✳ **J2785** Injection, regadenoson, **0.1 mg**

One billing unit equal to 0.1 mg of regadenoson

⚙ **J2788** Injection, Rho D immune globulin, human, minidose, **50 mcg (250 IU)**

NDC: Bay Rho-D, MicRhoGAM

Other: HypRho-D, RhoGam

IOM: 100-02, 15, 50

⚙ **J2790** Injection, Rho D immune globulin, human, full dose, **300 mcg (1500 IU)**

Administered to pregnant female to prevent hemolistic disease of newborn. Report 90384 to private payer

NDC: Hyperrho S/D, RhoGAM

Other: Gamulin Rh, HypRho-D, Rhesonativ

IOM: 100-02, 15, 50

⚙ **J2791** Injection, Rho(D) immune globulin (human), (Rhophylac), intramuscular or intravenous, **100 IU**

Agent must be billed per 100 IU in both physician office and hospital outpatient settings

IOM: 100-02, 15, 50

⚙ **J2792** Injection, Rho D immune globulin intravenous, human, solvent detergent, **100 IU**

NDC: WinRHo-SDF

Other: Gamulin RH, Hyperrho S/D

IOM: 100-02, 15, 50

⚙ **J2793** Injection, rilonacept, **1 mg**

IOM: 100-02, 15, 50

✳ **J2794** Injection, risperidone, long acting, **0.5 mg**

NDC: Risperdal Costa

✳ **J2795** Injection, ropivacaine hydrochloride, **1 mg**

NDC: Naropin

▶ New → Revised ✔ Reinstated ~~deleted~~ Deleted

⚙ Special coverage instructions ◆ Not covered or valid by Medicare ✳ Carrier discretion

✳ **J2796** Injection, romiplostim, **10 micrograms**

Stimulates bone marrow megakarocytes to produce platelets (i.e., ITP).

NDC: Nplate

✪ **J2800** Injection, methocarbamol, **up to 10 ml**

NDC: Robaxin

IOM: 100-02, 15, 50

✳ **J2805** Injection, sincalide, **5 micrograms**

✪ **J2810** Injection, theophylline, **per 40 mg**

IOM: 100-02, 15, 50

✪ **J2820** Injection, sargramostim (GM-CSF), **50 mcg**

NDC: Leukine

Other: Prokine

IOM: 100-02, 15, 50

✪ **J2850** Injection, secretin, synthetic, human, **1 microgram**

NDC: Chirhostim

IOM: 100-02, 15, 50

✪ **J2910** Injection, aurothioglucose, **up to 50 mg**

Other: Solganal

IOM: 100-02, 15, 50

✪ **J2916** Injection, sodium ferric gluconate complex in sucrose injection, **12.5 mg**

NDC: Ferrlecit, Nulecit

IOM: 100-02, 15, 50

✪ **J2920** Injection, methylprednisolone sodium succinate, **up to 40 mg**

NDC: Solu-Medrol

Other: A-MethaPred

IOM: 100-02, 15, 50

✪ **J2930** Injection, methylprednisolone sodium succinate, **up to 125 mg**

NDC: Solu-Medrol

Other: A-MethaPred

IOM: 100-02, 15, 50

✪ **J2940** Injection, somatrem, **1 mg**

IOM: 100-02, 15, 50,

Medicare Statute 1861s2b

✪ **J2941** Injection, somatropin, **1 mg**

Other: Genotropin, Humatrope, Nutropin, Omnitrope, Saizen, Serostim, Zorbtive

IOM: 100-02, 15, 50,

Medicare Statute 1861s2b

✪ **J2950** Injection, promazine HCL, **up to 25 mg**

Other: Prozine-50, Sparine

IOM: 100-02, 15, 50

✪ **J2993** Injection, reteplase, **18.1 mg**

NDC: Retavase

IOM: 100-02, 15, 50

✪ **J2995** Injection, streptokinase, **per 250,000 IU**

Bill 1 unit for each 250,000 IU

Other: Kabikinase, Streptase

IOM: 100-02, 15, 50

✪ **J2997** Injection, alteplase recombinant, **1 mg**

Thrombolytic agent, treatment of occluded catheters. Bill units of 1 mg administered

NDC: Activase, Cathflo Activase

IOM: 100-02, 15, 50

✪ **J3000** Injection, streptomycin, **up to 1 gm**

IOM: 100-02, 15, 50

✪ **J3010** Injection, fentanyl citrate, **0.1 mg**

NDC: Sublimaze

IOM: 100-02, 15, 50

✪ **J3030** Injection, sumatriptan succinate, **6 mg** (Code may be used for Medicare when drug administered under the direct supervision of a physician, not for use when drug is self administered)

NDC: Imitrex, Sumavel Dosepro

IOM: 100-02, 15, 150

✪ **J3070** Injection, pentazocine, **30 mg**

NDC: Talwin

IOM: 100-02, 15, 50

✳ **J3095** Injection, televancin, **10 mg**

Prescribed for the treatment of adults with complicated skin and skin structure infections (cSSSI) of the following Gram-positive microorganisms: *Staphylococcus aureus*; *Streptococcus* pyogenes, *Streptococcus* agalactiae, *Streptococcus* anginosus group. Separately payable under the ASC payment system.

NDC: Vibativ

✳ **J3101** Injection, tenecteplase, **1 mg**

NDC: TNKase

✪ **J3105** Injection, terbutaline sulfate, **up to 1 mg**

Other: Brethine

IOM: 100-02, 15, 50

▶ New   → Revised   ✔ Reinstated   ~~deleted~~ Deleted

✪ Special coverage instructions   ◆ Not covered or valid by Medicare   ✳ Carrier discretion

⊛ **J3110** Injection, teriparatide, **10 mcg**

Other: Forteo

⊛ **J3120** Injection, testosterone enanthate, **up to 100 mg**

Other: Andro LA 200, Andropository 100, Andryl 200, Delatest, Delatestryl, Durathate-200, Everone, Testone LA, Testrin PA

IOM: 100-02, 15, 50

⊛ **J3130** Injection, testosterone enanthate, **up to 200 mg**

Other: Andro LA 200, Andropository 100, Andryl 200, Delatest, Delatestryl, Durathate-200, Everone, Testone LA, Testrin PA

IOM: 100-02, 15, 50

⊛ **J3140** Injection, testosterone suspension, **up to 50 mg**

Other: Adronaq-50, Histerone, Testaqua, Testro AQ, Testoject-50

IOM: 100-02, 15, 50

⊛ **J3150** Injection, testosterone propionate, **up to 100 mg**

Other: DepAndro 100, Testex

IOM: 100-02, 15, 50

⊛ **J3230** Injection, chlorpromazine HCL, **up to 50 mg**

Other: Ormazine, Thorazine

IOM: 100-02, 15, 50

⊛ **J3240** Injection, thyrotropin alfa, **0.9 mg provided in 1.1 mg vial**

NDC: Thyrogen

IOM: 100-02, 15, 50

✳ **J3243** Injection, tigecycline, **1 mg**

✳ **J3246** Injection, tirofiban HCL, **0.25 mg**

NDC: Aggrastat

⊛ **J3250** Injection, trimethobenzamide HCL, **up to 200 mg**

NDC: Ticon, Tigan

Other: Arrestin, Tiject 20

IOM: 100-02, 15, 50

⊛ **J3260** Injection, tobramycin sulfate, **up to 80 mg**

Other: Nebcin

IOM: 100-02, 15, 50

✳ **J3262** Injection, tocilizumab, **1 mg**

Indicated for the treatment of adult patients with moderately to severely active rheumatoid arthritis (RA) who have had an inadequate response to one or more tumor necrosis factor (TNF) antagonist therapies.

NDC: Actemra

⊛ **J3265** Injection, torsemide, **10 mg/ml**

Other: Demadex

IOM: 100-02, 15, 50

⊛ **J3280** Injection, thiethylperazine maleate, **up to 10 mg**

Other: Norzine, Torecan

IOM: 100-02, 15, 50

✳ **J3285** Injection, treprostinil, **1 mg**

NDC: Remodulin

⊛ **J3300** Injection, triamcinolone acetonide, preservative free, **1 mg**

⊛ **J3301** Injection, triamcinolone acetonide, not otherwise specified, **10 mg**

NDC: Kenalog

Other: Cenacort A-40, Kenaject-40, Triam A, Triesence, Tri-Kort, Trilog

IOM: 100-02, 15, 50

⊛ **J3302** Injection, triamcinolone diacetate, **per 5 mg**

NDC: Clincacort

Other: Amcort, Aristocort, Cenacort Forte, Triamcot, Trilone

IOM: 100-02, 15, 50

⊛ **J3303** Injection, triamcinolone hexacetonide, **per 5 mg**

NDC: Aristospan

IOM: 100-02, 15, 50

⊛ **J3305** Injection, trimetrexate glucuronate, **per 25 mg**

Other: NeuTrexin

IOM: 100-02, 15, 50

⊛ **J3310** Injection, perphenazine, **up to 5 mg**

Other: Trilafon

IOM: 100-02, 15, 50

⊛ **J3315** Injection, triptorelin pamoate, **3.75 mg**

NDC: Trelstar

IOM: 100-02, 15, 50

⊛ **J3320** Injection, spectinomycin dihydrochloride, **up to 2 gm**

Other: Trobicin

IOM: 100-02, 15, 50

▶ New   → Revised   ✔ Reinstated   ~~deleted~~ Deleted

⊛ Special coverage instructions   ◆ Not covered or valid by Medicare   ✳ Carrier discretion

✪ **J3350** Injection, urea, **up to 40 gm**

Other: Ureaphil

IOM: 100-02, 15, 50

✪ **J3355** Injection, urofollitropin, **75 IU**

NDC: Bravelle

Other: Metrodin

IOM: 100-02, 15, 50

✳ **J3357** Injection, ustekinumab, **1 mg**

NDC: Stelara

✪ **J3360** Injection, diazepam, **up to 5 mg**

Other: Valium, Zetran

IOM: 100-02, 15, 50

✪ **J3364** Injection, urokinase, **5000 IU vial**

NDC: Abbokinase

IOM: 100-02, 15, 50

✪ **J3365** Injection, IV, urokinase, **250,000 IU vial**

Other: Kinlytic

IOM: 100-02, 15, 50,

Cross Reference Q0089

✪ **J3370** Injection, vancomycin HCL, **500 mg**

NDC: Vancocin

Other: Vancoled

IOM: 100-02, 15, 50; 100-03, 4, 280.14

✳ **J3385** Injection, velaglucerase alfa, **100 units**

Enzyme replacement therapy in Gaucher Disease that results from a specific enzyme deficiency in the body, caused by a genetic mutation received from both parents. Type 1 is the most prevalent Ashkenazi Jewish genetic disease, occurring in one in every 1,000.

NDC: VPRIV

✪ **J3396** Injection, verteporfin, **0.1 mg**

NDC: Visudyne

IOM: 100-03, 1, 80.2; 100-03, 1, 80.3

✪ **J3400** Injection, triflupromazine HCL, **up to 20 mg**

Other: Vesprin

IOM: 100-02, 15, 50

✪ **J3410** Injection, hydroxyzine HCL, **up to 25 mg**

Other: Hyzine-50, Vistacot, Vistaject 25

IOM: 100-02, 15, 50

✳ **J3411** Injection, thiamine HCL, **100 mg**

✳ **J3415** Injection, pyridoxine HCL, **100 mg**

Other: Rodex

✪ **J3420** Injection, vitamin B-12 cyanocobalamin, **up to 1000 mcg**

Medicare carriers may have local coverage decisions regarding vitamin B_{12} injections that provide reimbursement only for patients with certain types of anemia and other conditions

Other: Cobolin-M, Hydroxocobalamin, Neuroforte-R, Redisol, Rubramin PC, Sytobex, Vita #12

IOM: 100-02, 15, 50; 100-03, 2, 150.6

✪ **J3430** Injection, phytonadione (vitamin K), **per 1 mg**

NDC: Vitamin K1

Other: Aqua-Mephyton, Konakion, Menadione, Synkavite

IOM: 100-02, 15, 50

✪ **J3465** Injection, voriconazole, **10 mg**

NDC: VFEND

IOM: 100-02, 15, 50

✪ **J3470** Injection, hyaluronidase, **up to 150 units**

NDC: Amphadase

Other: Vitrase, Wydase

IOM: 100-02, 15, 50

✪ **J3471** Injection, hyaluronidase, ovine, preservative free, **per 1 USP unit (up to 999 USP units)**

NDC: Vitrase

✪ **J3472** Injection, hyaluronidase, ovine, preservative free, **per 1000 USP units**

✪ **J3473** Injection, hyaluronidase, recombinant, **1 USP unit**

IOM: 100-02, 15, 50

✪ **J3475** Injection, magnesium sulfate, **per 500 mg**

IOM: 100-02, 15, 50

✪ **J3480** Injection, potassium chloride, **per 2 meq**

IOM: 100-02, 15, 50

✪ **J3485** Injection, zidovudine, **10 mg**

NDC: Retrovir

IOM: 100-02, 15, 50

✳ **J3486** Injection, ziprasidone mesylate, **10 mg**

NDC: Geodon

✳ **J3487** Injection, zoledronic acid (Zometa), **1 mg**

NDC: Zometa

▶ New → Revised ✔ Reinstated deleted Deleted
✪ Special coverage instructions ◆ Not covered or valid by Medicare ✳ Carrier discretion

⊕ **J3488**   Injection, zoledronic acid (Reclast),
1 mg

Physician to specify 5 units for
approved 5 mg dosing of Reclast

NDC: Reclast

⊕ **J3490**   Unclassified drugs

Bill on paper. Bill one unit. Identify drug
and total dosage in "Remarks" field.

*Other: Acthib, Aminocaproic Acid,
Baciim, Bacitracin, Benzocaine,
Betamethasone Acetate, Brevital Sodium,
Bumetanide, Bupivacaine, Cefotetan,
Cimetidine, Ciprofloxacin, Cleocin
Phosphate, Clindamycin, Cortisone
Acetate, Definity, Diprivan, Engerix-B,
Ethanolamine, Famotidine, Ganirelix,
Gonal-F, Hyaluronic Acid, Kineret,
Marcaine, Metronidazole, Nafcillin,
Naltrexone, Ovidrel, Pegasys, Peg-Intron,
Penicillin G Sodium, Prodrox, Propofol,
Protonix, Recombivax, Rifadin,
Rifampin, Sensorcaine-MPF, Smz-TMP,
Sodium Hyaluronate, Sufenta,
Sufentanil Citrate, Timentin, Treanda,
Twinrix, Valcyte, Veritas Collagen Matrix*

IOM: 100-02, 15, 50

◆ **J3520**   Edetate disodium, **per 150 mg**

*Other: Chealamide, Disotate, Endrate
ethylenediamine-tetra-acetic*

IOM: 100-03, 1, 20.21; 100-03, 1, 20.22

⊕ **J3530**   Nasal vaccine inhalation

IOM: 100-02, 15, 50

◆ **J3535**   Drug administered through a metered
dose inhaler

Other: Ipratropium bromide

IOM: 100-02, 15, 50

◆ **J3570**   Laetrile, amygdalin, vitamin B-17

IOM: 100-03, 1, 30.7

✳ **J3590**   Unclassified biologics

Bill local carrier

Bill on paper. Bill one unit. Identify
drug and total dosage in "Remarks"
field.

Other: Bayhep B, Hyperhep-B, NABI-HB

Miscellaneous Drugs and Solutions

⊕ **J7030**   Infusion, normal saline solution,
1000 cc

Bill local carrier if incident to a
physician's service or used in an
implanted infusion pump. If other, bill
DME/MAC

NDC: Sodium Chloride

IOM: 100-02, 15, 50

⊕ **J7040**   Infusion, normal saline solution, sterile
(500 ml=1 unit)

Bill local carrier if incident to a
physician's service or used in an
implanted infusion pump. If other, bill
DME/MAC

NDC: Sodium Chloride

IOM: 100-02, 15, 50

⊕ **J7042**   5% dextrose/normal saline
(500 ml = 1 unit)

Bill local carrier if incident to a
physician's service or used in an
implanted infusion pump. If other, bill
DME/MAC

NDC: Dextrose-Nacl

IOM: 100-02, 15, 50

⊕ **J7050**   Infusion, normal saline solution, **250 cc**

Bill local carrier if incident to a
physician's service or used in an
implanted infusion pump. If other, bill
DME/MAC

NDC: Sodium Chloride

IOM: 100-02, 15, 50

⊕ **J7060**   5% dextrose/water **(500 ml = 1 unit)**

Bill local carrier if incident to a
physician's service or used in an
implanted infusion pump. If other, bill
DME/MAC

IOM: 100-02, 15, 50

⊕ **J7070**   Infusion, D 5 W, **1000 cc**

Bill local carrier if incident to a
physician's service or used in an
implanted infusion pump. If other, bill
DME/MAC

NDC: Dextrose

IOM: 100-02, 15, 50

▶ New   → Revised   ✔ Reinstated   ~~deleted~~ Deleted
⊕ Special coverage instructions   ◆ Not covered or valid by Medicare   ✳ Carrier discretion

⚙ **J7100** Infusion, dextran 40, **500 ml**

Bill local carrier if incident to a physician's service or used in an implanted infusion pump. If other, bill DME/MAC

Other: Gentran, LMD, LMD in Dextrose, Rheomacrodex

IOM: 100-02, 15, 50

⚙ **J7110** Infusion, dextran 75, **500 ml**

Bill local carrier if incident to a physician's service or used in an implanted infusion pump. If other, bill DME/MAC

NDC: Dextran 70 w/NACL, Dextran 75 in D5W

Other: Gentran

IOM: 100-02, 15, 50

⚙ **J7120** Ringer's lactate infusion, **up to 1000 cc**

Bill local carrier if incident to a physician's service or used in an implanted infusion pump. If other, bill DME/MAC

Replacement fluid or electrolytes.

NDC: Lactated Ringers

IOM: 100-02, 15, 50

⚙ **J7131** Hypertonic saline solution, **1 ml**

IOM: 100-02, 15, 50

▶ ✱ **J7178** Injection, human fibrinogen concentrate, **1 mg**

✱ **J7180** Injection, factor XIII (antihemophilic factor, human), 1 i.u.

⚙ **J7183** Injection, von Willebrand factor complex (human), wilate, **1 i.u. vwf:rco**

IOM: 100-02, 15, 50

✱ **J7185** Injection, Factor VIII (antihemophilic factor, recombinant) (Xyntha), **per IU**

Reported in place of temporary code Q2023.

⚙ **J7186** Injection, anti-hemophilic factor VIII/von Willebrand factor complex (human), **per factor VIII IU**

Bill local carrier

NDC: Alphanate

IOM: 100-02, 15, 50

⚙ **J7187** Injection, von Willebrand factor complex (HUMATE-P), **per IU VWF:RCO**

Bill local carrier

NDC: Humate-P Low Dilutent

Other: Wilate

IOM: 100-02, 15, 50

⚙ **J7189** Factor VIIa (anti-hemophilic factor, recombinant), **per 1 microgram**

Bill local carrier

NDC: NovoSeven

IOM: 100-02, 15, 50

⚙ **J7190** Factor VIII anti-hemophilic factor, human, **per IU**

Bill local carrier

NDC: Alphanate/von Willebrand factor complex, Hemofil M, Koate DVI, Monoclate-P

Other: Koate-HP, Kogenate, Recombinate

IOM: 100-02, 15, 50

⚙ **J7191** Factor VIII, anti-hemophilic factor (porcine), **per IU**

Bill local carrier

Other: Hyate C, Koate-HP, Kogenate, Monoclate-P, Recombinate

IOM: 100-02, 15, 50

✱ **J7192** Factor VIII (anti-hemophilic factor, recombinant) **per IU,** not otherwise specified

Bill local carrier

NDC: Advate, Helixate FS, Kogenate FS, Recombinate

Other: Koate-HP, Refacto

IOM: 100-02, 15, 50

⚙ **J7193** Factor IX (anti-hemophilic factor, purified, non-recombinant) **per IU**

Bill local carrier

NDC: AlphaNine SD, Mononine, Profiline, Proplex T

IOM: 100-02, 15, 50

⚙ **J7194** Factor IX, complex, **per IU**

Bill local carrier

NDC: Bebulin VH, Profilnine SD

Other: Konyne-80, Profilnine Heat-treated, Proplex SX-T, Proplex T

IOM: 100-02, 15, 50

⚙ **J7195** Factor IX (anti-hemophilic factor, recombinant) **per IU**

Bill local carrier

NDC: Benefix

Other: Konyne 80, Profiline, Proplex T

IOM: 100-02, 15, 50

✱ **J7196** Injection, antithrombin recombinant, **50 i.u.**

Other: ATryn

▶ **New**   → **Revised**   ✔ **Reinstated**   ~~deleted~~ **Deleted**

⚙ **Special coverage instructions**   ◆ **Not covered or valid by Medicare**   ✱ **Carrier discretion**

⊙ **J7197** Anti-thrombin III (human), **per IU**

Bill local carrier

NDC: Thrombate III

IOM: 100-02, 15, 50

⊙ **J7198** Anti-inhibitor, **per IU**

Bill local carrier

Diagnosis examples: 286.0 Congenital Factor VIII disorder; 286.1 Congenital Factor IX disorder; 286.4 VonWillebrand's disease

NDC: Feiba VH Immuno

Other: Autoplex T, Hemophilia clotting factors

IOM: 100-02, 15, 50; 100-03, 2, 110.3

⊙ **J7199** Hemophilia clotting factor, not otherwise classified

Bill local carrier

Other: Autoplex T

IOM: 100-02, 15, 50; 100-03, 2, 110.3

◆ **J7300** Intrauterine copper contraceptive

Bill local carrier

Report IVD insertion with 58300. Bill usual and customary charge.

Other: Paragard T 380 A

Medicare Statute 1862a1

◆ **J7302** Levonorgestrel-releasing intrauterine contraceptive system, **52 mg**

Bill local carrier

Other: Mirena

Medicare Statute 1862a1

◆ **J7303** Contraceptive supply, hormone containing vaginal ring, each

Bill local carrier

Medicare Statute 1862.1

◆ **J7304** Contraceptive supply, hormone containing patch, each

Bill local carrier

Only billed by Family Planning Clinics

Medicare Statute 1862.1

◆ **J7306** Levonorgestrel (contraceptive) implant system, including implants and supplies

Bill local carrier

◆ **J7307** Etonogestrel (contraceptive) implant system, including implant and supplies

Bill local carrier

✳ **J7308** Aminolevulinic acid HCL for topical administration, 20%, single unit dosage form **(354 mg)**

Bill local carrier

NDC: Levulan Kerastick

⊙ **J7309** Methyl aminolevulinate (MAL) for topical administration, 16.8%, **1 gram**

NDC: Metvixia

⊙ **J7310** Ganciclovir, **4.5 mg,** long-acting implant

Bill local carrier

NDC: Vitrasert

IOM: 100-02, 15, 50

✳ **J7311** Fluocinolone acetonide, intravitreal implant

Bill local carrier

Treatment of chronic noninfectious posterior segment uveitis

Other: Retisert

✳ **J7312** Injection, dexamethasone, intravitreal implant, **0.1 mg**

To bill for Ozurdex services submit the following codes: J7312 and 67028 with the modifier -22 (for the increased work difficulty and increased risk). Indicated for the treatment of macular edema occurring after branch retinal vein occlusion (BRVO) or central retinal vein occlusion (CRVO) and non-infectious uveitis affecting the posterior segment of the eye.

MDC: Ozurdex

▶ ✳ **J7315** Mitomycin, ophthalmic, 0.2 mg

✳ **J7321** Hyaluronan or derivative, Hyalgan or Supartz, for intra-articular injection, **per dose**

Bill local carrier

Therapeutic goal is to restore visco-elasticity of synovial hyaluronan, thereby decreasing pain, improving mobility and restoring natural protective functions of hyaluronan in joint

✳ **J7323** Hyaluronan or derivative, Euflexxa, for intra-articular injection, **per dose**

Bill local carrier

✳ **J7324** Hyaluronan or derivative, Orthovisc, for intra-articular injection, **per dose**

Bill local carrier

✳ **J7325** Hyaluronan or derivative, Synvisc or Synvisc-One, for intra-articular injection, **1 mg**

▶ New → Revised ✔ Reinstated ~~deleted~~ Deleted

⊙ Special coverage instructions ◆ Not covered or valid by Medicare ✳ Carrier discretion

✳ **J7326** Hyaluronan or derivative, Gel-One, for intra-articular injection, **per dose**

✳ **J7330** Autologous cultured chondrocytes, **implant**

Bill local carrier

NDC: Carticel

✳ **J7335** Capsaicin 8% patch, **per 10 square centimeters**

NDC: Qutenza

Immunosuppressive Drugs (Includes Non-injectibles)

J7500-J7599: Bill local carrier if incident to a physician's service or used in an implanted infusion pump. If other, bill DME/MAC

☺ **J7500** Azathioprine, oral, **50 mg**

NDC: Azasan

Other: Imuran

IOM: 100-02, 15, 50

☺ **J7501** Azathioprine, parenteral, **100 mg**

Other: Imuran

IOM: 100-02, 15, 50

☺ **J7502** Cyclosporine, oral, **100 mg**

NDC: Gengraf, Neoral, Sandimmune

IOM: 100-02, 15, 50

☺ **J7504** Lymphocyte immune globulin, antithymocyte globulin, equine, parenteral, **250 mg**

NDC: Atgam

IOM: 100-02, 15, 50; 100-03, 2, 110.3

☺ **J7505** Muromonab-CD3, parenteral, **5 mg**

NDC: Orthoclone OKT3

Other: Monoclonal antibodies (parenteral)

IOM: 100-02, 15, 50

☺ **J7506** Prednisone, oral, **per 5 mg**

Unit billing example, fifty 10 mg prednisone tablets dispensed, report J7506, 100 units (1 unit of J7506 = 5 mg)

Other: Prednicot

IOM: 100-02, 15, 50

☺ **J7507** Tacrolimus, oral, **per 1 mg**

NDC: Prograf

Other: Hecoria

IOM: 100-02, 15, 50

☺ **J7509** Methylprednisolone oral, **per 4 mg**

Other: Medrol, Methylpred DP

IOM: 100-02, 15, 50

☺ **J7510** Prednisolone oral, **per 5 mg**

Other: Cotolone, Delta-Cortef, Orapred, Pediapred, Prelone

IOM: 100-02, 15, 50

✳ **J7511** Lymphocyte immune globulin, antithymocyte globulin, rabbit, parenteral, **25 mg**

NDC: Thymoglobulin

☺ **J7513** Daclizumab, parenteral, **25 mg**

NDC: Zenapax

IOM: 100-02, 15, 50

✳ **J7515** Cyclosporine, oral, **25 mg**

NDC: Gengraf, Neoral, Sandimmune

✳ **J7516** Cyclosporin, parenteral, **250 mg**

NDC: Sandimmune

✳ **J7517** Mycophenolate mofetil, oral, **250 mg**

NDC: CellCept

☺ **J7518** Mycophenolic acid, oral, **180 mg**

NDC: Myfortic

IOM: 100-04, 4, 240; 100-4, 17, 80.3.1

☺ **J7520** Sirolimus, oral, **1 mg**

NDC: Rapamune

IOM: 100-02, 15, 50

☺ **J7525** Tacrolimus, parenteral, **5 mg**

NDC: Prograf

IOM: 100-02, 15, 50

▶ ☺ **J7527** Everolimus, oral, 0.25 mg

Other: Zortress

IOM 100-02, 15, 50

☺ **J7599** Immunosuppressive drug, not otherwise classified

Bill on paper. Bill one unit. Identify drug and total dosage in "Remarks" field.

IOM: 100-02, 15, 50

Inhalation Solutions

J7604-J7799: If "incident to" a physician's service, do not bill; otherwise, bill DME/MAC.

✳ **J7604** Acetylcysteine, inhalation solution, compounded product, administered through DME, unit dose form, **per gram**

Other: Mucomyst (unit dose form), Mucosol, N-acetyl-L-cysteine

---

▶ New   → Revised   ✔ Reinstated   deleted Deleted

☺ Special coverage instructions   ◆ Not covered or valid by Medicare   ✳ Carrier discretion

✳ **J7605** Arformoterol, inhalation solution, FDA approved final product, non-compounded, administered through DME, unit dose form, **15 micrograms**

Maintenance treatment of bronchoconstriction in patients with chronic obstructive pulmonary disease (COPD)

Other: Brovana

✳ **J7606** Formoterol fumarate, inhalation solution, FDA approved final product, non-compounded, administered through DME, unit dose form, **20 micrograms**

NDC: Perforomist

✳ **J7607** Levalbuterol, inhalation solution, compounded product, administered through DME, concentrated form, **0.5 mg**

✪ **J7608** Acetylcysteine, inhalation solution, FDA-approved final product, non-compounded, administered through DME, unit dose form, **per gram**

Other: Mucomyst, Mucosol

✳ **J7609** Albuterol, inhalation solution, compounded product, administered through DME, unit dose, **1 mg**

Patient's home, medications—such as albuterol when administered through a nebulizer—are considered DME and are payable under Part B.

Other: Proventil, Xopenex, Ventolin

✳ **J7610** Albuterol, inhalation solution, compounded product, administered through DME, concentrated form, **1 mg**

Other: Proventil, Xopenex, Ventolin

✪ **J7611** Albuterol, inhalation solution, FDA-approved final product, non-compounded, administered through DME, concentrated form, **1 mg**

Report once for each milligram administered. For example, 2 mg of concentrated albuterol (usually diluted with saline), reported with J7611×2

Other: Proventil, Xopenex

✪ **J7612** Levalbuterol, inhalation solution, FDA-approved final product, non-compounded, administered through DME, concentrated form, **0.5 mg**

NDC: Xopenex

✪ **J7613** Albuterol, inhalation solution, FDA-approved final product, non-compounded, administered through DME, unit dose, **1 mg**

NDC: Accuneb, Proventil, Ventolin

✪ **J7614** Levalbuterol, inhalation solution, FDA-approved final product, non-compounded, administered through DME, unit dose, **0.5 mg**

NDC: Xopenex

✳ **J7615** Levalbuterol, inhalation solution, compounded product, administered through DME, unit dose, **0.5 mg**

✪ **J7620** Albuterol, **up to 2.5 mg** and ipratropium bromide, **up to 0.5 mg,** FDA-approved final product, non-compounded, administered through DME

NDC: DuoNeb

✳ **J7622** Beclomethasone, inhalation solution, compounded product, administered through DME, unit dose form, **per milligram**

✳ **J7624** Betamethasone, inhalation solution, compounded product, administered through DME, unit dose form, **per mg**

Other: Celestone Soluspan

✳ **J7626** Budesonide inhalation solution, FDA-approved final product, non-compounded, administered through DME, unit dose form, **up to 0.5 mg**

NDC: Pulmicort

✳ **J7627** Budesonide, inhalation solution, compounded product, administered through DME, unit dose form, **up to 0.5 mg**

Other: Pulmicort Respulses

✪ **J7628** Bitolterol mesylate, inhalation solution, compounded product, administered through DME, concentrated form, **per milligram**

Other: Tornalate

✪ **J7629** Bitolterol mesylate, inhalation solution, compounded product, administered through DME, unit dose form, **per milligram**

Other: Tornalate

▶ New → Revised ✔ Reinstated ~~deleted~~ Deleted

✪ Special coverage instructions ◆ Not covered or valid by Medicare ✳ Carrier discretion

✪ **J7631** Cromolyn sodium, inhalation solution, FDA-approved final product, non-compounded, administered through DME, unit dose form, **per 10 milligrams**

Other: Intal

✳ **J7632** Cromolyn sodium, inhalation solution, compounded product, administered through DME, unit dose form, **per 10 milligrams**

Other: Intal

✳ **J7633** Budesonide, inhalation solution, FDA-approved final product, non-compounded, administered through DME, concentrated form, **per 0.25 milligram**

Other: Pulmicort Respules

✳ **J7634** Budesonide, inhalation solution, compounded product, administered through DME, concentrated form, **per 0.25 milligram**

✪ **J7635** Atropine, inhalation solution, compounded product, administered through DME, concentrated form, **per milligram**

✪ **J7636** Atropine, inhalation solution, compounded product, administered through DME, unit dose form, **per milligram**

✪ **J7637** Dexamethasone, inhalation solution, compounded product, administered through DME, concentrated form, **per milligram**

✪ **J7638** Dexamethasone, inhalation solution, compounded product, administered through DME, unit dose form, **per milligram**

✪ **J7639** Dornase alfa, inhalation solution, FDA-approved final product, non-compounded, administered through DME, unit dose form, **per milligram**

NDC: Pulmozyme

✳ **J7640** Formoterol, inhalation solution, compounded product, administered through DME, unit dose form, **12 micrograms**

✳ **J7641** Flunisolide, inhalation solution, compounded product, administered through DME, unit dose, **per milligram**

✪ **J7642** Glycopyrrolate, inhalation solution, compounded product, administered through DME, concentrated form, **per milligram**

✪ **J7643** Glycopyrrolate, inhalation solution, compounded product, administered through DME, unit dose form, **per milligram**

Other: Robinul

✪ **J7644** Ipratropium bromide, inhalation solution, FDA-approved final product, non-compounded, administered through DME, **per milligram**

Other: Atrovent

✳ **J7645** Ipratropium bromide, inhalation solution, compounded product, administered through DME, unit dose form, **per milligram**

Other: Atrovent

✳ **J7647** Isoetharine HCL, inhalation solution, compounded product, administered through DME, concentrated form, **per milligram**

Other: Bronkosol

✪ **J7648** Isoetharine HCL, inhalation solution, FDA-approved final product, non-compounded, administered through DME, concentrated form, **per milligram**

Other: Bronkosol

✪ **J7649** Isoetharine HCL, inhalation solution, FDA-approved final product, non-compounded, administered through DME, unit dose form, **per milligram**

Other: Bronkosol

✳ **J7650** Isoetharine HCL, inhalation solution, compounded product, administered through DME, unit dose form, **per milligram**

Other: Bronkosol

✳ **J7657** Isoproterenol HCL, inhalation solution, compounded product, administered through DME, concentrated form, **per milligram**

Other: Isuprel

✪ **J7658** Isoproterenol HCL inhalation solution, FDA-approved final product, non-compounded, administered through DME, concentrated form, **per milligram**

Other: Isuprel

✪ **J7659** Isoproterenol HCL, inhalation solution, FDA-approved final product, non-compounded, administered through DME, unit dose form, **per milligram**

Other: Isuprel

▶ New   → Revised   ✔ Reinstated   ~~deleted~~ Deleted

✪ Special coverage instructions   ◆ Not covered or valid by Medicare   ✳ Carrier discretion

✳ **J7660** Isoproterenol HCL, inhalation solution, compounded product, administered through DME, unit dose form, **per milligram**

Other: Isuprel

→ ✳ **J7665** Mannitol, administered through an inhaler, **5 mg**

NDC: Aridol

✳ **J7667** Metaproterenol sulfate, inhalation solution, compounded product, concentrated form, **per 10 milligrams**

Other: Metaprel

❂ **J7668** Metaproterenol sulfate, inhalation solution, FDA-approved final product, non-compounded, administered through DME, concentrated form, **per 10 milligrams**

Other: Metaprel

❂ **J7669** Metaproterenol sulfate, inhalation solution, FDA-approved final product, non-compounded, administered through DME, unit dose form, **per 10 milligrams**

Other: Alupent, Metaprel

✳ **J7670** Metaproterenol sulfate, inhalation solution, compounded product, administered through DME, unit dose form, **per 10 milligrams**

Other: Metaprel

✳ **J7674** Methacholine chloride administered as inhalation solution through a nebulizer, **per 1 mg**

NDC: Provocholine

✳ **J7676** Pentamidine isethionate, inhalation solution, compounded product, administered through DME, unit dose form, **per 300 mg**

Other: NebuPent, Pentam

❂ **J7680** Terbutaline sulfate, inhalation solution, compounded product, administered through DME, concentrated form, **per milligram**

Other: Brethine

❂ **J7681** Terbutaline sulfate, inhalation solution, compounded product, administered through DME, unit dose form, **per milligram**

Other: Brethine

❂ **J7682** Tobramycin, inhalation solution, FDA-approved final product, non-compounded unit dose form, administered through DME, **per 300 milligrams**

NDC: Tobi

Other: Nebcin

❂ **J7683** Triamcinolone, inhalation solution, compounded product, administered through DME, concentrated form, **per milligram**

❂ **J7684** Triamcinolone, inhalation solution, compounded product, administered through DME, unit dose form, **per milligram**

Other: Triamcinolone acetonide

✳ **J7685** Tobramycin, inhalation solution, compounded product, administered through DME, unit dose form, **per 300 milligrams**

✳ **J7686** Treprostinil, inhalation solution, FDA-approved final product, non-compounded, administered through DME, unit dose form, **1.74 mg**

NDC: Tyvaso

❂ **J7699** NOC drugs, inhalation solution administered through DME

Other: Gentamicin Sulfate, Sodium chloride, Tyvaso

❂ **J7799** NOC drugs, other than inhalation drugs, administered through DME

Bill on paper. Bill one unit and identify drug and total dosage in the "Remark" field.

Other: Epinephrine, Mannitol, Osmitrol, Phenylephrine, Resectisol, Sodium chloride

IOM: 100-02, 15, 110.3

Other

❂ **J8498** Antiemetic drug, rectal/suppository, not otherwise specified

Bill DME/MAC

Other: Compazine, Compro, Phenadoz, Phenergan, Prochlorperazine, Promethazine, Promethegan, Thorazine

Medicare Statute 1861(s)2t

▶ New → Revised ✔ Reinstated ~~deleted~~ Deleted
❂ Special coverage instructions ◆ Not covered or valid by Medicare ✳ Carrier discretion

◆ **J8499** Prescription drug, oral, non chemotherapeutic, NOS

If "incident to" a physician's service, do not bill; otherwise, bill DME/MAC

Other: Acyclovir, Millipred, Zovirax

IOM: 100-02, 15, 50

⊗ **J8501** Aprepitant, oral, **5 mg**

Bill DME/MAC

NDC: Emend

⊗ **J8510** Busulfan; oral, **2 mg**

Bill DME/MAC

NDC: Myleran

IOM 100-02, 15, 50; 100-04, 4, 240; 100-04, 17, 80.1.1

◆ **J8515** Cabergoline, oral, **0.25 mg**

Bill DME/MAC

IOM: 100-02, 15, 50; 100-04, 4, 240

⊗ **J8520** Capecitabine, oral, **150 mg**

Bill DME/MAC

NDC: Xeloda

IOM: 100-02, 15, 50; 100-04, 4, 240; 100-04, 17, 80.1.1

⊗ **J8521** Capecitabine, oral, **500 mg**

Bill DME/MAC

NDC: Xeloda

IOM: 100-02, 15, 50; 100-04, 4, 240; 100-04, 17, 80.1.1

⊗ **J8530** Cyclophosphamide; oral, **25 mg**

Bill DME/MAC

Other: Cytoxan

IOM: 100-02, 15, 50; 100-04, 4, 240; 100-04, 17, 80.1.1

⊗ **J8540** Dexamethasone, oral, **0.25 mg**

Bill DME/MAC

Other: Decadron, Dexone, Dexpak

Medicare Statute 1861(s)2t

⊗ **J8560** Etoposide; oral, **50 mg**

Bill DME/MAC

NDC: VePesid

IOM: 100-02, 15, 50; 100-04, 4, 230.1; 100-04, 4, 240; 100-04, 17, 80.1.1

~~J8561~~ ~~Everolimus, oral, **0.25 mg**~~ ✖

✳ **J8562** Fludarabine phosphate, oral, **10 mg**

Bill DME/MAC

NDC: Oforta

◆ **J8565** Gefitinib, oral, **250 mg**

Bill DME/MAC

Other: Iressa

⊗ **J8597** Antiemetic drug, oral, not otherwise specified

Bill DME/MAC

Medicare Statute 1861(s)2t

⊗ **J8600** Melphalan; oral, **2 mg**

Bill DME/MAC

NDC: Alkeran

IOM: 100-02, 15, 50; 100-04, 4, 240; 100-04, 17, 80.1.1

⊗ **J8610** Methotrexate; oral, **2.5 mg**

Bill DME/MAC

NDC: Rheumatrex, Trexall

IOM: 100-02, 15, 50; 100-04, 4, 240; 100-04, 17, 80.1.1

✳ **J8650** Nabilone, oral, **1 mg**

Bill DME/MAC

⊗ **J8700** Temozolomide, oral, **5 mg**

Bill DME/MAC

NDC: Temodar

IOM: 100-02, 15, 50; 100-04, 4, 240

✳ **J8705** Topotecan, oral, **0.25 mg**

Bill DME/MAC

Treatment for ovarian and lung cancers, etc. Report J9350 (Topotecan, 4 mg) for intravenous version

⊗ **J8999** Prescription drug, oral, chemotherapeutic, NOS

Bill DME/MAC

Other: Arimidex, Aromasin, Ceenu, Droxia, Flutamide, Hydrea, Hydroxyurea, Leukeran, Malulane, Megace, Megestrol Acetate, Mercaptopurine, Nolvadex, Purinethol, Tamoxifen Citrate

IOM: 100-02, 15, 50; 100-04, 4, 250; 100-04, 17, 80.1.1; 100-04, 17, 80.1.2

▶ New   → Revised   ✔ Reinstated   ~~deleted~~ Deleted

⊗ Special coverage instructions   ◆ Not covered or valid by Medicare   ✳ Carrier discretion

DRUGS OTHER THAN CHEMOTHERAPY   J8499 – J8999

CHEMOTHERAPY DRUGS (J9000-J9999)

NOTE: These codes cover the cost of the chemotherapy drug only, not to include the administration

J9000-J9999:	Bill local carrier if incident to a physician's service or used in an implanted infusion pump. If other, bill DME/MAC

⊗ **J9000** Injection, doxorubicin hydrochloride, **10 mg**

NDC: Adriamycin

Other: Rubex

IOM: 100-02, 15, 50

J9001 Injection, doxorubicin hydrochloride, all lipid formulations, 10 mg ✖

▶ ⊗ **J9002** Injection, doxorubicin hydrochloride, liposomal, doxil, 10 mg

IOM 100-02, 15, 50

⊗ **J9010** Injection, alemtuzumab, **10 mg**

NDC: Campath

Medicare Statute 1833(t)

⊗ **J9015** Injection, aldesleukin, **per single use vial**

NDC: Proleukin

IOM: 100-02, 15, 50

✳ **J9017** Injection, arsenic trioxide, **1 mg**

NDC: Trisenox

▶ ⊗ **J9019** Injection, asparaginase (Erwinaze), 1,000 iu

IOM 100-02, 15, 50

→ ⊗ **J9020** Injection, asparaginase, not otherwise specified, **10,000 units**

NDC: Elspar

IOM: 100-02, 15, 50

✳ **J9025** Injection, azacitidine, **1 mg**

NDC: Vidaza

✳ **J9027** Injection, clofarabine, **1 mg**

NDC: Clolar

⊗ **J9031** BCG (intravesical), **per instillation**

NDC: TheraCys, Tice BCG

IOM: 100-02, 15, 50

✳ **J9033** Injection, bendamustine HCL, **1 mg**

Treatment for form of non-Hodgkin's lymphoma; standard administration time is as an intravenous infusion over 30 minutes

NDC: Treanda

✳ **J9035** Injection, bevacizumab, **10 mg**

For malignant neoplasm of breast, considered J9207.

NDC: Avastin

⊗ **J9040** Injection, bleomycin sulfate, **15 units**

Other: Blenoxane

IOM: 100-02, 15, 50

✳ **J9041** Injection, bortezomib, **0.1 mg**

NDC: Velcade

▶ ✳ **J9042** Injection, brentuximab vedotin, **1 mg**

✳ **J9043** Injection, cabazitaxel, **1 mg**

NDC: Jertana

⊗ **J9045** Injection, carboplatin, **50 mg**

Other: Paraplatin

IOM: 100-02, 15, 50

⊗ **J9050** Injection, carmustine, **100 mg**

NDC: BiCNU

IOM: 100-02, 15, 50

✳ **J9055** Injection, cetuximab, **10 mg**

NDC: Erbitux

⊗ **J9060** Injection, cisplatin, powder or solution, **10 mg**

Other: Plantinol AQ

IOM: 100-02, 15, 50

⊗ **J9065** Injection, cladribine, **per 1 mg**

NDC: Leustatin

IOM: 100-02, 15, 50

⊗ **J9070** Cyclophosphamide, **100 mg**

Other: Cytoxan, Neosar

IOM: 100-02, 15, 50

✳ **J9098** Injection, cytarabine liposome, **10 mg**

NDC: DepoCyt

◆ **J9100** Injection, cytarabine, **100 mg**

Other: Cytosar-U

IOM: 100-02, 15, 50

⊗ **J9120** Injection, dactinomycin, **0.5 mg**

NDC: Cosmegen

IOM: 100-02, 15, 50

▶ New	→ Revised	✔ Reinstated	deleted Deleted
⊗ Special coverage instructions	◆ Not covered or valid by Medicare		✳ Carrier discretion

⊛ **J9130**   Dacarbazine, **100 mg**
Other: DTIC-Dome
IOM: 100-02, 15, 50

⊛ **J9150**   Injection, daunorubicin, **10 mg**
NDC: Cerubidine
IOM: 100-02, 15, 50

⊛ **J9151**   Injection, daunorubicin citrate, liposomal formulation, **10 mg**
NDC: Daunoxome
IOM: 100-02, 15, 50

✳ **J9155**   Injection, degarelix, **1 mg**
Report 1 unit for every 1 mg.
NDC: Firmagon

✳ **J9160**   Injection, denileukin diftitox, **300 micrograms**
NDC: Ontak

⊛ **J9165**   Injection, diethylstilbestrol diphosphate, **250 mg**
Other: Stilphostrol
IOM: 100-02, 15, 50

⊛ **J9171**   Injection, docetaxel, **1 mg**
Report 1 unit for every 1 mg.
NDC: Docefrez, Taxotere
IOM: 100-02, 15, 50

⊛ **J9175**   Injection, Elliott's B solution, **1 ml**
NDC: Elliott's b
IOM: 100-02, 15, 50

✳ **J9178**   Injection, epirubicin HCL, **2 mg**
NDC: Ellence

✳ **J9179**   Injection, eribulin mesylate, **0.1 mg**
NDC: Halaven

→ ⊛ **J9181**   Injection, etoposide, **10 mg**
NDC: Etopophos, VePesid

⊛ **J9185**   Injection, fludarabine phosphate, **50 mg**
NDC: Fludara
IOM: 100-02, 15, 50

⊛ **J9190**   Injection, fluorouracil, **500 mg**
NDC: Adrucil
IOM: 100-02, 15, 50

⊛ **J9200**   Injection, floxuridine, **500 mg**
Other: FUDR
IOM: 100-02, 15, 50

⊛ **J9201**   Injection, gemcitabine hydrochloride, **200 mg**
NDC: Gemzar
IOM: 100-02, 15, 50

⊛ **J9202**   Goserelin acetate implant, **per 3.6 mg**
NDC: Zoladex
IOM: 100-02, 15, 50

⊛ **J9206**   Injection, irinotecan, **20 mg**
NDC: Camptosar
IOM: 100-02, 15, 50

✳ **J9207**   Injection, ixabepilone, **1 mg**

→ ⊛ **J9208**   Injection, ifosfamide, **1 gm**
NDC: Ifex
IOM: 100-02, 15, 50

⊛ **J9209**   Injection, mesna, **200 mg**
NDC: Mesnex
IOM: 100-02, 15, 50

⊛ **J9211**   Injection, idarubicin hydrochloride, **5 mg**
NDC: Idamycin PFS
IOM: 100-02, 15, 50

⊛ **J9212**   Injection, interferon alfacon-1, recombinant, **1 mcg**
Other: Infergen
IOM: 100-02, 15, 50

⊛ **J9213**   Injection, interferon, alfa-2a, recombinant, **3 million units**
IOM: 100-02, 15, 50

⊛ **J9214**   Injection, interferon, alfa-2b, recombinant, **1 million units**
NDC: Intron-A
IOM: 100-02, 15, 50

⊛ **J9215**   Injection, interferon, alfa-n3 (human leukocyte derived), **250,000 IU**
Other: Alferon N
IOM: 100-02, 15, 50

⊛ **J9216**   Injection, interferon, gamma-1B, **3 million units**
Other: Actimmune
IOM: 100-02, 15, 50

⊛ **J9217**   Leuprolide acetate (for depot suspension), **7.5 mg**
NDC: Eligard, Lupron Depot
IOM: 100-02, 15, 50

⊛ **J9218**   Leuprolide acetate, **per 1 mg**
Other: Lupron
IOM: 100-02, 15, 50

▶ **New**   → **Revised**   ✔ **Reinstated**   ~~deleted~~ **Deleted**
⊛ **Special coverage instructions**   ◆ **Not covered or valid by Medicare**   ✳ **Carrier discretion**

⊕ **J9219** Leuprolide acetate implant, **65 mg**
NDC: Viadur
IOM: 100-02, 15, 50

⊕ **J9225** Histrelin implant (Vantas), **50 mg**
IOM: 100-02, 15, 50

⊕ **J9226** Histrelin implant (Supprelin LA), **50 mg**
Other: Vantas
IOM: 100-02, 15, 50

✳ **J9228** Injection, ipilimumab, **1 mg**
NDC: Yervoy

⊕ **J9230** Injection, mechlorethamine hydrochloride, (nitrogen mustard), **10 mg**
NDC: Mustargen
IOM: 100-02, 15, 50

⊕ **J9245** Injection, melphalan hydrochloride, **50 mg**
NDC: Alkeran
IOM: 100-02, 15, 50

⊕ **J9250** Methotrexate sodium, **5 mg**
Other: Folex
IOM: 100-02, 15, 50

⊕ **J9260** Methotrexate sodium, **50 mg**
Other: Folex
IOM: 100-02, 15, 50

✳ **J9261** Injection, nelarabine, **50 mg**
NDC: Arranon

✳ **J9263** Injection, oxaliplatin, **0.5 mg**
Eloxatin, platinum-based anticancer drug that destroys cancer cells
NDC: Eloxatin

✳ **J9264** Injection, paclitaxel protein-bound particles, **1 mg**
NDC: Abraxane

⊕ **J9265** Injection, paclitaxel, **30 mg**
Other: Taxol
IOM: 100-02, 15, 50

⊕ **J9266** Injection, pegaspargase, **per single dose vial**
NDC: Oncaspar
IOM: 100-02, 15, 50

⊕ **J9268** Injection, pentostatin, **10 mg**
NDC: Nipent
IOM: 100-02, 15, 50

⊕ **J9270** Injection, plicamycin, **2.5 mg**
Other: Mithracin
IOM: 100-02, 15, 50

→ ⊕ **J9280** Injection, mitomycin, **5 mg**
NDC: Mutamycin
IOM: 100-02, 15, 50

⊕ **J9293** Injection, mitoxantrone hydrochloride, **per 5 mg**
Other: Novantrone
IOM: 100-02, 15, 50

✳ **J9300** Injection, gemtuzumab ozogamicin, **5 mg**
NDC: Mylotarg

✳ **J9302** Injection, ofatumumab, **10 mg**
NDC: Arzerra
Other: Doulinum

✳ **J9303** Injection, panitumumab, **10 mg**
Other: Vectibix

✳ **J9305** Injection, pemetrexed, **10 mg**
NDC: Alimta

✳ **J9307** Injection, pralatrexate, **1 mg**
NDC: Folotyn

⊕ **J9310** Injection, rituximab, **100 mg**
NDC: RituXan
IOM: 100-02, 15, 50

✳ **J9315** Injection, romidepsin, **1 mg**
NDC: Istodax

⊕ **J9320** Injection, streptozocin, **1 gram**
NDC: Zanosar
IOM: 100-02, 15, 50

✳ **J9328** Injection, temozolomide, **1 mg**
Intravenous formulation, not for oral administration
NDC: Temodar

✳ **J9330** Injection, temsirolimus, **1 mg**
Treatment for advanced renal cell carcinoma; standard administration is intravenous infusion greater than 30-60 minutes
Other: Torisel

⊕ **J9340** Injection, thiotepa, **15 mg**
Other: Thiethylenethiophosphoramide/T
IOM: 100-02, 15, 50

✳ **J9351** Injection, topotecan, **0.1 mg**
NDC: Hycamtin

▶ New → Revised ✔ Reinstated deleted Deleted
⊕ Special coverage instructions ◆ Not covered or valid by Medicare ✳ Carrier discretion

✳ **J9355** Injection, trastuzumab, **10 mg**

NDC: Herceptin

⊛ **J9357** Injection, valrubicin, intravesical, **200 mg**

NDC: Valstar

IOM: 100-02, 15, 50

⊛ **J9360** Injection, vinblastine sulfate, **1 mg**

Other: Alkaban-AQ, Velban, Velsar

IOM: 100-02, 15, 50

⊛ **J9370** Vincristine sulfate, **1 mg**

Other: Oncovin, Vincasar PFS

IOM: 100-02, 15, 50

⊛ **J9390** Injection, vinorelbine tartrate, **10 mg**

NDC: Navelbine

IOM: 100-02, 15, 50

✳ **J9395** Injection, fulvestrant, **25 mg**

NDC: Faslodex

⊛ **J9600** Injection, porfimer sodium, **75 mg**

Other: Photofrin

IOM: 100-02, 15, 50

⊛ **J9999** Not otherwise classified, antineoplastic drugs

Bill on paper, bill one unit, and identify drug and total dosage in "Remarks" field. Include invoice of cost or NDC number in "Remarks" field.

Other: Allopurinol Sodium, Ifosfamide/Mesna

IOM: 100-02, 15, 50; 100-03, 2, 110.2

▶ New   → Revised   ✔ Reinstated   ~~deleted~~ Deleted

⊛ Special coverage instructions   ◆ Not covered or valid by Medicare   ✳ Carrier discretion

TEMPORARY CODES ASSIGNED TO DME REGIONAL CARRIERS (K0000-K9999)

Wheelchairs and Accessories

NOTE: This section contains national codes assigned by CMS on a temporary basis and for the exclusive use of the durable medical equipment regional carriers (DMERC).

* **K0001** Standard wheelchair

  Bill DME/MAC

  Capped rental

* **K0002** Standard hemi (low seat) wheelchair

  Bill DME/MAC

  Capped rental

* **K0003** Lightweight wheelchair

  Bill DME/MAC

  Capped rental

* **K0004** High strength, lightweight wheelchair

  Bill DME/MAC

  Capped rental

* **K0005** Ultralightweight wheelchair

  Bill DME/MAC

  Capped rental. Inexpensive and routinely purchased DME

* **K0006** Heavy duty wheelchair

  Bill DME/MAC

  Capped rental

* **K0007** Extra heavy duty wheelchair

  Bill DME/MAC

  Capped rental

* **K0009** Other manual wheelchair/base

  Not Otherwise Classified.

* **K0010** Standard - weight frame motorized/ power wheelchair

  Capped rental. Codes K0010-K0014 are not for manual wheelchairs with add-on power packs. Use the appropriate code for the manual wheelchair base provided (K0001-K0009) and code K0460

* **K0011** Standard - weight frame motorized/ power wheelchair with programmable control parameters for speed adjustment, tremor dampening, acceleration control and braking

  Capped rental. A patient who requires a power wheelchair usually is totally nonambulatory and has severe weakness of the upper extremities due to a neurologic or muscular disease/ condition

* **K0012** Lightweight portable motorized/power wheelchair

  Capped rental

* **K0014** Other motorized/power wheelchair base

  Capped rental

* **K0015** Detachable, non-adjustable height armrest, each

  Inexpensive and routinely purchased DME

* **K0017** Detachable, adjustable height armrest, base, each

  Inexpensive and routinely purchased DME

* **K0018** Detachable, adjustable height armrest, upper portion, each

  Inexpensive and routinely purchased DME

* **K0019** Arm pad, each

  Inexpensive and routinely purchased DME

* **K0020** Fixed, adjustable height armrest, pair

  Inexpensive and routinely purchased DME

* **K0037** High mount flip-up footrest, each

  Inexpensive and routinely purchased DME

* **K0038** Leg strap, each

  Inexpensive and routinely purchased DME

* **K0039** Leg strap, H style, each

  Inexpensive and routinely purchased DME

* **K0040** Adjustable angle footplate, each

  Inexpensive and routinely purchased DME

* **K0041** Large size footplate, each

  Inexpensive and routinely purchased DME

▶ New → Revised ✔ Reinstated ~~deleted~~ Deleted

☉ Special coverage instructions ◆ Not covered or valid by Medicare * Carrier discretion

* **K0042** Standard size footplate, each

Inexpensive and routinely purchased DME

* **K0043** Footrest, lower extension tube, each

Inexpensive and routinely purchased DME

* **K0044** Footrest, upper hanger bracket, each

Inexpensive and routinely purchased DME

* **K0045** Footrest, complete assembly

Inexpensive and routinely purchased DME

* **K0046** Elevating legrest, lower extension tube, each

Inexpensive and routinely purchased DME

* **K0047** Elevating legrest, upper hanger bracket, each

Inexpensive and routinely purchased DME

* **K0050** Ratchet assembly

Inexpensive and routinely purchased DME

* **K0051** Cam release assembly, footrest or legrests, each

Inexpensive and routinely purchased DME

* **K0052** Swing-away, detachable footrests, each

Inexpensive and routinely purchased DME

* **K0053** Elevating footrests, articulating (telescoping), each

Inexpensive and routinely purchased DME

* **K0056** Seat height less than 17″ or equal to or greater than 21″ for a high strength, lightweight, or ultralightweight wheelchair

Inexpensive and routinely purchased DME

* **K0065** Spoke protectors, each

Inexpensive and routinely purchased DME

* **K0069** Rear wheel assembly, complete, with solid tire, spokes or molded, each

Inexpensive and routinely purchased DME

* **K0070** Rear wheel assembly, complete, with pneumatic tire, spokes or molded, each

Inexpensive and routinely purchased DME

* **K0071** Front caster assembly, complete, with pneumatic tire, each

Caster assembly includes a caster fork (E2396), wheel rim, and tire. Inexpensive and routinely purchased DME

* **K0072** Front caster assembly, complete, with semi-pneumatic tire, each

Inexpensive and routinely purchased DME

* **K0073** Caster pin lock, each

Inexpensive and routinely purchased DME

* **K0077** Front caster assembly, complete, with solid tire, each

* **K0098** Drive belt for power wheelchair

Inexpensive and routinely purchased DME

* **K0105** IV hanger, each

Inexpensive and routinely purchased DME

* **K0108** Wheelchair component or accessory, not otherwise specified

⊚ **K0195** Elevating leg rests, pair (for use with capped rental wheelchair base)

Bill DME/MAC

Medically necessary replacement items are covered if rollabout chair or transport chair covered

IOM: 100-03, 4, 280.1

⊚ **K0455** Infusion pump used for uninterrupted parenteral administration of medication (e.g., epoprostenol or treprostinol)

Bill DME/MAC

An EIP may also be referred to as an external insulin pump, ambulatory pump, or mini-infuser. CMN/DIF required. Frequent and substantial service DME

IOM: 100-03, 1, 50.3

⊚ **K0462** Temporary replacement for patient owned equipment being repaired, any type

Bill DME/MAC

Only report for maintenance and service for an item for which initial claim was paid. The term power mobility device (PMD) includes power operated vehicles (POVs) and power wheelchairs (PWCs). Not Otherwise Classified.

IOM: 100-04, 20, 40.1

▶ **New**   → **Revised**   ✔ **Reinstated**   deleted **Deleted**

⊚ **Special coverage instructions**   ◆ **Not covered or valid by Medicare**   * **Carrier discretion**

⊙ **K0552** Supplies for external drug infusion pump, syringe type cartridge, sterile, each

Bill DME/MAC

Supplies.

IOM: 100-03, 1, 50.3

✳ **K0601** Replacement battery for external infusion pump owned by patient, silver oxide, 1.5 volt, each

Bill DME/MAC

Inexpensive and routinely purchased DME

✳ **K0602** Replacement battery for external infusion pump owned by patient, silver oxide, 3 volt, each

Bill DME/MAC

Inexpensive and routinely purchased DME

✳ **K0603** Replacement battery for external infusion pump owned by patient, alkaline, 1.5 volt, each

Bill DME/MAC

Inexpensive and routinely purchased DME

✳ **K0604** Replacement battery for external infusion pump owned by patient, lithium, 3.6 volt, each

Bill DME/MAC

Inexpensive and routinely purchased DME

✳ **K0605** Replacement battery for external infusion pump owned by patient, lithium, 4.5 volt, each

Bill DME/MAC

Inexpensive and routinely purchased DME

✳ **K0606** Automatic external defibrillator, with integrated electrocardiogram analysis, garment type

Bill DME/MAC

Capped rental

✳ **K0607** Replacement battery for automated external defibrillator, garment type only, each

Bill DME/MAC

Inexpensive and routinely purchased DME

✳ **K0608** Replacement garment for use with automated external defibrillator, each

Bill DME/MAC

Inexpensive and routinely purchased DME

✳ **K0609** Replacement electrodes for use with automated external defibrillator, garment type only, each

Bill DME/MAC

Supplies.

✳ **K0669** Wheelchair accessory, wheelchair seat or back cushion, does not meet specific code criteria or no written coding verification from DME PDAC

Bill DME/MAC

Inexpensive and routinely purchased DME

✳ **K0672** Addition to lower extremity orthosis, removable soft interface, all components, replacement only, each

Bill DME/MAC

Prosthetics/Orthotics

✳ **K0730** Controlled dose inhalation drug delivery system

Bill DME/MAC

Inexpensive and routinely purchased DME

✳ **K0733** Power wheelchair accessory, 12 to 24 amp hour sealed lead acid battery, each (e.g., gel cell, absorbed glassmat)

Bill DME/MAC

Inexpensive and routinely purchased DME

✳ **K0738** Portable gaseous oxygen system, rental; home compressor used to fill portable oxygen cylinders; includes portable containers, regulator, flowmeter, humidifier, cannula or mask, and tubing

Bill DME/MAC

Oxygen and oxygen equipment

✳ **K0739** Repair or nonroutine service for durable medical equipment other than oxygen equipment requiring the skill of a technician, labor component, per 15 minutes

Local carrier if used with implanted DME. If other, bill DME/MAC.

▶ New   → Revised   ✔ Reinstated   ~~deleted~~ Deleted

⊙ Special coverage instructions   ◆ Not covered or valid by Medicare   ✳ Carrier discretion

◆ **K0740** Repair or nonroutine service for oxygen equipment requiring the skill of a technician, labor component, per 15 minutes

Bill DME/MAC

~~K0741~~ ~~Portable gaseous oxygen system,~~ ✖
~~rental, includes portable container,~~
~~regulator, flowmeter, humidifier,~~
~~cannula or mask, and tubing, for~~
~~cluster headaches~~

~~K0742~~ ~~Portable oxygen contents, gaseous,~~ ✖
~~1 month's supply = 1 unit, for cluster~~
~~headaches, for initial months supply or~~
~~to replace used contents~~

✳ **K0743** Suction pump, home model, portable, for use on wounds

Bill DME/MAC

✳ **K0744** Absorptive wound dressing for use with suction pump, home model, portable, pad size 16 square inches or less

Bill DME/MAC

✳ **K0745** Absorptive wound dressing for use with suction pump, home model, portable, pad size more than 16 square inches but less than or equal to 48 square inches

Bill DME/MAC

✳ **K0746** Absorptive wound dressing for use with suction pump, home model, portable, pad size greater than 48 square inches

Bill DME/MAC

✳ **K0800** Power operated vehicle, group 1 standard, patient weight capacity up to and including 300 pounds

Bill DME/MAC

Power mobility device (PMD) includes power operated vehicles (POVs) and power wheelchairs (PWCs). Inexpensive and routinely purchased DME

✳ **K0801** Power operated vehicle, group 1 heavy duty, patient weight capacity 301 to 450 pounds

Bill DME/MAC

Inexpensive and routinely purchased DME

✳ **K0802** Power operated vehicle, group 1 very heavy duty, patient weight capacity 451 to 600 pounds

Bill DME/MAC

Inexpensive and routinely purchased DME

✳ **K0806** Power operated vehicle, group 2 standard, patient weight capacity up to and including 300 pounds

Bill DME/MAC

Inexpensive and routinely purchased DME

✳ **K0807** Power operated vehicle, group 2 heavy duty, patient weight capacity 301 to 450 pounds

Bill DME/MAC

Inexpensive and routinely purchased DME

✳ **K0808** Power operated vehicle, group 2 very heavy duty, patient weight capacity 451 to 600 pounds

Bill DME/MAC

Inexpensive and routinely purchased DME

✳ **K0812** Power operated vehicle, not otherwise classified

Bill DME/MAC

Not Otherwise Classified.

✳ **K0813** Power wheelchair, group 1 standard, portable, sling/solid seat and back, patient weight capacity up to and including 300 pounds

Bill DME/MAC

Capped rental

✳ **K0814** Power wheelchair, group 1 standard, portable, captains chair, patient weight capacity up to and including 300 pounds

Bill DME/MAC

Capped rental

✳ **K0815** Power wheelchair, group 1 standard, sling/solid seat and back, patient weight capacity up to and including 300 pounds

Bill DME/MAC

Capped rental

✳ **K0816** Power wheelchair, group 1 standard, captains chair, patient weight capacity up to and including 300 pounds

Bill DME/MAC

Capped rental

✳ **K0820** Power wheelchair, group 2 standard, portable, sling/solid seat/back, patient weight capacity up to and including 300 pounds

Bill DME/MAC

Capped rental

▶ New → Revised ✔ Reinstated ~~deleted~~ Deleted

☺ Special coverage instructions ◆ Not covered or valid by Medicare ✳ Carrier discretion

* **K0821** Power wheelchair, group 2 standard, portable, captains chair, patient weight capacity up to and including 300 pounds

  Bill DME/MAC

  Capped rental

* **K0822** Power wheelchair, group 2 standard, sling/solid seat/back, patient weight capacity up to and including 300 pounds

  Bill DME/MAC

  Capped rental

* **K0823** Power wheelchair, group 2 standard, captains chair, patient weight capacity up to and including 300 pounds

  Bill DME/MAC

  Capped rental

* **K0824** Power wheelchair, group 2 heavy duty, sling/solid seat/back, patient weight capacity 301 to 450 pounds

  Bill DME/MAC

  Capped rental

* **K0825** Power wheelchair, group 2 heavy duty, captains chair, patient weight capacity 301 to 450 pounds

  Bill DME/MAC

  Capped rental

* **K0826** Power wheelchair, group 2 very heavy duty, sling/solid seat/back, patient weight capacity 451 to 600 pounds

  Bill DME/MAC

  Capped rental

* **K0827** Power wheelchair, group 2 very heavy duty, captains chair, patient weight capacity 451 to 600 pounds

  Bill DME/MAC

  Capped rental

* **K0828** Power wheelchair, group 2 extra heavy duty, sling/solid seat/back, patient weight capacity 601 pounds or more

  Bill DME/MAC

  Capped rental

* **K0829** Power wheelchair, group 2 extra heavy duty, captains chair, patient weight 601 pounds or more

  Bill DME/MAC

  Capped rental

* **K0830** Power wheelchair, group 2 standard, seat elevator, sling/solid seat/back, patient weight capacity up to and including 300 pounds

  Bill DME/MAC

  Capped rental

* **K0831** Power wheelchair, group 2 standard, seat elevator, captains chair, patient weight capacity up to and including 300 pounds

  Bill DME/MAC

* **K0835** Power wheelchair, group 2 standard, single power option, sling/solid seat/back, patient weight capacity up to and including 300 pounds

  Bill DME/MAC

  Capped rental

* **K0836** Power wheelchair, group 2 standard, single power option, captains chair, patient weight capacity up to and including 300 pounds

  Bill DME/MAC

  Capped rental

* **K0837** Power wheelchair, group 2 heavy duty, single power option, sling/solid seat/back, patient weight capacity 301 to 450 pounds

  Bill DME/MAC

  Capped rental

* **K0838** Power wheelchair, group 2 heavy duty, single power option, captains chair, patient weight capacity 301 to 450 pounds

  Bill DME/MAC

  Capped rental

* **K0839** Power wheelchair, group 2 very heavy duty, single power option sling/solid seat/back, patient weight capacity 451 to 600 pounds

  Bill DME/MAC

  Capped rental

* **K0840** Power wheelchair, group 2 extra heavy duty, single power option, sling/solid seat/back, patient weight capacity 601 pounds or more

  Bill DME/MAC

  Capped rental

▶ New → Revised ✔ Reinstated ~~deleted~~ Deleted

☉ Special coverage instructions ◆ Not covered or valid by Medicare ✳ Carrier discretion

＊ **K0841** Power wheelchair, group 2 standard, multiple power option, sling/solid seat/back, patient weight capacity up to and including 300 pounds

Bill DME/MAC

Capped rental

＊ **K0842** Power wheelchair, group 2 standard, multiple power option, captains chair, patient weight capacity up to and including 300 pounds

Bill DME/MAC

Capped rental

＊ **K0843** Power wheelchair, group 2 heavy duty, multiple power option, sling/solid seat/back, patient weight capacity 301 to 450 pounds

Bill DME/MAC

Capped rental

＊ **K0848** Power wheelchair, group 3 standard, sling/solid seat/back, patient weight capacity up to and including 300 pounds

Bill DME/MAC

Capped rental

＊ **K0849** Power wheelchair, group 3 standard, captains chair, patient weight capacity up to and including 300 pounds

Bill DME/MAC

Capped rental

＊ **K0850** Power wheelchair, group 3 heavy duty, sling/solid seat/back, patient weight capacity 301 to 450 pounds

Bill DME/MAC

Capped rental

＊ **K0851** Power wheelchair, group 3 heavy duty, captains chair, patient weight capacity 301 to 450 pounds

Bill DME/MAC

Capped rental

＊ **K0852** Power wheelchair, group 3 very heavy duty, sling/solid seat/back, patient weight capacity 451 to 600 pounds

Bill DME/MAC

Capped rental

＊ **K0853** Power wheelchair, group 3 very heavy duty, captains chair, patient weight capacity 451 to 600 pounds

Bill DME/MAC

Capped rental

＊ **K0854** Power wheelchair, group 3 extra heavy duty, sling/solid seat/back, patient weight capacity 601 pounds or more

Bill DME/MAC

Capped rental

＊ **K0855** Power wheelchair, group 3 extra heavy duty, captains chair, patient weight capacity 601 pounds or more

Bill DME/MAC

Capped rental

＊ **K0856** Power wheelchair, group 3 standard, single power option, sling/solid seat/back, patient weight capacity up to and including 300 pounds

Bill DME/MAC

Capped rental

＊ **K0857** Power wheelchair, group 3 standard, single power option, captains chair, patient weight capacity up to and including 300 pounds

Bill DME/MAC

Capped rental

＊ **K0858** Power wheelchair, group 3 heavy duty, single power option, sling/solid seat/back, patient weight 301 to 450 pounds

Bill DME/MAC

Capped rental

＊ **K0859** Power wheelchair, group 3 heavy duty, single power option, captains chair, patient weight capacity 301 to 450 pounds

Bill DME/MAC

Capped rental

＊ **K0860** Power wheelchair, group 3 very heavy duty, single power option, sling/solid seat/back, patient weight capacity 451 to 600 pounds

Bill DME/MAC

Capped rental

＊ **K0861** Power wheelchair, group 3 standard, multiple power option, sling/solid seat/back, patient weight capacity up to and including 300 pounds

Bill DME/MAC

Capped rental

▶ New　→ Revised　✔ Reinstated　-deleted- Deleted

◎ Special coverage instructions　◆ Not covered or valid by Medicare　＊ Carrier discretion

* **K0862**   Power wheelchair, group 3 heavy duty, multiple power option, sling/solid seat/back, patient weight capacity 301 to 450 pounds

Bill DME/MAC

Capped rental

* **K0863**   Power wheelchair, group 3 very heavy duty, multiple power option, sling/solid seat/back, patient weight capacity 451 to 600 pounds

Bill DME/MAC

Capped rental

* **K0864**   Power wheelchair, group 3 extra heavy duty, multiple power option, sling/solid seat/back, patient weight capacity 601 pounds or more

Bill DME/MAC

Capped rental

* **K0868**   Power wheelchair, group 4 standard, sling/solid seat/back, patient weight capacity up to and including 300 pounds

Bill DME/MAC

Capped rental

* **K0869**   Power wheelchair, group 4 standard, captains chair, patient weight capacity up to and including 300 pounds

Bill DME/MAC

Capped rental

* **K0870**   Power wheelchair, group 4 heavy duty, sling/solid seat/back, patient weight capacity 301 to 450 pounds

Bill DME/MAC

Capped rental

* **K0871**   Power wheelchair, group 4 very heavy duty, sling/solid seat/back, patient weight capacity 451 to 600 pounds

Bill DME/MAC

Capped rental

* **K0877**   Power wheelchair, group 4 standard, single power option, sling/solid seat/back, patient weight capacity up to and including 300 pounds

Bill DME/MAC

Capped rental

* **K0878**   Power wheelchair, group 4 standard, single power option, captains chair, patient weight capacity up to and including 300 pounds

Bill DME/MAC

Capped rental

* **K0879**   Power wheelchair, group 4 heavy duty, single power option, sling/solid seat/back, patient weight capacity 301 to 450 pounds

Bill DME/MAC

Capped rental

* **K0880**   Power wheelchair, group 4 very heavy duty, single power option, sling/solid seat/back, patient weight 451 to 600 pounds

Bill DME/MAC

Capped rental

* **K0884**   Power wheelchair, group 4 standard, multiple power option, sling/solid seat/back, patient weight capacity up to and including 300 pounds

Bill DME/MAC

Capped rental

* **K0885**   Power wheelchair, group 4 standard, multiple power option, captains chair, patient weight capacity up to and including 300 pounds

Bill DME/MAC

Capped rental

* **K0886**   Power wheelchair, group 4 heavy duty, multiple power option, sling/solid seat/back, patient weight capacity 301 to 450 pounds

Bill DME/MAC

Capped rental

* **K0890**   Power wheelchair, group 5 pediatric, single power option, sling/solid seat/back, patient weight capacity up to and including 125 pounds

Bill DME/MAC

Capped rental

* **K0891**   Power wheelchair, group 5 pediatric, multiple power option, sling/solid seat/back, patient weight capacity up to and including 125 pounds

Bill DME/MAC

Capped rental

* **K0898**   Power wheelchair, not otherwise classified

Bill DME/MAC

* **K0899**   Power mobility device, not coded by DME PDAC or does not meet criteria

Bill DME/MAC

▶ New   → Revised   ✔ Reinstated   ~~deleted~~ Deleted

⊙ Special coverage instructions   ◆ Not covered or valid by Medicare   * Carrier discretion

228

ORTHOTICS (L0100-L4999)

DMEPOS fee schedule:
www.cms.gov/DMEPOSFeeSched/LSDMEPOSFEE/
list.asp#TopOfPage

Orthotic Devices: Spinal

Cervical

L0112-L0220:   Bill DME/MAC

✳ **L0112**   Cranial cervical orthosis, congenital torticollis type, with or without soft interface material, adjustable range of motion joint, custom fabricated

✳ **L0113**   Cranial cervical orthosis, torticollis type, with or without joint, with or without soft interface material, prefabricated, includes fitting and adjustment

✳ **L0120**   Cervical, flexible, non-adjustable (foam collar)

Cervical orthoses, including soft and rigid devices may be used as nonoperative management for cervical trauma

✳ **L0130**   Cervical, flexible, thermoplastic collar, molded to patient

✳ **L0140**   Cervical, semi-rigid, adjustable (plastic collar)

✳ **L0150**   Cervical, semi-rigid, adjustable molded chin cup (plastic collar with mandibular/occipital piece)

✳ **L0160**   Cervical, semi-rigid, wire frame occipital/mandibular support

✳ **L0170**   Cervical, collar, molded to patient model

✳ **L0172**   Cervical, collar, semi-rigid thermoplastic foam, two piece

✳ **L0174**   Cervical, collar, semi-rigid, thermoplastic foam, two piece with thoracic extension

Multiple Post Collar

✳ **L0180**   Cervical, multiple post collar, occipital/mandibular supports, adjustable

✳ **L0190**   Cervical, multiple post collar, occipital/mandibular supports, adjustable cervical bars (SOMI, Guilford, Taylor types)

✳ **L0200**   Cervical, multiple post collar, occipital/mandibular supports, adjustable cervical bars, and thoracic extension

Thoracic

✳ **L0220**   Thoracic, rib belt, custom fabricated

Thoracic-Lumbar-Sacral

Anterior-Posterior-Lateral Rotary-Control

L0430-L0492:   Bill DME/MAC

✳ **L0430**   Spinal orthosis, anterior-posterior-lateral control, with interface material, custom fitted (Dewall posture protector only)

✳ **L0450**   TLSO, flexible, provides trunk support, upper thoracic region, produces intracavitary pressure to reduce load on the intervertebral disks with rigid stays or panel(s), includes shoulder straps and closures, prefabricated, includes fitting and adjustment

Used to immobilize specified area of spine, and is generally worn under clothing

✳ **L0452**   TLSO, flexible, provides trunk support, upper thoracic region, produces intracavitary pressure to reduce load on the intervertebral disks with rigid stays or panel(s), includes shoulder straps and closures, custom fabricated

✳ **L0454**   TLSO flexible, provides trunk support, extends from sacrococcygeal junction to above T-9 vertebra, restricts gross trunk motion in the sagittal plane, produces intracavitary pressure to reduce load on the intervertebral disks with rigid stays or panel(s), includes shoulder straps and closures, prefabricated, includes fitting and adjustment

Used to immobilize specified areas of spine; and is generally designed to be worn under clothing; not specifically designed for patients in wheelchairs

✳ **L0456**   TLSO, flexible, provides trunk support, thoracic region, rigid posterior panel and soft anterior apron, extends from the sacrococcygeal junction and terminates just inferior to the scapular spine, restricts gross trunk motion in the sagittal plane, produces intracavitary pressure to reduce load on the intervertebral disks, includes straps and closures, prefabricated, includes fitting and adjustment

---

▶ New   ➔ Revised   ✔ Reinstated   ~~deleted~~ Deleted
☺ Special coverage instructions   ◆ Not covered or valid by Medicare   ✳ Carrier discretion

✳ **L0458**   TLSO, triplanar control, modular segmented spinal system, two rigid plastic shells, posterior extends from the sacrococcygeal junction and terminates just inferior to the scapular spine, anterior extends from the symphysis pubis to the xiphoid, soft liner, restricts gross trunk motion in the sagittal, coronal, and transverse planes, lateral strength is provided by overlapping plastic and stabilizing closures, includes straps and closures, prefabricated, includes fitting and adjustment

To meet Medicare's definition of body jacket, orthosis has to have rigid plastic shell that circles trunk with overlapping edges and stabilizing closures, and entire circumference of shell must be made of same rigid material

✳ **L0460**   TLSO, triplanar control, modular segmented spinal system, two rigid plastic shells, posterior extends from the sacrococcygeal junction and terminates just inferior to the scapular spine, anterior extends from the symphysis pubis to the sternal notch, soft liner, restricts gross trunk motion in the sagittal, coronal, and transverse planes, lateral strength is provided by overlapping plastic and stabilizing closures, includes straps and closures, prefabricated, includes fitting and adjustment

✳ **L0462**   TLSO, triplanar control, modular segmented spinal system, three rigid plastic shells, posterior extends from the sacrococcygeal junction and terminates just inferior to the scapular spine, anterior extends from the symphysis pubis to the sternal notch, soft liner, restricts gross trunk motion in the sagittal, coronal, and transverse planes, lateral strength is provided by overlapping plastic and stabilizing closures, includes straps and closures, prefabricated, includes fitting and adjustment

✳ **L0464**   TLSO, triplanar control, modular segmented spinal system, four rigid plastic shells, posterior extends from sacrococcygeal junction and terminates just inferior to scapular spine, anterior extends from symphysis pubis to the sternal notch, soft liner, restricts gross trunk motion in sagittal, coronal, and transverse planes, lateral strength is provided by overlapping plastic and stabilizing closures, includes straps and closures, prefabricated, includes fitting and adjustment

✳ **L0466**   TLSO, sagittal control, rigid posterior frame and flexible soft anterior apron with straps, closures and padding, restricts gross trunk motion in sagittal plane, produces intracavitary pressure to reduce load on intervertebral disks, includes fitting and shaping the frame, prefabricated, includes fitting and adjustment

✳ **L0468**   TLSO, sagittal-coronal control, rigid posterior frame and flexible soft anterior apron with straps, closures and padding, extends from sacrococcygeal junction over scapulae, lateral strength provided by pelvic, thoracic, and lateral frame pieces, restricts gross trunk motion in sagittal, and coronal planes, produces intracavitary pressure to reduce load on intervertebral disks, includes fitting and shaping the frame, prefabricated, includes fitting and adjustment

✳ **L0470**   TLSO, triplanar control, rigid posterior frame and flexible soft anterior apron with straps, closures and padding, extends from sacrococcygeal junction to scapula, lateral strength provided by pelvic, thoracic, and lateral frame pieces, rotational strength provided by subclavicular extensions, restricts gross trunk motion in sagittal, coronal, and transverse planes, provides intracavitary pressure to reduce load on the intervertebral disks, includes fitting and shaping the frame, prefabricated, includes fitting and adjustment

✳ **L0472**   TLSO, triplanar control, hyperextension, rigid anterior and lateral frame extends from symphysis pubis to sternal notch with two anterior components (one pubic and one sternal), posterior and lateral pads with straps and closures, limits spinal flexion, restricts gross trunk motion in sagittal, coronal, and transverse planes, includes fitting and shaping the frame, prefabricated, includes fitting and adjustment

✳ **L0480**   TLSO, triplanar control, one piece rigid plastic shell without interface liner, with multiple straps and closures, posterior extends from sacrococcygeal junction and terminates just inferior to scapular spine, anterior extends from symphysis pubis to sternal notch, anterior or posterior opening, restricts gross trunk motion in sagittal, coronal, and transverse planes, includes a carved plaster or CAD-CAM model, custom fabricated

---

▶ New   → Revised   ✔ Reinstated   ‑deleted‑ Deleted

⊛ Special coverage instructions   ◆ Not covered or valid by Medicare   ✳ Carrier discretion

✳ **L0482** TLSO, triplanar control, one piece rigid plastic shell with interface liner, multiple straps and closures, posterior extends from sacrococcygeal junction and terminates just inferior to scapular spine, anterior extends from symphysis pubis to sternal notch, anterior or posterior opening, restricts gross trunk motion in sagittal, coronal, and transverse planes, includes a carved plaster or CAD-CAM model, custom fabricated

✳ **L0484** TLSO, triplanar control, two piece rigid plastic shell without interface liner, with multiple straps and closures, posterior extends from sacrococcygeal junction and terminates just inferior to scapular spine, anterior extends from symphysis pubis to sternal notch, lateral strength is enhanced by overlapping plastic, restricts gross trunk motion in the sagittal, coronal, and transverse planes, includes a carved plaster or CAD-CAM model, custom fabricated

✳ **L0486** TLSO, triplanar control, two piece rigid plastic shell with interface liner, multiple straps and closures, posterior extends from sacrococcygeal junction and terminates just inferior to scapular spine, anterior extends from symphysis pubis to sternal notch, lateral strength is enhanced by overlapping plastic, restricts gross trunk motion in the sagittal, coronal, and transverse planes, includes a carved plaster or CAD-CAM model, custom fabricated

✳ **L0488** TLSO, triplanar control, one piece rigid plastic shell with interface liner, multiple straps and closures, posterior extends from sacrococcygeal junction and terminates just inferior to scapular spine, anterior extends from symphysis pubis to sternal notch, anterior or posterior opening, restricts gross trunk motion in sagittal, coronal, and transverse planes, prefabricated, includes fitting and adjustment

✳ **L0490** TLSO, sagittal-coronal control, one piece rigid plastic shell, with overlapping reinforced anterior, with multiple straps and closures, posterior extends from sacrococcygeal junction and terminates at or before the T-9 vertebra, anterior extends from symphysis pubis to xiphoid, anterior opening, restricts gross trunk motion in sagittal and coronal planes, prefabricated, includes fitting and adjustment

✳ **L0491** TLSO, sagittal-coronal control, modular segmented spinal system, two rigid plastic shells, posterior extends from the sacrococcygeal junction and terminates just inferior to the scapular spine, anterior extends from the symphysis pubis to the xiphoid, soft liner, restricts gross trunk motion in the sagittal and coronal planes, lateral strength is provided by overlapping plastic and stabilizing closures, includes straps and closures, prefabricated, includes fitting and adjustment

✳ **L0492** TLSO, sagittal-coronal control, modular segmented spinal system, three rigid plastic shells, posterior extends from the sacrococcygeal junction and terminates just inferior to the scapular spine, anterior extends from the symphysis pubis to the xiphoid, soft liner, restricts gross trunk motion in the sagittal and coronal planes, lateral strength is provided by overlapping plastic and stabilizing closures, includes straps and closures, prefabricated, includes fitting and adjustment

Sacroilliac, Lumbar, Sacral Orthosis

L0621-L0640: Bill DME/MAC

✳ **L0621** Sacroiliac orthosis, flexible, provides pelvic-sacral support, reduces motion about the sacroiliac joint, includes straps, closures, may include pendulous abdomen design, prefabricated, includes fitting and adjustment

✳ **L0622** Sacroiliac orthosis, flexible, provides pelvic-sacral support, reduces motion about the sacroiliac joint, includes straps, closures, may include pendulous abdomen design, custom fabricated

Type of custom-fabricated device for which impression of specific body part is made (e.g., by means of plaster cast, or CAD-CAM [computer-aided design] technology); impression then used to make specific patient model

✳ **L0623** Sacroiliac orthosis, provides pelvic-sacral support, with rigid or semi-rigid panels over the sacrum and abdomen, reduces motion about the sacroiliac joint, includes straps, closures, may include pendulous abdomen design, prefabricated, includes fitting and adjustment

▶ New　→ Revised　✔ Reinstated　deleted Deleted

☺ Special coverage instructions　◆ Not covered or valid by Medicare　✳ Carrier discretion

* **L0624**   Sacroiliac orthosis, provides pelvic-sacral support, with rigid or semi-rigid panels placed over the sacrum and abdomen, reduces motion about the sacroiliac joint, includes straps, closures, may include pendulous abdomen design, custom fabricated

Custom fitted

* **L0625**   Lumbar orthosis, flexible, provides lumbar support, posterior extends from L-1 to below L-5 vertebra, produces intracavitary pressure to reduce load on the intervertebral discs, includes straps, closures, may include pendulous abdomen design, shoulder straps, stays, prefabricated, includes fitting and adjustment

* **L0626**   Lumbar orthosis, sagittal control, with rigid posterior panel(s), posterior extends from L-1 to below L-5 vertebra, produces intracavitary pressure to reduce load on the intervertebral discs, includes straps, closures, may include padding, stays, shoulder straps, pendulous abdomen design, prefabricated, includes fitting and adjustment

* **L0627**   Lumbar orthosis, sagittal control, with rigid anterior and posterior panels, posterior extends from L-1 to below L-5 vertebra, produces intracavitary pressure to reduce load on the intervertebral discs, includes straps, closures, may include padding, shoulder straps, pendulous abdomen design, prefabricated, includes fitting and adjustment

* **L0628**   Lumbar-sacral orthosis, flexible, provides lumbo-sacral support, posterior extends from sacrococcygeal junction to T-9 vertebra, produces intracavitary pressure to reduce load on the intervertebral discs, includes straps, closures, may include stays, shoulder straps, pendulous abdomen design, prefabricated, includes fitting and adjustment

* **L0629**   Lumbar-sacral orthosis, flexible, provides lumbo-sacral support, posterior extends from sacrococcygeal junction to T-9 vertebra, produces intracavitary pressure to reduce load on the intervertebral discs, includes straps, closures, may include stays, shoulder straps, pendulous abdomen design, custom fabricated

Custom fitted

* **L0630**   Lumbar-sacral orthosis, sagittal control, with rigid posterior panel(s), posterior extends from sacrococcygeal junction to T-9 vertebra, produces intracavitary pressure to reduce load on the intervertebral discs, includes straps, closures, may include padding, stays, shoulder straps, pendulous abdomen design, prefabricated, includes fitting and adjustment

* **L0631**   Lumbar-sacral orthosis, sagittal control, with rigid anterior and posterior panels, posterior extends from sacrococcygeal junction to T-9 vertebra, produces intracavitary pressure to reduce load on the intervertebral discs, includes straps, closures, may include padding, shoulder straps, pendulous abdomen design, prefabricated, includes fitting and adjustment

* **L0632**   Lumbar-sacral orthosis, sagittal control, with rigid anterior and posterior panels, posterior extends from sacrococcygeal junction to T-9 vertebra, produces intracavitary pressure to reduce load on the intervertebral discs, includes straps, closures, may include padding, shoulder straps, pendulous abdomen design, custom fabricated

Custom fitted

* **L0633**   Lumbar-sacral orthosis, sagittal-coronal control, with rigid posterior frame/panel(s), posterior extends from sacrococcygeal junction to T-9 vertebra, lateral strength provided by rigid lateral frame/panels, produces intracavitary pressure to reduce load on intervertebral discs, includes straps, closures, may include padding, stays, shoulder straps, pendulous abdomen design, prefabricated, includes fitting and adjustment

* **L0634**   Lumbar-sacral orthosis, sagittal-coronal control, with rigid posterior frame/panel(s), posterior extends from sacrococcygeal junction to T-9 vertebra, lateral strength provided by rigid lateral frame/panel(s), produces intracavitary pressure to reduce load on intervertebral discs, includes straps, closures, may include padding, stays, shoulder straps, pendulous abdomen design, custom fabricated

Custom fitted

▶ **New**   → **Revised**   ✔ **Reinstated**   ~~deleted~~ **Deleted**

○ **Special coverage instructions**   ◆ **Not covered or valid by Medicare**   * **Carrier discretion**

✳ **L0635** Lumbar-sacral orthosis, sagittal-coronal control, lumbar flexion, rigid posterior frame/panel(s), lateral articulating design to flex the lumbar spine, posterior extends from sacrococcygeal junction to T-9 vertebra, lateral strength provided by rigid lateral frame/panel(s), produces intracavitary pressure to reduce load on intervertebral discs, includes straps, closures, may include padding, anterior panel, pendulous abdomen design, prefabricated, includes fitting and adjustment

✳ **L0636** Lumbar sacral orthosis, sagittal-coronal control, lumbar flexion, rigid posterior frame/panels, lateral articulating design to flex the lumbar spine, posterior extends from sacrococcygeal junction to T-9 vertebra, lateral strength provided by rigid lateral frame/panels, produces intracavitary pressure to reduce load on intervertebral discs, includes straps, closures, may include padding, anterior panel, pendulous abdomen design, custom fabricated

Custom fitted

✳ **L0637** Lumbar-sacral orthosis, sagittal-coronal control, with rigid anterior and posterior frame/panels, posterior extends from sacrococcygeal junction to T-9 vertebra, lateral strength provided by rigid lateral frame/panels, produces intracavitary pressure to reduce load on intervertebral discs, includes straps, closures, may include padding, shoulder straps, pendulous abdomen design, prefabricated, includes fitting and adjustment

✳ **L0638** Lumbar-sacral orthosis, sagittal-coronal control, with rigid anterior and posterior frame/panels, posterior extends from sacrococcygeal junction to T-9 vertebra, lateral strength provided by rigid lateral frame/panels, produces intracavitary pressure to reduce load on intervertebral discs, includes straps, closures, may include padding, shoulder straps, pendulous abdomen design, custom fabricated

✳ **L0639** Lumbar-sacral orthosis, sagittal-coronal control, rigid shell(s)/panel(s), posterior extends from sacrococcygeal junction to T-9 vertebra, anterior extends from symphysis pubis to xyphoid, produces intracavitary pressure to reduce load on the intervertebral discs, overall strength is provided by overlapping rigid material and stabilizing closures, includes straps, closures may include soft interface, pendulous abdomen design, prefabricated, includes fitting and adjustment

Characterized by rigid plastic shell that encircles trunk with overlapping edges and stabilizing closures and provides high degree of immobility

✳ **L0640** Lumbar-sacral orthosis, sagittal-coronal control, rigid shell(s)/panel(s), posterior extends from sacrococcygeal junction to T-9 vertebra, anterior extends from symphysis pubis to xyphoid, produces intracavitary pressure to reduce load on the intervertebral discs, overall strength is provided by overlapping rigid material and stabilizing closures, includes straps, closures, may include soft interface, pendulous abdomen design, custom fabricated

Custom fitted

Cervical-Thoracic-Lumbar-Sacral

Anterior-Posterior-Lateral Control

L0700-L0710: Bill DME/MAC

✳ **L0700** Cervical-thoracic-lumbar-sacral-orthoses (CTLSO), anterior-posterior-lateral control, molded to patient model, (Minerva type)

✳ **L0710** CTLSO, anterior-posterior-lateral-control, molded to patient model, with interface material, (Minerva type)

HALO Procedure

L0810-L0861: Bill DME/MAC

✳ **L0810** HALO procedure, cervical halo incorporated into jacket vest

✳ **L0820** HALO procedure, cervical halo incorporated into plaster body jacket

✳ **L0830** HALO procedure, cervical halo incorporated into Milwaukee type orthosis

▶ New → Revised ✔ Reinstated deleted Deleted ✪ Special coverage instructions ◆ Not covered or valid by Medicare ✳ Carrier discretion

ORTHOTICS L0635 – L0830

233

* **L0859** Addition to HALO procedure, magnetic resonance image compatible systems, rings and pins, any material

* **L0861** Addition to HALO procedure, replacement liner/interface material

Additions to Spinal Orthoses

L0970-L0999: Bill DME/MAC

TLSO - Thoraci-lumbar-sacral orthoses

Spinal orthoses may be prefabricated, prefitted, or custom fabricated. Conservative treatment for back pain may include the use of spinal orthoses.

* **L0970** TLSO, corset front

* **L0972** LSO, corset front

* **L0974** TLSO, full corset

* **L0976** LSO, full corset

* **L0978** Axillary crutch extension

* **L0980** Peroneal straps, pair

* **L0982** Stocking supporter grips, set of four (4)

Convenience item

* **L0984** Protective body sock, each

Convenience item

Garment made of cloth or similar material that is worn under spinal orthosis and is not primarily medical in nature

* **L0999** Addition to spinal orthosis, not otherwise specified

Orthotic Devices: Scoliosis Procedures (L1000-L1520)

NOTE: Orthotic care of scoliosis differs from other orthotic care in that the treatment is more dynamic in nature and uses ongoing continual modification of the orthosis to the patient's changing condition. This coding structure uses the proper names, or eponyms, of the procedures because they have historic and universal acceptance in the profession. It should be recognized that variations to the basic procedures described by the founders/developers are accepted in various medical and orthotic practices throughout the country. All procedures include a model of patient when indicated.

Scoliosis: Cervical-Thoracic-Lumbar-Sacral (CTLSO) (Milwaukee)

L1000-L1520: Bill DME/MAC

* **L1000** Cervical-thoracic-lumbar-sacral orthosis (CTLSO) (Milwaukee), inclusive of furnishing initial orthosis, including model

* **L1001** Cervical thoracic lumbar sacral orthosis, immobilizer, infant size, prefabricated, includes fitting and adjustment

* **L1005** Tension based scoliosis orthosis and accessory pads, includes fitting and adjustment

* **L1010** Addition to cervical-thoracic-lumbar-sacral orthosis (CTLSO) or scoliosis orthosis, axilla sling

Correction Pads

* **L1020** Addition to CTLSO or scoliosis orthosis, kyphosis pad

* **L1025** Addition to CTLSO or scoliosis orthosis, kyphosis pad, floating

* **L1030** Addition to CTLSO or scoliosis orthosis, lumbar bolster pad

* **L1040** Addition to CTLSO or scoliosis orthosis, lumbar or lumbar rib pad

* **L1050** Addition to CTLSO or scoliosis orthosis, sternal pad

* **L1060** Addition to CTLSO or scoliosis orthosis, thoracic pad

* **L1070** Addition to CTLSO or scoliosis orthosis, trapezius sling

* **L1080** Addition to CTLSO or scoliosis orthosis, outrigger

* **L1085** Addition to CTLSO or scoliosis orthosis, outrigger, bilateral with vertical extensions

* **L1090** Addition to CTLSO or scoliosis orthosis, lumbar sling

* **L1100** Addition to CTLSO or scoliosis orthosis, ring flange, plastic or leather

* **L1110** Addition to CTLSO or scoliosis orthosis, ring flange, plastic or leather, molded to patient model

* **L1120** Addition to CTLSO, scoliosis orthosis, cover for upright, each

---

Scoliosis: Thoracic-Lumbar-Sacral (Low Profile)

* **L1200** Thoracic-lumbar-sacral-orthosis (TLSO), inclusive of furnishing initial orthosis only

* **L1210** Addition to TLSO, (low profile), lateral thoracic extension

* **L1220** Addition to TLSO, (low profile), anterior thoracic extension

* **L1230** Addition to TLSO, (low profile), Milwaukee type superstructure

* **L1240** Addition to TLSO, (low profile), lumbar derotation pad

* **L1250** Addition to TLSO, (low profile), anterior ASIS pad

* **L1260** Addition to TLSO, (low profile), anterior thoracic derotation pad

* **L1270** Addition to TLSO, (low profile), abdominal pad

* **L1280** Addition to TLSO, (low profile), rib gusset (elastic), each

* **L1290** Addition to TLSO, (low profile), lateral trochanteric pad

Other Scoliosis Procedures

* **L1300** Other scoliosis procedure, body jacket molded to patient model

* **L1310** Other scoliosis procedure, postoperative body jacket

* **L1499** Spinal orthosis, not otherwise specified

Orthotic Devices: Lower Limb

NOTE: the procedures in L1600-L2999 are considered as *base* or *basic procedures* and may be modified by listing procedure from the Additions Sections and adding them to the base procedure.

Hip: Flexible

L1600-L2999: Bill DME/MAC

* **L1600** Hip orthosis (HO), abduction control of hip joints, flexible, Frejka type with cover, prefabricated, includes fitting and adjustment

* **L1610** Hip orthosis, abduction control of hip joints, flexible, (Frejka cover only) prefabricated, includes fitting and adjustment

* **L1620** Hip orthosis, abduction control of hip joints, flexible, (Pavlik harness), prefabricated, includes fitting and adjustment

* **L1630** Hip orthosis, abduction control of hip joints, semi-flexible (Von Rosen type), custom-fabricated

* **L1640** Hip orthosis, abduction control of hip joints, static, pelvic band or spreader bar, thigh cuffs, custom-fabricated

* **L1650** Hip orthosis, abduction control of hip joints, static, adjustable, (Ilfled type), prefabricated, includes fitting and adjustment

* **L1652** Hip orthosis, bilateral thigh cuffs with adjustable abductor spreader bar, adult size, prefabricated, includes fitting and adjustment, any type

* **L1660** Hip orthosis, abduction control of hip joints, static, plastic, prefabricated, includes fitting and adjustment

* **L1680** Hip orthosis, abduction control of hip joints, dynamic, pelvic control, adjustable hip motion control, thigh cuffs (Rancho hip action type), custom fabrication

* **L1685** Hip orthosis, abduction control of hip joint, postoperative hip abduction type, custom fabricated

* **L1686** Hip orthosis, abduction control of hip joint, postoperative hip abduction type, prefabricated, includes fitting and adjustment

* **L1690** Combination, bilateral, lumbo-sacral, hip, femur orthosis providing adduction and internal rotation control, prefabricated, includes fitting and adjustment

Legg Perthes

* **L1700** Legg-Perthes orthosis, (Toronto type), custom-fabricated

* **L1710** Legg-Perthes orthosis, (Newington type), custom-fabricated

* **L1720** Legg-Perthes orthosis, trilateral, (Tachdjian type), custom-fabricated

* **L1730** Legg-Perthes orthosis, (Scottish Rite type), custom-fabricated

* **L1755** Legg-Perthes orthosis, (Patten bottom type), custom-fabricated

Knee (KO)

* **L1810** Knee orthosis, elastic with joints, prefabricated, includes fitting and adjustment

---

▶ New   → Revised   ✔ Reinstated   ~~deleted~~ Deleted

☺ Special coverage instructions   ◆ Not covered or valid by Medicare   * Carrier discretion

* **L1820** Knee orthosis, elastic with condylar pads and joints, with or without patellar control, prefabricated, includes fitting and adjustment

* **L1830** Knee orthosis, immobilizer, canvas longitudinal, prefabricated, includes fitting and adjustment

* **L1831** Knee orthosis, locking knee joint(s), positional orthosis, prefabricated, includes fitting and adjustment

* **L1832** Knee orthrosis, adjustable knee joints (unicentric or polycentric), positional orthosis, rigid support, prefabricated, includes fitting and adjustment

* **L1834** Knee orthosis, without knee joint, rigid, custom-fabricated

* **L1836** Knee orthosis, rigid, without joint(s), includes soft interface material, prefabricated, includes fitting and adjustment

* **L1840** Knee orthosis, derotation, medial-lateral, anterior cruciate ligament, custom fabricated

* **L1843** Knee orthosis, single upright, thigh and calf, with adjustable flexion and extension joint (unicentric or polycentric), medial-lateral and rotation control, with or without varus/valgus adjustment; prefabricated, includes fitting and adjustment

* **L1844** Knee orthosis, single upright, thigh and calf, with adjustable flexion and extension joint (unicentric or polycentric), medial-lateral and rotation control, with or without varus/valgus adjustment, custom fabricated

* **L1845** Knee orthrosis, double upright, thigh and calf, with adjustable flexion and extension joint (unicentric or polycentric), medial-lateral and rotation control, with or without varus/valgus adjustment, prefabricated, includes fitting and adjustment

* **L1846** Knee orthrosis, double upright, thigh and calf, with adjustable flexion and extension joint (unicentric or polycentric), medial-lateral and rotation control, with or without varus/valgus adjustment, custom fabricated

* **L1847** Knee orthosis, double upright with adjustable joint, with inflatable air support chambers, prefabricated, includes fitting and adjustment

* **L1850** Knee orthosis, Swedish type, prefabricated, includes fitting and adjustment

* **L1860** Knee orthosis, modification of supracondylar prosthetic socket, custom fabricated (SK)

Ankle-Foot (AFO)

* **L1900** Ankle foot orthosis (AFO), spring wire, dorsiflexion assist calf band, custom-fabricated

* **L1902** Ankle foot orthosis, ankle gauntlet, prefabricated, includes fitting and adjustment

* **L1904** Ankle foot orthosis, molded ankle gauntlet, custom-fabricated

* **L1906** Ankle-foot orthosis, multiligamentus ankle support, prefabricated, includes fitting and adjustment

* **L1907** AFO, supramalleolar with straps, with or without interface/pads, custom fabricated

* **L1910** Ankle foot orthosis, posterior, single bar, clasp attachment to shoe counter, prefabricated, includes fitting and adjustment

* **L1920** Ankle foot orthosis, single upright with static or adjustable stop (Phelps or Perlstein type), custom-fabricated

* **L1930** Ankle-foot orthosis, plastic or other material, prefabricated, includes fitting and adjustment

* **L1932** AFO, rigid anterior tibial section, total carbon fiber or equal material, prefabricated, includes fitting and adjustment

* **L1940** Ankle foot orthosis, plastic or other material, custom-fabricated

* **L1945** Ankle foot orthosis, plastic, rigid anterior tibial section (floor reaction), custom-fabricated

* **L1950** Ankle foot orthosis, spiral, (Institute of Rehabilitation Medicine type), plastic, custom-fabricated

* **L1951** Ankle foot orthosis, spiral, (Institute of Rehabilitative Medicine type), plastic or other material, prefabricated, includes fitting and adjustment

* **L1960** Ankle foot orthosis, posterior solid ankle, plastic, custom-fabricated

* **L1970** Ankle foot orthosis, plastic, with ankle joint, custom-fabricated

* **L1971** Ankle foot orthosis, plastic or other material with ankle joint, prefabricated, includes fitting and adjustment

---

▶ New   → Revised   ✔ Reinstated   ~~deleted~~ Deleted

☺ **Special coverage instructions**   ◆ **Not covered or valid by Medicare**   ✳ **Carrier discretion**

* **L1980** Ankle foot orthosis, single upright free plantar dorsiflexion, solid stirrup, calf band/cuff (single bar 'BK' orthosis), custom-fabricated

* **L1990** Ankle foot orthosis, double upright free plantar dorsiflexion, solid stirrup, calf band/cuff (double bar 'BK' orthosis), custom-fabricated

Hip-Knee-Ankle-Foot (or Any Combination)

NOTE: L2000, L2020, and L2036 are base procedures to be used with any knee joint. L2010 and L2030 are to be used only with no knee joint.

* **L2000** Knee ankle foot orthosis, single upright, free knee, free ankle, solid stirrup, thigh and calf bands/cuffs (single bar 'AK' orthosis), custom-fabricated

* **L2005** Knee ankle foot orthosis, any material, single or double upright, stance control, automatic lock and swing phase release, any type activation; includes ankle joint, any type, custom fabricated

* **L2010** Knee ankle foot orthosis, single upright, free ankle, solid stirrup, thigh and calf bands/cuffs (single bar 'AK' orthosis), without knee joint, custom-fabricated

* **L2020** Knee ankle foot orthosis, double upright, free knee, free ankle, solid stirrup, thigh and calf bands/cuffs (double bar 'AK' orthosis), custom-fabricated

* **L2030** Knee ankle foot orthosis, double upright, free ankle, solid stirrup, thigh and calf bands/cuffs (double bar 'AK' orthosis), without knee joint, custom fabricated

* **L2034** Knee ankle foot orthosis, full plastic, single upright, with or without free motion knee, medial lateral rotation control, with or without free motion ankle, custom fabricated

* **L2035** Knee ankle foot orthosis, full plastic, static (pediatric size), without free motion ankle, prefabricated, includes fitting and adjustment

* **L2036** Knee ankle foot orthosis, full plastic, double upright, with or without free motion knee, with or without free motion ankle, custom fabricated

* **L2037** Knee ankle foot orthosis, full plastic, single upright, with or without free motion knee, with or without free motion ankle, custom fabricated

* **L2038** Knee ankle foot orthosis, full plastic, with or without free motion knee, multi-axis ankle, custom fabricated

Torsion Control

* **L2040** Hip knee ankle foot orthosis, torsion control, bilateral rotation straps, pelvic band/belt, custom fabricated

* **L2050** Hip knee ankle foot orthosis, torsion control, bilateral torsion cables, hip joint, pelvic band/belt, custom-fabricated

* **L2060** Hip knee ankle foot orthosis, torsion control, bilateral torsion cables, ball bearing hip joint, pelvic band/belt, custom-fabricated

* **L2070** Hip knee ankle foot orthosis, torsion control, unilateral rotation straps, pelvic band/belt, custom-fabricated

* **L2080** Hip knee ankle foot orthosis, torsion control, unilateral torsion cable, hip joint, pelvic band/belt, custom-fabricated

* **L2090** Hip knee ankle foot orthosis, torsion control, unilateral torsion cable, ball bearing hip joint, pelvic band/belt, custom-fabricated

Fracture Orthoses

* **L2106** Ankle foot orthosis, fracture orthosis, tibial fracture cast orthosis, thermoplastic type casting material, custom-fabricated

* **L2108** Ankle foot orthosis, fracture orthosis, tibial fracture cast orthosis, custom-fabricated

* **L2112** Ankle foot orthosis, fracture orthosis, tibial fracture orthosis, soft, prefabricated, includes fitting and adjustment

* **L2114** Ankle foot orthosis, fracture orthosis, tibial fracture orthosis, semi-rigid, prefabricated, includes fitting and adjustment

* **L2116** Ankle foot orthosis, fracture orthosis, tibial fracture orthosis, rigid, prefabricated, includes fitting and adjustment

* **L2126** Knee ankle foot orthosis, fracture orthosis, femoral fracture cast orthosis, thermoplastic type casting material, custom-fabricated

---

▶ New → Revised ✔ Reinstated ~~deleted~~ Deleted

⊘ Special coverage instructions ◆ Not covered or valid by Medicare * Carrier discretion

✳ **L2128** Knee ankle foot orthosis, fracture orthosis, femoral fracture cast orthosis, custom-fabricated

✳ **L2132** KAFO, femoral fracture cast orthosis, soft, prefabricated, includes fitting and adjustment

✳ **L2134** KAFO, femoral fracture cast orthosis, semi-rigid, prefabricated, includes fitting and adjustment

✳ **L2136** KAFO, fracture orthosis, femoral fracture cast orthosis, rigid, prefabricated, includes fitting and adjustment

Additions to Fracture Orthosis

✳ **L2180** Addition to lower extremity fracture orthosis, plastic shoe insert with ankle joints

✳ **L2182** Addition to lower extremity fracture orthosis, drop lock knee joint

✳ **L2184** Addition to lower extremity fracture orthosis, limited motion knee joint

✳ **L2186** Addition to lower extremity fracture orthosis, adjustable motion knee joint, Lerman type

✳ **L2188** Addition to lower extremity fracture orthosis, quadrilateral brim

✳ **L2190** Addition to lower extremity fracture orthosis, waist belt

✳ **L2192** Addition to lower extremity fracture orthosis, hip joint, pelvic band, thigh flange, and pelvic belt

Additions to Lower Extremity Orthosis
Shoe-Ankle-Shin-Knee

✳ **L2200** Addition to lower extremity, limited ankle motion, each joint

✳ **L2210** Addition to lower extremity, dorsiflexion assist (plantar flexion resist), each joint

✳ **L2220** Addition to lower extremity, dorsiflexion and plantar flexion assist/resist, each joint

✳ **L2230** Addition to lower extremity, split flat caliper stirrups and plate attachment

✳ **L2232** Addition to lower extremity orthosis, rocker bottom for total contact ankle foot orthosis, for custom fabricated orthosis only

✳ **L2240** Addition to lower extremity, round caliper and plate attachment

✳ **L2250** Addition to lower extremity, foot plate, molded to patient model, stirrup attachment

✳ **L2260** Addition to lower extremity, reinforced solid stirrup (Scott-Craig type)

✳ **L2265** Addition to lower extremity, long tongue stirrup

✳ **L2270** Addition to lower extremity, varus/valgus correction ('T') strap, padded/lined or malleolus pad

✳ **L2275** Addition to lower extremity, varus/valgus correction, plastic modification, padded/lined

✳ **L2280** Addition to lower extremity, molded inner boot

✳ **L2300** Addition to lower extremity, abduction bar (bilateral hip involvement), jointed, adjustable

✳ **L2310** Addition to lower extremity, abduction bar-straight

✳ **L2320** Addition to lower extremity, non-molded lacer, for custom fabricated orthosis only

✳ **L2330** Addition to lower extremity, lacer molded to patient model, for custom fabricated orthosis only

Used whether closure is lacer or Velcro

✳ **L2335** Addition to lower extremity, anterior swing band

✳ **L2340** Addition to lower extremity, pre-tibial shell, molded to patient model

✳ **L2350** Addition to lower extremity, prosthetic type, (BK) socket, molded to patient model, (used for 'PTB' and 'AFO' orthoses)

✳ **L2360** Addition to lower extremity, extended steel shank

✳ **L2370** Addition to lower extremity, Patten bottom

✳ **L2375** Addition to lower extremity, torsion control, ankle joint and half solid stirrup

✳ **L2380** Addition to lower extremity, torsion control, straight knee joint, each joint

✳ **L2385** Addition to lower extremity, straight knee joint, heavy duty, each joint

✳ **L2387** Addition to lower extremity, polycentric knee joint, for custom fabricated knee ankle foot orthosis, each joint

✳ **L2390** Addition to lower extremity, offset knee joint, each joint

✳ **L2395** Addition to lower extremity, offset knee joint, heavy duty, each joint

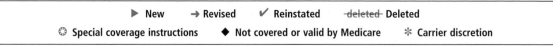

▶ New → Revised ✔ Reinstated deleted Deleted
☉ Special coverage instructions ◆ Not covered or valid by Medicare ✳ Carrier discretion

⁎ **L2397**   Addition to lower extremity orthosis, suspension sleeve

Additions to Straight Knee or Offset Knee Joints

⁎ **L2405**   Addition to knee joint, drop lock, each

⁎ **L2415**   Addition to knee lock with integrated release mechanism (bail, cable, or equal), any material, each joint

⁎ **L2425**   Addition to knee joint, disc or dial lock for adjustable knee flexion, each joint

⁎ **L2430**   Addition to knee joint, ratchet lock for active and progressive knee extension, each joint

⁎ **L2492**   Addition to knee joint, lift loop for drop lock ring

Additions to Thigh/Weight Bearing

Gluteal/Ischial Weight Bearing

⁎ **L2500**   Addition to lower extremity, thigh/ weight bearing, gluteal/ischial weight bearing, ring

⁎ **L2510**   Addition to lower extremity, thigh/ weight bearing, quadri-lateral brim, molded to patient model

⁎ **L2520**   Addition to lower extremity, thigh/ weight bearing, quadri-lateral brim, custom fitted

⁎ **L2525**   Addition to lower extremity, thigh/ weight bearing, ischial containment/ narrow M-L brim molded to patient model

⁎ **L2526**   Addition to lower extremity, thigh/ weight bearing, ischial containment/ narrow M-L brim, custom fitted

⁎ **L2530**   Addition to lower extremity, thigh-weight bearing, lacer, non-molded

⁎ **L2540**   Addition to lower extremity, thigh/ weight bearing, lacer, molded to patient model

⁎ **L2550**   Addition to lower extremity, thigh/ weight bearing, high roll cuff

Additions to Pelvic and Thoracic Control

⁎ **L2570**   Addition to lower extremity, pelvic control, hip joint, Clevis type two position joint, each

⁎ **L2580**   Addition to lower extremity, pelvic control, pelvic sling

⁎ **L2600**   Addition to lower extremity, pelvic control, hip joint, Clevis type, or thrust bearing, free, each

⁎ **L2610**   Addition to lower extremity, pelvic control, hip joint, Clevis or thrust bearing, lock, each

⁎ **L2620**   Addition to lower extremity, pelvic control, hip joint, heavy duty, each

⁎ **L2622**   Addition to lower extremity, pelvic control, hip joint, adjustable flexion, each

⁎ **L2624**   Addition to lower extremity, pelvic control, hip joint, adjustable flexion, extension, abduction control, each

⁎ **L2627**   Addition to lower extremity, pelvic control, plastic, molded to patient model, reciprocating hip joint and cables

⁎ **L2628**   Addition to lower extremity, pelvic control, metal frame, reciprocating hip joint and cables

⁎ **L2630**   Addition to lower extremity, pelvic control, band and belt, unilateral

⁎ **L2640**   Addition to lower extremity, pelvic control, band and belt, bilateral

⁎ **L2650**   Addition to lower extremity, pelvic and thoracic control, gluteal pad, each

⁎ **L2660**   Addition to lower extremity, thoracic control, thoracic band

⁎ **L2670**   Addition to lower extremity, thoracic control, paraspinal uprights

⁎ **L2680**   Addition to lower extremity, thoracic control, lateral support uprights

General Additions

⁎ **L2750**   Addition to lower extremity orthosis, plating chrome or nickel, per bar

⁎ **L2755**   Addition to lower extremity orthosis, high strength, lightweight material, all hybrid lamination/prepreg composite, per segment, for custom fabricated orthosis only

⁎ **L2760**   Addition to lower extremity orthosis, extension, per extension, per bar (for lineal adjustment for growth)

⁎ **L2768**   Orthotic side bar disconnect device, per bar

⁎ **L2780**   Addition to lower extremity orthosis, non-corrosive finish, per bar

⁎ **L2785**   Addition to lower extremity orthosis, drop lock retainer, each

⁎ **L2795**   Addition to lower extremity orthosis, knee control, full kneecap

▶ New   → Revised   ✔ Reinstated   deleted Deleted
☉ Special coverage instructions   ◆ Not covered or valid by Medicare   ⁎ Carrier discretion

✳ **L2800** Addition to lower extremity orthosis, knee control, knee cap, medial or lateral pull, for use with custom fabricated orthosis only

✳ **L2810** Addition to lower extremity orthosis, knee control, condylar pad

✳ **L2820** Addition to lower extremity orthosis, soft interface for molded plastic, below knee section

Only report if soft interface provided, either leather or other material

✳ **L2830** Addition to lower extremity orthosis, soft interface for molded plastic, above knee section

✳ **L2840** Addition to lower extremity orthosis, tibial length sock, fracture or equal, each

✳ **L2850** Addition to lower extremity orthosis, femoral length sock, fracture or equal, each

◆ **L2861** Addition to lower extremity joint, knee or ankle, concentric adjustable torsion style mechanism for custom fabricated orthotics only, each

✳ **L2999** Lower extremity orthoses, not otherwise specified

Foot (Orthopedic Shoes)

Insert, Removable, Molded to Patient Model

L3000-L3649: Bill DME/MAC

⚙ **L3000** Foot, insert, removable, molded to patient model, 'UCB' type, Berkeley shell, each

If both feet casted and supplied with an orthosis, bill L3000-LT and L3000-RT

IOM: 100-02, 15, 290

⚙ **L3001** Foot, insert, removable, molded to patient model, Spenco, each

IOM: 100-02, 15, 290

⚙ **L3002** Foot, insert, removable, molded to patient model, Plastazote or equal, each

IOM: 100-02, 15, 290

⚙ **L3003** Foot, insert, removable, molded to patient model, silicone gel, each

IOM: 100-02, 15, 290

⚙ **L3010** Foot, insert, removable, molded to patient model, longitudinal arch support, each

IOM: 100-02, 15, 290

⚙ **L3020** Foot, insert, removable, molded to patient model, longitudinal/metatarsal support, each

IOM: 100-02, 15, 290

⚙ **L3030** Foot, insert, removable, formed to patient foot, each

IOM: 100-02, 15, 290

✳ **L3031** Foot, insert/plate, removable, addition to lower extremity orthosis, high strength, lightweight material, all hybrid lamination/prepreg composite, each

Arch Support, Removable, Premolded

⚙ **L3040** Foot, arch support, removable, premolded, longitudinal, each

IOM: 100-02, 15, 290

⚙ **L3050** Foot, arch support, removable, premolded, metatarsal, each

IOM: 100-02, 15, 290

⚙ **L3060** Foot, arch support, removable, premolded, longitudinal/metatarsal, each

IOM: 100-02, 15, 290

Arch Support, Non-removable, Attached to Shoe

⚙ **L3070** Foot, arch support, non-removable attached to shoe, longitudinal, each

IOM: 100-02, 15, 290

⚙ **L3080** Foot, arch support, non-removable attached to shoe, metatarsal, each

IOM: 100-02, 15, 290

⚙ **L3090** Foot, arch support, non-removable attached to shoe, longitudinal/metatarsal, each

IOM: 100-02, 15, 290

⚙ **L3100** Hallus-valgus night dynamic splint

IOM: 100-02, 15, 290

Abduction and Rotation Bars

⚙ **L3140** Foot, abduction rotation bar, including shoes

IOM: 100-02, 15, 290

⚙ **L3150** Foot, abduction rotation bar, without shoes

IOM: 100-02, 15, 290

✳ **L3160** Foot, adjustable shoe-styled positioning device

▶ New → Revised ✔ Reinstated deleted Deleted

⚙ Special coverage instructions ◆ Not covered or valid by Medicare ✳ Carrier discretion

⊗ **L3170** Foot, plastic, silicone or equal, heel stabilizer, each
IOM: 100-02, 15, 290

Orthopedic Footwear

⊗ **L3201** Orthopedic shoe, oxford with supinator or pronator, infant
IOM: 100-02, 15, 290

⊗ **L3202** Orthopedic shoe, oxford with supinator or pronator, child
IOM: 100-02, 15, 290

⊗ **L3203** Orthopedic shoe, oxford with supinator or pronator, junior
IOM: 100-02, 15, 290

⊗ **L3204** Orthopedic shoe, hightop with supinator or pronator, infant
IOM: 100-02, 15, 290

⊗ **L3206** Orthopedic shoe, hightop with supinator or pronator, child
IOM: 100-02, 15, 290

⊗ **L3207** Orthopedic shoe, hightop with supinator or pronator, junior
IOM: 100-02, 15, 290

⊗ **L3208** Surgical boot, infant, each
IOM: 100-02, 15, 100

⊗ **L3209** Surgical boot, each, child
IOM: 100-02, 15, 100

⊗ **L3211** Surgical boot, each, junior
IOM: 100-02, 15, 100

⊗ **L3212** Benesch boot, pair, infant
IOM: 100-02, 15, 100

⊗ **L3213** Benesch boot, pair, child
IOM: 100-02, 15, 100

⊗ **L3214** Benesch boot, pair, junior
IOM: 100-02, 15, 100

◆ **L3215** Orthopedic footwear, ladies shoe, oxford, each
Medicare Statute 1862a8

◆ **L3216** Orthopedic footwear, ladies shoe, depth inlay, each
Medicare Statute 1862a8

◆ **L3217** Orthopedic footwear, ladies shoe, hightop, depth inlay, each
Medicare Statute 1862a8

◆ **L3219** Orthopedic footwear, mens shoe, oxford, each
Medicare Statute 1862a8

◆ **L3221** Orthopedic footwear, mens shoe, depth inlay, each
Medicare Statute 1862a8

◆ **L3222** Orthopedic footwear, mens shoe, hightop, depth inlay, each
Medicare Statute 1862a8

⊗ **L3224** Orthopedic footwear, ladies shoe, oxford, used as an integral part of a brace (orthosis)
IOM: 100-02, 15, 290

⊗ **L3225** Orthopedic footwear, mens shoe, oxford, used as an integral part of a brace (orthosis)
IOM: 100-02, 15, 290

⊗ **L3230** Orthopedic footwear, custom shoe, depth inlay, each
IOM: 100-02, 15, 290

⊗ **L3250** Orthopedic footwear, custom molded shoe, removable inner mold, prosthetic shoe, each
IOM: 100-02, 15, 290

⊗ **L3251** Foot, shoe molded to patient model, silicone shoe, each
IOM: 100-02, 15, 290

⊗ **L3252** Foot, shoe molded to patient model, Plastazote (or similar), custom fabricated, each
IOM: 100-02, 15, 290

⊗ **L3253** Foot, molded shoe Plastazote (or similar), custom fitted, each
IOM: 100-02, 15, 290

⊗ **L3254** Non-standard size or width
IOM: 100-02, 15, 290

⊗ **L3255** Non-standard size or length
IOM: 100-02, 15, 290

⊗ **L3257** Orthopedic footwear, additional charge for split size
IOM: 100-02, 15, 290

⊗ **L3260** Surgical boot/shoe, each
IOM: 100-02, 15, 100

✳ **L3265** Plastazote sandal, each

Shoe Modifications
Lifts

⊗ **L3300** Lift, elevation, heel, tapered to metatarsals, per inch
IOM: 100-02, 15, 290

▶ New   → Revised   ✔ Reinstated   ~~deleted~~ Deleted

⊗ Special coverage instructions   ◆ Not covered or valid by Medicare   ✳ Carrier discretion

☼ **L3310** Lift, elevation, heel and sole, Neoprene, per inch
IOM: 100-02, 15, 290

☼ **L3320** Lift, elevation, heel and sole, cork, per inch
IOM: 100-02, 15, 290

☼ **L3330** Lift, elevation, metal extension (skate)
IOM: 100-02, 15, 290

☼ **L3332** Lift, elevation, inside shoe, tapered, up to one-half inch
IOM: 100-02, 15, 290

☼ **L3334** Lift, elevation, heel, per inch
IOM: 100-02, 15, 290

Wedges

☼ **L3340** Heel wedge, SACH
IOM: 100-02, 15, 290

☼ **L3350** Heel wedge
IOM: 100-02, 15, 290

☼ **L3360** Sole wedge, outside sole
IOM: 100-02, 15, 290

☼ **L3370** Sole wedge, between sole
IOM: 100-02, 15, 290

☼ **L3380** Clubfoot wedge
IOM: 100-02, 15, 290

☼ **L3390** Outflare wedge
IOM: 100-02, 15, 290

☼ **L3400** Metatarsal bar wedge, rocker
IOM: 100-02, 15, 290

☼ **L3410** Metatarsal bar wedge, between sole
IOM: 100-02, 15, 290

☼ **L3420** Full sole and heel wedge, between sole
IOM: 100-02, 15, 290

Heels

☼ **L3430** Heel, counter, plastic reinforced
IOM: 100-02, 15, 290

☼ **L3440** Heel, counter, leather reinforced
IOM: 100-02, 15, 290

☼ **L3450** Heel, SACH cushion type
IOM: 100-02, 15, 290

☼ **L3455** Heel, new leather, standard
IOM: 100-02, 15, 290

☼ **L3460** Heel, new rubber, standard
IOM: 100-02, 15, 290

☼ **L3465** Heel, Thomas with wedge
IOM: 100-02, 15, 290

☼ **L3470** Heel, Thomas extended to ball
IOM: 100-02, 15, 290

☼ **L3480** Heel, pad and depression for spur
IOM: 100-02, 15, 290

☼ **L3485** Heel, pad, removable for spur
IOM: 100-02, 15, 290

Additions to Orthopedic Shoes

☼ **L3500** Orthopedic shoe addition, insole, leather
IOM: 100-02, 15, 290

☼ **L3510** Orthopedic shoe addition, insole, rubber
IOM: 100-02, 15, 290

☼ **L3520** Orthopedic shoe addition, insole, felt covered with leather
IOM: 100-02, 15, 290

☼ **L3530** Orthopedic shoe addition, sole, half
IOM: 100-02, 15, 290

☼ **L3540** Orthopedic shoe addition, sole, full
IOM: 100-02, 15, 290

☼ **L3550** Orthopedic shoe addition, toe tap standard
IOM: 100-02, 15, 290

☼ **L3560** Orthopedic shoe addition, toe tap, horseshoe
IOM: 100-02, 15, 290

☼ **L3570** Orthopedic shoe addition, special extension to instep (leather with eyelets)
IOM: 100-02, 15, 290

☼ **L3580** Orthopedic shoe addition, convert instep to Velcro closure
IOM: 100-02, 15, 290

☼ **L3590** Orthopedic shoe addition, convert firm shoe counter to soft counter
IOM: 100-02, 15, 290

☼ **L3595** Orthopedic shoe addition, March bar
IOM: 100-02, 15, 290

▶ New   → Revised   ✔ Reinstated   ~~deleted~~ Deleted

☼ Special coverage instructions   ◆ Not covered or valid by Medicare   ✳ Carrier discretion

Transfer or Replacement

⊛ **L3600**   Transfer of an orthosis from one shoe to another, caliper plate, existing

IOM: 100-02, 15, 290

⊛ **L3610**   Transfer of an orthosis from one shoe to another, caliper plate, new

IOM: 100-02, 15, 290

⊛ **L3620**   Transfer of an orthosis from one shoe to another, solid stirrup, existing

IOM: 100-02, 15, 290

⊛ **L3630**   Transfer of an orthosis from one shoe to another, solid stirrup, new

IOM: 100-02, 15, 290

⊛ **L3640**   Transfer of an orthosis from one shoe to another, Dennis Browne splint (Riveton), both shoes

IOM: 100-02, 15, 290

⊛ **L3649**   Orthopedic shoe, modification, addition or transfer, not otherwise specified

IOM: 100-02, 15, 290

Orthotic Devices: Upper Limb

NOTE: The procedures in this section are considered as *base* or *basic procedures* and may be modified by listing procedures from the Additions section and adding them to the base procedure.

L3650-L3956:   Bill DME/MAC

Shoulder

✳ **L3650**   Shoulder orthosis, (SO), figure of eight design abduction restrainer, prefabricated, includes fitting and adjustment

✳ **L3660**   Shoulder orthosis, figure of eight design abduction restrainer, canvas and webbing, prefabricated, includes fitting and adjustment

✳ **L3670**   Shoulder orthosis, acromio/clavicular (canvas and webbing type), prefabricated, includes fitting and adjustment

✳ **L3671**   Shoulder orthosis, shoulder joint design, without joints, may include soft interface, straps, custom fabricated, includes fitting and adjustment

✳ **L3674**   Shoulder orthosis, abduction positioning (airplane design), thoracic component and support bar, with or without nontorsion joint/turnbuckle, may include soft interface, straps, custom fabricated, includes fitting and adjustment

✳ **L3675**   Shoulder orthosis, vest type abduction restrainer, canvas webbing type or equal, prefabricated, includes fitting and adjustment

⊛ **L3677**   Shoulder orthosis, shoulder joint design, without joints, may include soft interface, straps, pre-fabricated, includes fitting and adjustment

Elbow

✳ **L3702**   Elbow orthosis, without joints, may include soft interface, straps, custom fabricated, includes fitting and adjustment

✳ **L3710**   Elbow orthosis, elastic with metal joints, prefabricated, includes fitting and adjustment

✳ **L3720**   Elbow orthosis, double upright with forearm/arm cuffs, free motion, custom-fabricated

✳ **L3730**   Elbow orthosis, double upright with forearm/arm cuffs, extension/flexion assist, custom-fabricated

✳ **L3740**   Elbow orthosis, double upright with forearm/arm cuffs, adjustable position lock with active control, custom-fabricated

✳ **L3760**   Elbow orthosis, with adjustable position locking joint(s), prefabricated, includes fitting and adjustments, any type

✳ **L3762**   Elbow orthosis, rigid, without joints, includes soft interface material, prefabricated, includes fitting and adjustment

✳ **L3763**   Elbow wrist hand orthosis, rigid, without joints, may include soft interface, straps, custom fabricated, includes fitting and adjustment

✳ **L3764**   Elbow wrist hand orthosis, includes one or more nontorsion joints, elastic bands, turnbuckles, may include soft interface, straps, custom fabricated, includes fitting and adjustment

✳ **L3765**   Elbow wrist hand finger orthosis, rigid, without joints, may include soft interface, straps, custom fabricated, includes fitting and adjustment

---

▶ New	→ Revised	✔ Reinstated	deleted Deleted
⊛ Special coverage instructions		◆ Not covered or valid by Medicare	✳ Carrier discretion

* **L3766** Elbow wrist hand finger orthosis, includes one or more nontorsion joints, elastic bands, turnbuckles, may include soft interface, straps, custom fabricated, includes fitting and adjustment

Wrist-Hand-Finger Orthosis (WHFO)

* **L3806** Wrist hand finger orthosis, includes one or more nontorsion joint(s), turnbuckles, elastic bands/springs, may include soft interface material, straps, custom fabricated, includes fitting and adjustment

* **L3807** Wrist hand finger orthosis, without joint(s), prefabricated, includes fitting and adjustments, any type

* **L3808** Wrist hand finger orthosis, rigid without joints, may include soft interface material; straps, custom fabricated, includes fitting and adjustment

Additions and Extensions

◆ **L3891** Addition to upper extremity joint, wrist or elbow, concentric adjustable torsion style mechanism for custom fabricated orthotics only, each

* **L3900** Wrist hand finger orthosis, dynamic flexor hinge, reciprocal wrist extension/flexion, finger flexion/extension, wrist or finger driven, custom-fabricated

* **L3901** Wrist hand finger orthosis, dynamic flexor hinge, reciprocal wrist extension/flexion, finger flexion/extension, cable driven, custom-fabricated

External Power

* **L3904** Wrist hand finger orthosis, external powered, electric, custom-fabricated

* **L3905** Wrist hand orthosis, includes one or more nontorsion joints, elastic bands, turnbuckles, may include soft interface, straps, custom fabricated, includes fitting and adjustment

Other Wrist-Hand-Finger Orthoses: Custom Fitted

* **L3906** Wrist hand orthosis, without joints, may include soft interface, straps, custom fabricated, includes fitting and adjustment

* **L3908** Wrist hand orthosis, wrist extension control cock-up, non molded, prefabricated, includes fitting and adjustment

* **L3912** Hand finger orthosis, flexion glove with elastic finger control, prefabricated, includes fitting and adjustment

* **L3913** Hand finger orthosis, without joints, may include soft interface, straps, custom fabricated, includes fitting and adjustment

* **L3915** Wrist hand orthosis, includes one or more nontorsion joint(s), elastic bands, turnbuckles, may include soft interface, straps, prefabricated, includes fitting and adjustment

* **L3917** Hand orthosis, metacarpal fracture orthosis, prefabricated, includes fitting and adjustment

* **L3919** Hand orthosis, without joints, may include soft interface, straps, custom fabricated, includes fitting and adjustment

* **L3921** Hand finger orthosis, includes one or more nontorsion joints, elastic bands, turnbuckles, may include soft interface, straps, custom fabricated, includes fitting and adjustment

* **L3923** Hand finger orthosis, without joints, may include soft interface, straps, prefabricated, includes fitting and adjustments

* **L3925** Finger orthosis, proximal interphalangeal (PIP)/distal interphalangeal (DIP), non torsion joint/spring, extension/flexion, may include soft interface material, prefabricated, includes fitting and adjustment

* **L3927** Finger orthosis, proximal interphalangeal (PIP)/distal interphalangeal (DIP), without joint/spring, extension/flexion (e.g. static or ring type), may include soft interface material, prefabricated, includes fitting and adjustment

* **L3929** Hand finger orthosis, includes one or more nontorsion joint(s), turnbuckles, elastic bands/springs, may include soft interface material, straps, prefabricated, includes fitting and adjustment

---

▶ New   → Revised   ✔ Reinstated   ~~deleted~~ Deleted

☉ Special coverage instructions   ◆ Not covered or valid by Medicare   ✳ Carrier discretion

✳ **L3931** Wrist hand finger orthosis, includes one or more nontorsion joint(s), turnbuckles, elastic bands/springs, may include soft interface material, straps, prefabricated, includes fitting and adjustment

✳ **L3933** Finger orthosis, without joints, may include soft interface, custom fabricated, includes fitting and adjustment

✳ **L3935** Finger orthosis, nontorsion joint, may include soft interface, custom fabricated, includes fitting and adjustment

✳ **L3956** Addition of joint to upper extremity orthosis, any material, per joint

Shoulder-Elbow-Wrist-Hand Orthosis (SEWHO)

Abduction Positioning: Custom Fitted

L3960-L4631: Bill DME/MAC

✳ **L3960** Shoulder elbow wrist hand orthosis, abduction positioning, airplane design, prefabricated, includes fitting and adjustment

✳ **L3961** Shoulder elbow wrist hand orthosis, shoulder cap design, without joints, may include soft interface, straps, custom fabricated, includes fitting and adjustment

✳ **L3962** Shoulder elbow wrist hand orthosis, abduction positioning, Erbs palsy design, prefabricated, includes fitting and adjustment

✳ **L3967** Shoulder elbow wrist hand orthosis, abduction positioning (airplane design), thoracic component and support bar, without joints, may include soft interface, straps, custom fabricated, includes fitting and adjustment

Additions to Mobile Arm Supports and SEWHO

✳ **L3971** Shoulder elbow wrist hand orthosis, shoulder cap design, includes one or more nontorsion joints, elastic bands, turnbuckles, may include soft interface, straps, custom fabricated, includes fitting and adjustment

✳ **L3973** Shoulder elbow wrist hand orthosis, abduction positioning (airplane design), thoracic component and support bar, includes one or more nontorsion joints, elastic bands, turnbuckles, may include soft interface, straps, custom fabricated, includes fitting and adjustment

✳ **L3975** Shoulder elbow wrist hand finger orthosis, shoulder cap design, without joints, may include soft interface, straps, custom fabricated, includes fitting and adjustment

✳ **L3976** Shoulder elbow wrist hand finger orthosis, abduction positioning (airplane design), thoracic component and support bar, without joints, may include soft interface, straps, custom fabricated, includes fitting and adjustment

✳ **L3977** Shoulder elbow wrist hand finger orthosis, shoulder cap design, includes one or more nontorsion joints, elastic bands, turnbuckles, may include soft interface, straps, custom fabricated, includes fitting and adjustment

✳ **L3978** Shoulder elbow wrist hand finger orthosis, abduction positioning (airplane design), thoracic component and support bar, includes one or more nontorsion joints, elastic bands, turnbuckles, may include soft interface, straps, custom fabricated, includes fitting and adjustment

Fracture Orthoses

✳ **L3980** Upper extremity fracture orthosis, humeral, prefabricated, includes fitting and adjustment

✳ **L3982** Upper extremity fracture orthosis, radius/ulnar, prefabricated, includes fitting and adjustment

✳ **L3984** Upper extremity fracture orthosis, wrist, prefabricated, includes fitting and adjustment

✳ **L3995** Addition to upper extremity orthosis, sock, fracture or equal, each

✳ **L3999** Upper limb orthosis, not otherwise specified

Specific Repair

* **L4000** Replace girdle for spinal orthosis (CTLSO or SO)

* **L4002** Replacement strap, any orthosis, includes all components, any length, any type

* **L4010** Replace trilateral socket brim

* **L4020** Replace quadrilateral socket brim, molded to patient model

* **L4030** Replace quadrilateral socket brim, custom fitted

* **L4040** Replace molded thigh lacer, for custom fabricated orthosis only

* **L4045** Replace non-molded thigh lacer, for custom fabricated orthosis only

* **L4050** Replace molded calf lacer, for custom fabricated orthosis only

* **L4055** Replace non-molded calf lacer, for custom fabricated orthosis only

* **L4060** Replace high roll cuff

* **L4070** Replace proximal and distal upright for KAFO

* **L4080** Replace metal bands KAFO, proximal thigh

* **L4090** Replace metal bands KAFO-AFO, calf or distal thigh

* **L4100** Replace leather cuff KAFO, proximal thigh

* **L4110** Replace leather cuff KAFO-AFO, calf or distal thigh

* **L4130** Replace pretibial shell

Repairs

⊚ **L4205** Repair of orthotic device, labor component, per 15 minutes
    IOM: 100-02, 15, 110.2

⊚ **L4210** Repair of orthotic device, repair or replace minor parts
    IOM: 100-02, 15, 110.2; 100-02, 15, 120

Ancillary Orthotic Services

* **L4350** Ankle control orthosis, stirrup style, rigid, includes any type interface (e.g., pneumatic, gel), prefabricated, includes fitting and adjustment

* **L4360** Walking boot, pneumatic, and/or vacuum, with or without joints, with or without interface material, prefabricated, includes fitting and adjustment
    Noncovered when walking boots used primarily to relieve pressure, especially on sole of foot, or are used for patients with foot ulcers

* **L4370** Pneumatic full leg splint, prefabricated, includes fitting and adjustment

* **L4386** Walking boot, non-pneumatic, with or without joints, with or without interface material, prefabricated, includes fitting and adjustment

* **L4392** Replacement, soft interface material, static AFO

* **L4394** Replace soft interface material, foot drop splint

* **L4396** Static or dynamic ankle foot orthosis, including soft interface material, adjustable for fit, for positioning, may be used for minimal ambulation, prefabricated, includes fitting and adjustment

* **L4398** Foot drop splint, recumbent positioning device, prefabricated, includes fitting and adjustment

* **L4631** Ankle foot orthosis, walking boot type, varus/valgus correction, rocker bottom, anterior tibial shell, soft interface, custom arch support, plastic or other material, includes straps and closures, custom fabricated

PROSTHETICS (L5000-L9999)

Lower Limb (L5000-L5999)

NOTE: The procedures in this section are considered as *base* or *basic procedures* and may be modified by listing items/procedures or special materials from the Additions section and adding them to the base procedure.

Partial Foot

L5000-L5999: Bill DME/MAC

⊚ **L5000** Partial foot, shoe insert with longitudinal arch, toe filler
    IOM: 100-02, 15, 290

⊚ **L5010** Partial foot, molded socket, ankle height, with toe filler
    IOM: 100-02, 15, 290

▶ New   → Revised   ✔ Reinstated   ~~deleted~~ Deleted
⊚ Special coverage instructions   ◆ Not covered or valid by Medicare   * Carrier discretion

⊘ **L5020**   Partial foot, molded socket, tibial tubercle height, with toe filler

IOM: 100-02, 15, 290

Ankle

✳ **L5050**   Ankle, Symes, molded socket, SACH foot

✳ **L5060**   Ankle, Symes, metal frame, molded leather socket, articulated ankle/foot

Below Knee

✳ **L5100**   Below knee, molded socket, shin, SACH foot

✳ **L5105**   Below knee, plastic socket, joints and thigh lacer, SACH foot

Knee Disarticulation

✳ **L5150**   Knee disarticulation (or through knee), molded socket, external knee joints, shin, SACH foot

✳ **L5160**   Knee disarticulation (or through knee), molded socket, bent knee configuration, external knee joints, shin, SACH foot

Above Knee

✳ **L5200**   Above knee, molded socket, single axis constant friction knee, shin, SACH foot

✳ **L5210**   Above knee, short prosthesis, no knee joint ('stubbies'), with foot blocks, no ankle joints, each

✳ **L5220**   Above knee, short prosthesis, no knee joint ('stubbies'), with articulated ankle/foot, dynamically aligned, each

✳ **L5230**   Above knee, for proximal femoral focal deficiency, constant friction knee, shin, SACH foot

Hip Disarticulation

✳ **L5250**   Hip disarticulation, Canadian type; molded socket, hip joint, single axis constant friction knee, shin, SACH foot

✳ **L5270**   Hip disarticulation, tilt table type; molded socket, locking hip joint, single axis constant friction knee, shin, SACH foot

Hemipelvectomy

✳ **L5280**   Hemipelvectomy, Canadian type; molded socket, hip joint, single axis constant friction knee, shin, SACH foot

Endoskeleton: Below Knee

✳ **L5301**   Below knee, molded socket, shin, SACH foot, endoskeletal system

✳ **L5312**   Knee disarticulation (or through knee), molded socket, single axis knee, pylon, sach foot, endoskeletal system

Endoskeletal: Above Knee

✳ **L5321**   Above knee, molded socket, open end, SACH foot, endoskeletal system, single axis knee

Endoskeletal: Hip Disarticulation

✳ **L5331**   Hip disarticulation, Canadian type, molded socket, endoskeletal system, hip joint, single axis knee, SACH foot

Endoskeletal: Hemipelvectomy

✳ **L5341**   Hemipelvectomy, Canadian type, molded socket, endoskeletal system, hip joint, single axis knee, SACH foot

Immediate Postsurgical or Early Fitting Procedures

✳ **L5400**   Immediate post surgical or early fitting, application of initial rigid dressing, including fitting, alignment, suspension, and one cast change, below knee

✳ **L5410**   Immediate post surgical or early fitting, application of initial rigid dressing, including fitting, alignment and suspension, below knee, each additional cast change and realignment

✳ **L5420**   Immediate post surgical or early fitting, application of initial rigid dressing, including fitting, alignment and suspension and one cast change 'AK' or knee disarticulation

---

▶ New   → Revised   ✔ Reinstated   ~~deleted~~ Deleted
⊘ Special coverage instructions   ◆ Not covered or valid by Medicare   ✳ Carrier discretion

* **L5430** Immediate postsurgical or early fitting, application of initial rigid dressing, including fitting, alignment, and suspension, 'AK' or knee disarticulation, each additional cast change and realignment

* **L5450** Immediate post surgical or early fitting, application of non-weight bearing rigid dressing, below knee

* **L5460** Immediate post surgical or early fitting, application of non-weight bearing rigid dressing, above knee

Initial Prosthesis

* **L5500** Initial, below knee 'PTB' type socket, non-alignable system, pylon, no cover, SACH foot, plaster socket, direct formed

* **L5505** Initial, above knee–knee disarticulation, ischial level socket, non-alignable system, pylon, no cover, SACH foot, plaster socket, direct formed

Preparatory Prosthesis

* **L5510** Preparatory, below knee 'PTB' type socket, non-alignable system, pylon, no cover, SACH foot, plaster socket, molded to model

* **L5520** Preparatory, below knee 'PTB' type socket, non-alignable system, pylon, no cover, SACH foot, thermoplastic or equal, direct formed

* **L5530** Preparatory, below knee 'PTB' type socket, non-alignable system, pylon, no cover, SACH foot, thermoplastic or equal, molded to model

* **L5535** Preparatory, below knee 'PTB' type socket, non-alignable system, no cover, SACH foot, prefabricated, adjustable open end socket

* **L5540** Preparatory, below knee 'PTB' type socket, non-alignable system, pylon, no cover, SACH foot, laminated socket, molded to model

* **L5560** Preparatory, above knee - knee disarticulation, ischial level socket, non-alignable system, pylon, no cover, SACH foot, plaster socket, molded to model

* **L5570** Preparatory, above knee - knee disarticulation, ischial level socket, non-alignable system, pylon, no cover, SACH foot, thermoplastic or equal, direct formed

* **L5580** Preparatory, above knee - knee disarticulation, ischial level socket, non-alignable system, pylon, no cover, SACH foot, thermoplastic or equal, molded to model

* **L5585** Preparatory, above knee - knee disarticulation, ischial level socket, non-alignable system, pylon, no cover, SACH foot, prefabricated adjustable open end socket

* **L5590** Preparatory, above knee - knee disarticulation, ischial level socket, non-alignable system, pylon, no cover, SACH foot, laminated socket, molded to model

* **L5595** Preparatory, hip disarticulation-hemipelvectomy, pylon, no cover, SACH foot, thermoplastic or equal, molded to patient model

* **L5600** Preparatory, hip disarticulation-hemipelvectomy, pylon, no cover, SACH foot, laminated socket, molded to patient model

Additions to Lower Extremity

* **L5610** Addition to lower extremity, endoskeletal system, above knee, hydracadence system

* **L5611** Addition to lower extremity, endoskeletal system, above knee-knee disarticulation, 4 bar linkage, with friction swing phase control

* **L5613** Addition to lower extremity, endoskeletal system, above knee-knee disarticulation, 4 bar linkage, with hydraulic swing phase control

* **L5614** Addition to lower extremity, exoskeletal system, above knee-knee disarticulation, 4 bar linkage, with pneumatic swing phase control

* **L5616** Addition to lower extremity, endoskeletal system, above knee, universal multiplex system, friction swing phase control

* **L5617** Addition to lower extremity, quick change self-aligning unit, above knee or below knee, each

Additions to Test Sockets

* **L5618** Addition to lower extremity, test socket, Symes

* **L5620** Addition to lower extremity, test socket, below knee

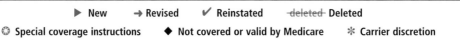

▶ New → Revised ✔ Reinstated ~~deleted~~ Deleted
☺ Special coverage instructions ◆ Not covered or valid by Medicare ✳ Carrier discretion

* **L5622** Addition to lower extremity, test socket, knee disarticulation

* **L5624** Addition to lower extremity, test socket, above knee

* **L5626** Addition to lower extremity, test socket, hip disarticulation

* **L5628** Addition to lower extremity, test socket, hemipelvectomy

* **L5629** Addition to lower extremity, below knee, acrylic socket

Additions to Socket Variations

* **L5630** Addition to lower extremity, Symes type, expandable wall socket

* **L5631** Addition to lower extremity, above knee or knee disarticulation, acrylic socket

* **L5632** Addition to lower extremity, Symes type, 'PTB' brim design socket

* **L5634** Addition to lower extremity, Symes type, posterior opening (Canadian) socket

* **L5636** Addition to lower extremity, Symes type, medial opening socket

* **L5637** Addition to lower extremity, below knee, total contact

* **L5638** Addition to lower extremity, below knee, leather socket

* **L5639** Addition to lower extremity, below knee, wood socket

* **L5640** Addition to lower extremity, knee disarticulation, leather socket

* **L5642** Addition to lower extremity, above knee, leather socket

* **L5643** Addition to lower extremity, hip disarticulation, flexible inner socket, external frame

* **L5644** Addition to lower extremity, above knee, wood socket

* **L5645** Addition to lower extremity, below knee, flexible inner socket, external frame

* **L5646** Addition to lower extremity, below knee, air, fluid, gel or equal, cushion socket

* **L5647** Addition to lower extremity, below knee, suction socket

* **L5648** Addition to lower extremity, above knee, air, fluid, gel or equal, cushion socket

* **L5649** Addition to lower extremity, ischial containment/narrow M-L socket

* **L5650** Additions to lower extremity, total contact, above knee or knee disarticulation socket

* **L5651** Addition to lower extremity, above knee, flexible inner socket, external frame

* **L5652** Addition to lower extremity, suction suspension, above knee or knee disarticulation socket

* **L5653** Addition to lower extremity, knee disarticulation, expandable wall socket

Additions to Socket Insert and Suspension

* **L5654** Addition to lower extremity, socket insert, Symes, (Kemblo, Pelite, Aliplast, Plastazote or equal)

* **L5655** Addition to lower extremity, socket insert, below knee (Kemblo, Pelite, Aliplast, Plastazote or equal)

* **L5656** Addition to lower extremity, socket insert, knee disarticulation (Kemblo, Pelite, Aliplast, Plastazote or equal)

* **L5658** Addition to lower extremity, socket insert, above knee (Kemblo, Pelite, Aliplast, Plastazote or equal)

* **L5661** Addition to lower extremity, socket insert, multi-durometer Symes

* **L5665** Addition to lower extremity, socket insert, multi-durometer, below knee

* **L5666** Addition to lower extremity, below knee, cuff suspension

* **L5668** Addition to lower extremity, below knee, molded distal cushion

* **L5670** Addition to lower extremity, below knee, molded supracondylar suspension ('PTS' or similar)

* **L5671** Addition to lower extremity, below knee/above knee suspension locking mechanism (shuttle, lanyard or equal), excludes socket insert

* **L5672** Addition to lower extremity, below knee, removable medial brim suspension

* **L5673** Addition to lower extremity, below knee/above knee, custom fabricated from existing mold or prefabricated, socket insert, silicone gel, elastomeric or equal, for use with locking mechanism

* **L5676** Additions to lower extremity, below knee, knee joints, single axis, pair

* **L5677** Additions to lower extremity, below knee, knee joints, polycentric, pair

---

▶ New   → Revised   ✔ Reinstated   ~~deleted~~ Deleted

⊙ Special coverage instructions   ◆ Not covered or valid by Medicare   ✳ Carrier discretion

* **L5678** Additions to lower extremity, below knee, joint covers, pair

* **L5679** Addition to lower extremity, below knee/above knee, custom fabricated from existing mold or prefabricated, socket insert, silicone gel, elastomeric or equal, not for use with locking mechanism

* **L5680** Addition to lower extremity, below knee, thigh lacer, nonmolded

* **L5681** Addition to lower extremity, below knee/above knee, custom fabricated socket insert for congenital or atypical traumatic amputee, silicone gel, elastomeric or equal, for use with or without locking mechanism, initial only (for other than initial, use code L5673 or L5679)

* **L5682** Addition to lower extremity, below knee, thigh lacer, gluteal/ischial, molded

* **L5683** Addition to lower extremity, below knee/above knee, custom fabricated socket insert for other than congenital or atypical traumatic amputee, silicone gel, elastomeric, or equal, for use with or without locking mechanism, initial only (for other than initial, use code L5673 or L5679)

* **L5684** Addition to lower extremity, below knee, fork strap

* **L5685** Addition to lower extremity prosthesis, below knee, suspension/sealing sleeve, with or without valve, any material, each

* **L5686** Addition to lower extremity, below knee, back check (extension control)

* **L5688** Addition to lower extremity, below knee, waist belt, webbing

* **L5690** Addition to lower extremity, below knee, waist belt, padded and lined

* **L5692** Addition to lower extremity, above knee, pelvic control belt, light

* **L5694** Addition to lower extremity, above knee, pelvic control belt, padded and lined

* **L5695** Addition to lower extremity, above knee, pelvic control, sleeve suspension, neoprene or equal, each

* **L5696** Addition to lower extremity, above knee or knee disarticulation, pelvic joint

* **L5697** Addition to lower extremity, above knee or knee disarticulation, pelvic band

* **L5698** Addition to lower extremity, above knee or knee disarticulation, Silesian bandage

* **L5699** All lower extremity prostheses, shoulder harness

Additions/Replacements to Feet-Ankle Units

* **L5700** Replacement, socket, below knee, molded to patient model

* **L5701** Replacement, socket, above knee/knee disarticulation, including attachment plate, molded to patient model

* **L5702** Replacement, socket, hip disarticulation, including hip joint, molded to patient model

* **L5703** Ankle, Symes, molded to patient model, socket without solid ankle cushion heel (SACH) foot, replacement only

* **L5704** Custom shaped protective cover, below knee

* **L5705** Custom shaped protective cover, above knee

* **L5706** Custom shaped protective cover, knee disarticulation

* **L5707** Custom shaped protective cover, hip disarticulation

Additions to Exoskeletal–Knee-Shin System

* **L5710** Addition, exoskeletal knee-shin system, single axis, manual lock

* **L5711** Additions exoskeletal knee-shin system, single axis, manual lock, ultra-light material

* **L5712** Addition, exoskeletal knee-shin system, single axis, friction swing and stance phase control (safety knee)

* **L5714** Addition, exoskeletal knee-shin system, single axis, variable friction swing phase control

* **L5716** Addition, exoskeletal knee-shin system, polycentric, mechanical stance phase lock

* **L5718** Addition, exoskeletal knee-shin system, polycentric, friction swing and stance phase control

* **L5722** Addition, exoskeletal knee-shin system, single axis, pneumatic swing, friction stance phase control

* **L5724** Addition, exoskeletal knee-shin system, single axis, fluid swing phase control

* **L5726** Addition, exoskeletal knee-shin system, single axis, external joints, fluid swing phase control

* **L5728** Addition, exoskeletal knee-shin system, single axis, fluid swing and stance phase control

▶ New   → Revised   ✔ Reinstated   -deleted- Deleted

◎ Special coverage instructions   ◆ Not covered or valid by Medicare   * Carrier discretion

* **L5780** Addition, exoskeletal knee-shin system, single axis, pneumatic/hydra pneumatic swing phase control

* **L5781** Addition to lower limb prosthesis, vacuum pump, residual limb volume management and moisture evacuation system

* **L5782** Addition to lower limb prosthesis, vacuum pump, residual limb volume management and moisture evacuation system, heavy duty

Component Modification

* **L5785** Addition, exoskeletal system, below knee, ultra-light material (titanium, carbon fiber, or equal)

* **L5790** Addition, exoskeletal system, above knee, ultra-light material (titanium, carbon fiber, or equal)

* **L5795** Addition, exoskeletal system, hip disarticulation, ultra-light material (titanium, carbon fiber, or equal)

Endoskeletal

* **L5810** Addition, endoskeletal knee-shin system, single axis, manual lock

* **L5811** Addition, endoskeletal knee-shin system, single axis, manual lock, ultralight material

* **L5812** Addition, endoskeletal knee-shin system, single axis, friction swing and stance phase control (safety knee)

* **L5814** Addition, endoskeletal knee-shin system, polycentric, hydraulic swing phase control, mechanical stance phase lock

* **L5816** Addition, endoskeletal knee-shin system, polycentric, mechanical stance phase lock

* **L5818** Addition, endoskeletal knee-shin system, polycentric, friction swing, and stance phase control

* **L5822** Addition, endoskeletal knee-shin system, single axis, pneumatic swing, friction stance phase control

* **L5824** Addition, endoskeletal knee-shin system, single axis, fluid swing phase control

* **L5826** Addition, endoskeletal knee-shin system, single axis, hydraulic swing phase control, with miniature high activity frame

* **L5828** Addition, endoskeletal knee-shin system, single axis, fluid swing and stance phase control

* **L5830** Addition, endoskeletal knee-shin system, single axis, pneumatic/swing phase control

* **L5840** Addition, endoskeletal knee/shin system, 4-bar linkage or multiaxial, pneumatic swing phase control

* **L5845** Addition, endoskeletal, knee-shin system, stance flexion feature, adjustable

* **L5848** Addition to endoskeletal, knee-shin system, fluid stance extension, dampening feature, with or without adjustability

* **L5850** Addition, endoskeletal system, above knee or hip disarticulation, knee extension assist

* **L5855** Addition, endoskeletal system, hip disarticulation, mechanical hip extension assist

* **L5856** Addition to lower extremity prosthesis, endoskeletal knee-shin system, microprocessor control feature, swing and stance phase; includes electronic sensor(s), any type

* **L5857** Addition to lower extremity prosthesis, endoskeletal knee-shin system, microprocessor control feature, swing phase only; includes electronic sensor(s), any type

* **L5858** Addition to lower extremity prosthesis, endoskeletal knee shin system, microprocessor control feature, stance phase only, includes electronic sensor(s), any type

▶ * **L5859** Addition to lower extremity prosthesis, endoskeletal knee-shin system, powered and programmable flexion/extension assist control, includes any type motor(s)

* **L5910** Addition, endoskeletal system, below knee, alignable system

* **L5920** Addition, endoskeletal system, above knee or hip disarticulation, alignable system

* **L5925** Addition, endoskeletal system, above knee, knee disarticulation or hip disarticulation, manual lock

* **L5930** Addition, endoskeletal system, high activity knee control frame

* **L5940** Addition, endoskeletal system, below knee, ultra-light material (titanium, carbon fiber or equal)

▶ New → Revised ✔ Reinstated ~~deleted~~ Deleted
◎ Special coverage instructions ◆ Not covered or valid by Medicare * Carrier discretion

* **L5950** Addition, endoskeletal system, above knee, ultra-light material (titanium, carbon fiber or equal)

* **L5960** Addition, endoskeletal system, hip disarticulation, ultra-light material (titanium, carbon fiber, or equal)

* **L5961** Addition, endoskeletal system, polycentric hip joint, pneumatic or hydraulic control, rotation control, with or without flexion, and/or extension control

* **L5962** Addition, endoskeletal system, below knee, flexible protective outer surface covering system

* **L5964** Addition, endoskeletal system, above knee, flexible protective outer surface covering system

* **L5966** Addition, endoskeletal system, hip disarticulation, flexible protective outer surface covering system

* **L5968** Addition to lower limb prosthesis, multiaxial ankle with swing phase active dorsiflexion feature

* **L5970** All lower extremity prostheses, foot, external keel, SACH foot

* **L5971** All lower extremity prosthesis, solid ankle cushion keel (SACH) foot, replacement only

→ * **L5972** All lower extremity prostheses (foot, flexible keel)

* **L5973** Endoskeletal ankle foot system, microprocessor controlled feature, dorsiflexion and/or plantar flexion control, includes power source

* **L5974** All lower extremity prostheses, foot, single axis ankle/foot

* **L5975** All lower extremity prostheses, combination single axis ankle and flexible keel foot

* **L5976** All lower extremity prostheses, energy storing foot (Seattle Carbon Copy II or equal)

* **L5978** All lower extremity prostheses, foot, multiaxial ankle/foot

* **L5979** All lower extremity prostheses, multiaxial ankle, dynamic response foot, one piece system

* **L5980** All lower extremity prostheses, flex foot system

* **L5981** All lower extremity prostheses, flexwalk system or equal

* **L5982** All exoskeletal lower extremity prostheses, axial rotation unit

* **L5984** All endoskeletal lower extremity prostheses, axial rotation unit, with or without adjustability

* **L5985** All endoskeletal lower extremity prostheses, dynamic prosthetic pylon

* **L5986** All lower extremity prostheses, multiaxial rotation unit ('MCP' or equal)

* **L5987** All lower extremity prostheses, shank foot system with vertical loading pylon

* **L5988** Addition to lower limb prosthesis, vertical shock reducing pylon feature

* **L5990** Addition to lower extremity prosthesis, user adjustable heel height

* **L5999** Lower extremity prosthesis, not otherwise specified

Upper Limb

NOTE: The procedures in L6000-L6599 are considered as base or basic procedures and may be modified by listing procedures from the additions sections. The base procedures include only standard friction wrist and control cable system unless otherwise specified.

Partial Hand

L6000-L6698:   Bill DME/MAC

* **L6000** Partial hand, thumb remaining

* **L6010** Partial hand, little and/or ring finger remaining

* **L6020** Partial hand, no finger remaining

* **L6025** Transcarpal/metacarpal or partial hand disarticulation prosthesis, external power, self-suspended, inner socket with removable forearm section, electrodes and cables, two batteries, charger, myoelectric control of terminal device

Wrist Disarticulation

* **L6050** Wrist disarticulation, molded socket, flexible elbow hinges, triceps pad

* **L6055** Wrist disarticulation, molded socket with expandable interface, flexible elbow hinges, triceps pad

Below Elbow

* **L6100** Below elbow, molded socket, flexible elbow hinge, triceps pad

* **L6110** Below elbow, molded socket, (Muenster or Northwestern suspension types)

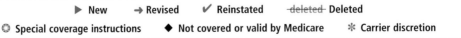

▶ New   → Revised   ✔ Reinstated   deleted Deleted
✪ Special coverage instructions   ◆ Not covered or valid by Medicare   * Carrier discretion

* **L6120**   Below elbow, molded double wall split socket, step-up hinges, half cuff

* **L6130**   Below elbow, molded double wall split socket, stump activated locking hinge, half cuff

Elbow Disarticulation

* **L6200**   Elbow disarticulation, molded socket, outside locking hinge, forearm

* **L6205**   Elbow disarticulation, molded socket with expandable interface, outside locking hinges, forearm

Above Elbow

* **L6250**   Above elbow, molded double wall socket, internal locking elbow, forearm

Shoulder Disarticulation

* **L6300**   Shoulder disarticulation, molded socket, shoulder bulkhead, humeral section, internal locking elbow, forearm

* **L6310**   Shoulder disarticulation, passive restoration (complete prosthesis)

* **L6320**   Shoulder disarticulation, passive restoration (shoulder cap only)

Interscapular Thoracic

* **L6350**   Interscapular thoracic, molded socket, shoulder bulkhead, humeral section, internal locking elbow, forearm

* **L6360**   Interscapular thoracic, passive restoration (complete prosthesis)

* **L6370**   Interscapular thoracic, passive restoration (shoulder cap only)

Immediate and Early Postsurgical Procedures

* **L6380**   Immediate post surgical or early fitting, application of initial rigid dressing, including fitting alignment and suspension of components, and one cast change, wrist disarticulation or below elbow

* **L6382**   Immediate post surgical or early fitting, application of initial rigid dressing including fitting alignment and suspension of components, and one cast change, elbow disarticulation or above elbow

* **L6384**   Immediate post surgical or early fitting, application of initial rigid dressing including fitting alignment and suspension of components, and one cast change, shoulder disarticulation or interscapular thoracic

* **L6386**   Immediate post surgical or early fitting, each additional cast change and realignment

* **L6388**   Immediate post surgical or early fitting, application of rigid dressing only

Endoskeletal: Below Elbow

* **L6400**   Below elbow, molded socket, endoskeletal system, including soft prosthetic tissue shaping

Endoskeletal: Elbow Disarticulation

* **L6450**   Elbow disarticulation, molded socket, endoskeletal system, including soft prosthetic tissue shaping

Endoskeletal: Above Elbow

* **L6500**   Above elbow, molded socket, endoskeletal system, including soft prosthetic tissue shaping

Endoskeletal: Shoulder Disarticulation

* **L6550**   Shoulder disarticulation, molded socket, endoskeletal system, including soft prosthetic tissue shaping

Endoskeletal: Interscapular Thoracic

* **L6570**   Interscapular thoracic, molded socket, endoskeletal system, including soft prosthetic tissue shaping

* **L6580**   Preparatory, wrist disarticulation or below elbow, single wall plastic socket, friction wrist, flexible elbow hinges, figure of eight harness, humeral cuff, Bowden cable control, USMC or equal pylon, no cover, molded to patient model

* **L6582**   Preparatory, wrist disarticulation or below elbow, single wall socket, friction wrist, flexible elbow hinges, figure of eight harness, humeral cuff, Bowden cable control, USMC or equal pylon, no cover, direct formed

---

▶ New   → Revised   ✔ Reinstated   ~~deleted~~ Deleted

✪ Special coverage instructions   ◆ Not covered or valid by Medicare   * Carrier discretion

✳ **L6584**   Preparatory, elbow disarticulation or above elbow, single wall plastic socket, friction wrist, locking elbow, figure of eight harness, fair lead cable control, USMC or equal pylon, no cover, molded to patient model

✳ **L6586**   Preparatory, elbow disarticulation or above elbow, single wall socket, friction wrist, locking elbow, figure of eight harness, fair lead cable control, USMC or equal pylon, no cover, direct formed

✳ **L6588**   Preparatory, shoulder disarticulation or interscapular thoracic, single wall plastic socket, shoulder joint, locking elbow, friction wrist, chest strap, fair lead cable control, USMC or equal pylon, no cover, molded to patient model

✳ **L6590**   Preparatory, shoulder disarticulation or interscapular thoracic, single wall socket, shoulder joint, locking elbow, friction wrist, chest strap, fair lead cable control, USMC or equal pylon, no cover, direct formed

Additions to Upper Limb

NOTE: The following procedures/modifications/ components may be added to other base procedures. The items in this section should reflect the additional complexity of each modification procedure, in addition to base procedure, at the time of the original order.

✳ **L6600**   Upper extremity additions, polycentric hinge, pair

✳ **L6605**   Upper extremity additions, single pivot hinge, pair

✳ **L6610**   Upper extremity additions, flexible metal hinge, pair

✳ **L6611**   Addition to upper extremity prosthesis, external powered, additional switch, any type

✳ **L6615**   Upper extremity addition, disconnect locking wrist unit

✳ **L6616**   Upper extremity addition, additional disconnect insert for locking wrist unit, each

✳ **L6620**   Upper extremity addition, flexion/ extension wrist unit, with or without friction

✳ **L6621**   Upper extremity prosthesis addition, flexion/extension wrist with or without friction, for use with external powered terminal device

✳ **L6623**   Upper extremity addition, spring assisted rotational wrist unit with latch release

✳ **L6624**   Upper extremity addition, flexion/ extension and rotation wrist unit

✳ **L6625**   Upper extremity addition, rotation wrist unit with cable lock

✳ **L6628**   Upper extremity addition, quick disconnect hook adapter, Otto Bock or equal

✳ **L6629**   Upper extremity addition, quick disconnect lamination collar with coupling piece, Otto Bock or equal

✳ **L6630**   Upper extremity addition, stainless steel, any wrist

✳ **L6632**   Upper extremity addition, latex suspension sleeve, each

✳ **L6635**   Upper extremity addition, lift assist for elbow

✳ **L6637**   Upper extremity addition, nudge control elbow lock

✳ **L6638**   Upper extremity addition to prosthesis, electric locking feature, only for use with manually powered elbow

✳ **L6640**   Upper extremity additions, shoulder abduction joint, pair

✳ **L6641**   Upper extremity addition, excursion amplifier, pulley type

✳ **L6642**   Upper extremity addition, excursion amplifier, lever type

✳ **L6645**   Upper extremity addition, shoulder flexion-abduction joint, each

✳ **L6646**   Upper extremity addition, shoulder joint, multipositional locking, flexion, adjustable abduction friction control, for use with body powered or external powered system

✳ **L6647**   Upper extremity addition, shoulder lock mechanism, body powered actuator

✳ **L6648**   Upper extremity addition, shoulder lock mechanism, external powered actuator

✳ **L6650**   Upper extremity addition, shoulder universal joint, each

✳ **L6655**   Upper extremity addition, standard control cable, extra

✳ **L6660**   Upper extremity addition, heavy duty control cable

✳ **L6665**   Upper extremity addition, Teflon, or equal, cable lining

✳ **L6670**   Upper extremity addition, hook to hand, cable adapter

---

▶ New   → Revised   ✔ Reinstated   ~~deleted~~ Deleted

⊚ Special coverage instructions   ◆ Not covered or valid by Medicare   ✳ Carrier discretion

✳ **L6672** Upper extremity addition, harness, chest or shoulder, saddle type

✳ **L6675** Upper extremity addition, harness, (e.g. figure of eight type), single cable design

✳ **L6676** Upper extremity addition, harness, (e.g. figure of eight type), dual cable design

✳ **L6677** Upper extremity addition, harness, triple control, simultaneous operation of terminal device and elbow

✳ **L6680** Upper extremity addition, test socket, wrist disarticulation or below elbow

✳ **L6682** Upper extremity addition, test socket, elbow disarticulation or above elbow

✳ **L6684** Upper extremity addition, test socket, shoulder disarticulation or interscapular thoracic

✳ **L6686** Upper extremity addition, suction socket

✳ **L6687** Upper extremity addition, frame type socket, below elbow or wrist disarticulation

✳ **L6688** Upper extremity addition, frame type socket, above elbow or elbow disarticulation

✳ **L6689** Upper extremity addition, frame type socket, shoulder disarticulation

✳ **L6690** Upper extremity addition, frame type socket, interscapular-thoracic

✳ **L6691** Upper extremity addition, removable insert, each

✳ **L6692** Upper extremity addition, silicone gel insert or equal, each

✳ **L6693** Upper extremity addition, locking elbow, forearm counterbalance

✳ **L6694** Addition to upper extremity prosthesis, below elbow/above elbow, custom fabricated from existing mold or prefabricated, socket insert, silicone gel, elastomeric or equal, for use with locking mechanism

✳ **L6695** Addition to upper extremity prosthesis, below elbow/above elbow, custom fabricated from existing mold or prefabricated, socket insert, silicone gel, elastomeric or equal, not for use with locking mechanism

✳ **L6696** Addition to upper extremity prosthesis, below elbow/above elbow, custom fabricated socket insert for congenital or atypical traumatic amputee, silicone gel, elastomeric or equal, for use with or without locking mechanism, initial only (for other than initial, use code L6694 or L6695)

✳ **L6697** Addition to upper extremity prosthesis, below elbow/above elbow, custom fabricated socket insert for other than congenital or atypical traumatic amputee, silicone gel, elastomeric or equal, for use with or without locking mechanism, initial only (for other than initial, use code L6694 or L6695)

✳ **L6698** Addition to upper extremity prosthesis, below elbow/above elbow, lock mechanism, excludes socket insert

Terminal Devices

Hooks

L6703-L6915: Bill DME/MAC

✳ **L6703** Terminal device, passive hand/mitt, any material, any size

✳ **L6704** Terminal device, sport/recreational/work attachment, any material, any size

✳ **L6706** Terminal device, hook, mechanical, voluntary opening, any material, any size, lined or unlined

✳ **L6707** Terminal device, hook, mechanical, voluntary closing, any material, any size, lined or unlined

✳ **L6708** Terminal device, hand, mechanical, voluntary opening, any material, any size

✳ **L6709** Terminal device, hand, mechanical, voluntary closing, any material, any size

✳ **L6711** Terminal device, hook, mechanical, voluntary opening, any material, any size, lined or unlined, pediatric

✳ **L6712** Terminal device, hook, mechanical, voluntary closing, any material, any size, lined or unlined, pediatric

✳ **L6713** Terminal device, hand, mechanical, voluntary opening, any material, any size, pediatric

---

▶ New → Revised ✔ Reinstated ~~deleted~~ Deleted
⊘ Special coverage instructions ◆ Not covered or valid by Medicare ✳ Carrier discretion

* **L6714** Terminal device, hand, mechanical, voluntary closing, any material, any size, pediatric

* **L6715** Terminal device, multiple articulating digit, includes motor(s), initial issue or replacement

* **L6721** Terminal device, hook or hand, heavy duty, mechanical, voluntary opening, any material, any size, lined or unlined

* **L6722** Terminal device, hook or hand, heavy duty, mechanical, voluntary closing, any material, any size, lined or unlined

☉ **L6805** Addition to terminal device, modifier wrist unit

IOM: 100-02, 15, 120; 100-04, 3, 10.4

☉ **L6810** Addition to terminal device, precision pinch device

IOM: 100-02, 15, 120; 100-04, 3, 10.4

Hands

* **L6880** Electric hand, switch or myoelectric controlled, independently articulating digits, any grasp pattern or combination of grasp patterns, includes motor(s)

* **L6881** Automatic grasp feature, addition to upper limb electric prosthetic terminal device

☉ **L6882** Microprocessor control feature, addition to upper limb prosthetic terminal device

IOM: 100-02, 15, 120; 100-04, 3, 10.4

Replacement Sockets

* **L6883** Replacement socket, below elbow/wrist disarticulation, molded to patient model, for use with or without external power

* **L6884** Replacement socket, above elbow/elbow disarticulation, molded to patient model, for use with or without external power

* **L6885** Replacement socket, shoulder disarticulation/interscapular thoracic, molded to patient model, for use with or without external power

Gloves for Above Hands

* **L6890** Addition to upper extremity prosthesis, glove for terminal device, any material, prefabricated, includes fitting and adjustment

* **L6895** Addition to upper extremity prosthesis, glove for terminal device, any material, custom fabricated

Hand Restoration

* **L6900** Hand restoration (casts, shading and measurements included), partial hand, with glove, thumb or one finger remaining

* **L6905** Hand restoration (casts, shading and measurements included), partial hand, with glove, multiple fingers remaining

* **L6910** Hand restoration (casts, shading and measurements included), partial hand, with glove, no fingers remaining

* **L6915** Hand restoration (shading, and measurements included), replacement glove for above

External Power

Base Devices

* **L6920** Wrist disarticulation, external power, self-suspended inner socket, removable forearm shell, Otto Bock or equal switch, cables, two batteries and one charger, switch control of terminal device

Bill DME/MAC

* **L6925** Wrist disarticulation, external power, self-suspended inner socket, removable forearm shell, Otto Bock or equal electrodes, cables, two batteries and one charger, myoelectronic control of terminal device

Bill DME/MAC

* **L6930** Below elbow, external power, self-suspended inner socket, removable forearm shell, Otto Bock or equal switch, cables, two batteries and one charger, switch control of terminal device

Bill DME/MAC

▶ New   → Revised   ✔ Reinstated   ~~deleted~~ Deleted
☉ Special coverage instructions   ◆ Not covered or valid by Medicare   * Carrier discretion

⚹ **L6935** Below elbow, external power, self-suspended inner socket, removable forearm shell, Otto Bock or equal electrodes, cables, two batteries and one charger, myoelectronic control of terminal device

Bill DME/MAC

⚹ **L6940** Elbow disarticulation, external power, molded inner socket, removable humeral shell, outside locking hinges, forearm, Otto Bock or equal switch, cables, two batteries and one charger, switch control of terminal device

Bill DME/MAC

⚹ **L6945** Elbow disarticulation, external power, molded inner socket, removable humeral shell, outside locking hinges, forearm, Otto Bock or equal electrodes, cables, two batteries and one charger, myoelectronic control of terminal device

Bill DME/MAC

⚹ **L6950** Above elbow, external power, molded inner socket, removable humeral shell, internal locking elbow, forearm, Otto Bock or equal switch, cables, two batteries and one charger, switch control of terminal device

Bill DME/MAC

⚹ **L6955** Above elbow, external power, molded inner socket, removable humeral shell, internal locking elbow, forearm, Otto Bock or equal electrodes, cables, two batteries and one charger, myoelectronic control of terminal device

Bill DME/MAC

⚹ **L6960** Shoulder disarticulation, external power, molded inner socket, removable shoulder shell, shoulder bulkhead, humeral section, mechanical elbow, forearm, Otto Bock or equal switch, cables, two batteries and one charger, switch control of terminal device

Bill DME/MAC

⚹ **L6965** Shoulder disarticulation, external power, molded inner socket, removable shoulder shell, shoulder bulkhead, humeral section, mechanical elbow, forearm, Otto Bock or equal electrodes, cables, two batteries and one charger, myoelectronic control of terminal device

Bill DME/MAC

⚹ **L6970** Interscapular-thoracic, external power, molded inner socket, removable shoulder shell, shoulder bulkhead, humeral section, mechanical elbow, forearm, Otto Bock or equal switch, cables, two batteries and one charger, switch control of terminal device

Bill DME/MAC

⚹ **L6975** Interscapular-thoracic, external power, molded inner socket, removable shoulder shell, shoulder bulkhead, humeral section, mechanical elbow, forearm, Otto Bock or equal electrodes, cables, two batteries and one charger, myoelectronic control of terminal device

Bill DME/MAC

Terminal Devices

⚹ **L7007** Electric hand, switch or myoelectric controlled, adult

Bill DME/MAC

⚹ **L7008** Electric hand, switch or myoelectric controlled, pediatric

Bill DME/MAC

⚹ **L7009** Electric hook, switch or myoelectric controlled, adult

Bill DME/MAC

⚹ **L7040** Prehensile actuator, switch controlled

Bill DME/MAC

⚹ **L7045** Electric hook, switch or myoelectric controlled, pediatric

Bill DME/MAC

Elbow

⚹ **L7170** Electronic elbow, Hosmer or equal, switch controlled

Bill DME/MAC

⚹ **L7180** Electronic elbow, microprocessor sequential control of elbow and terminal device

Bill DME/MAC

⚹ **L7181** Electronic elbow, microprocessor simultaneous control of elbow and terminal device

Bill DME/MAC

⚹ **L7185** Electronic elbow, adolescent, Variety Village or equal, switch controlled

Bill DME/MAC

▶ New   → Revised   ✔ Reinstated   deleted Deleted

☺ Special coverage instructions   ◆ Not covered or valid by Medicare   ⚹ Carrier discretion

* **L7186** Electronic elbow, child, Variety Village or equal, switch controlled

Bill DME/MAC

* **L7190** Electronic elbow, adolescent, Variety Village or equal, myoelectronically controlled

Bill DME/MAC

* **L7191** Electronic elbow, child, Variety Village or equal, myoelectronically controlled

Bill DME/MAC

* **L7260** Electronic wrist rotator, Otto Bock or equal

Bill DME/MAC

* **L7261** Electronic wrist rotator, for Utah arm

Bill DME/MAC

Battery Components

* **L7360** Six volt battery, each

Bill DME/MAC

* **L7362** Battery charger, six volt, each

Bill DME/MAC

* **L7364** Twelve volt battery, each

Bill DME/MAC

* **L7366** Battery charger, twelve volt, each

Bill DME/MAC

* **L7367** Lithium ion battery, replacement

Bill DME/MAC

* **L7368** Lithium ion battery charger, replacement only

Bill DME/MAC

Other/Repair

* **L7400** Addition to upper extremity prosthesis, below elbow/wrist disarticulation, ultralight material (titanium, carbon fiber or equal)

Bill DME/MAC

* **L7401** Addition to upper extremity prosthesis, above elbow disarticulation, ultralight material (titanium, carbon fiber or equal)

Bill DME/MAC

* **L7402** Addition to upper extremity prosthesis, shoulder disarticulation/interscapular thoracic, ultralight material (titanium, carbon fiber or equal)

Bill DME/MAC

* **L7403** Addition to upper extremity prosthesis, below elbow/wrist disarticulation, acrylic material

Bill DME/MAC

* **L7404** Addition to upper extremity prosthesis, above elbow disarticulation, acrylic material

Bill DME/MAC

* **L7405** Addition to upper extremity prosthesis, shoulder disarticulation/interscapular thoracic, acrylic material

Bill DME/MAC

* **L7499** Upper extremity prosthesis, not otherwise specified

Bill DME/MAC

◎ **L7510** Repair of prosthetic device, repair or replace minor parts

Bill local carrier if repair of implanted prosthetic device. If other, bill DME/MAC

IOM: 100-02, 15, 110.2; 100-02, 15, 120; 100-04, 32, 100

* **L7520** Repair prosthetic device, labor component, per 15 minutes

Bill local carrier if repair of implanted prosthetic device. If other, bill DME/MAC

◆ **L7600** Prosthetic donning sleeve, any material, each

Bill DME/MAC

Medicare Statute 1862(1)(a)

General

* **L7900** Male vacuum erection system

Bill DME/MAC

▶ * **L7902** Tension ring, for vacuum erection device, any type, replacement only, each

Breast Prostheses

→ ◎ **L8000** Breast prosthesis, mastectomy bra, without integrated breast prosthesis form, any size, any type

Bill DME/MAC

IOM: 100-02, 15, 120

→ ◎ **L8001** Breast prosthesis, mastectomy bra, with integrated breast prosthesis form, unilateral, any size, any type

Bill DME/MAC

IOM: 100-02, 15, 120

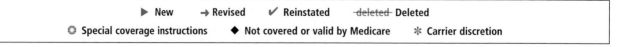

▶ New   → Revised   ✔ Reinstated   ~~deleted~~ Deleted   ◎ Special coverage instructions   ◆ Not covered or valid by Medicare   * Carrier discretion

→ ⊚ **L8002** Breast prosthesis, mastectomy bra, with integrated breast prosthesis form, bilateral, any size, any type

Bill DME/MAC

IOM: 100-02, 15, 120

⊚ **L8010** Breast prosthesis, mastectomy sleeve

Bill DME/MAC

IOM: 100-02, 15, 120

⊚ **L8015** External breast prosthesis garment, with mastectomy form, post mastectomy

Bill DME/MAC

IOM: 100-02, 15, 120

⊚ **L8020** Breast prosthesis, mastectomy form

Bill DME/MAC

IOM: 100-02, 15, 120

✳ **L8030** Breast prosthesis, silicone or equal, without integral adhesive

Bill DME/MAC

IOM: 100-02, 15, 120

⊚ **L8031** Breast prosthesis, silicone or equal, with integral adhesive

Bill DME/MAC

IOM: 100-02, 15, 120

✳ **L8032** Nipple prosthesis, reusable, any type, each

Bill DME/MAC

⊚ **L8035** Custom breast prosthesis, post mastectomy, molded to patient model

Bill DME/MAC

IOM: 100-02, 15, 120

✳ **L8039** Breast prosthesis, not otherwise specified

Bill DME/MAC

Nasal, Orbital, Auricular Prosthesis

✳ **L8040** Nasal prosthesis, provided by a non-physician

Bill DME/MAC

✳ **L8041** Midfacial prosthesis, provided by a non-physician

Bill DME/MAC

✳ **L8042** Orbital prosthesis, provided by a non-physician

Bill DME/MAC

✳ **L8043** Upper facial prosthesis, provided by a non-physician

Bill DME/MAC

✳ **L8044** Hemi-facial prosthesis, provided by a non-physician

Bill DME/MAC

✳ **L8045** Auricular prosthesis, provided by a non-physician

Bill DME/MAC

✳ **L8046** Partial facial prosthesis, provided by a non-physician

Bill DME/MAC

✳ **L8047** Nasal septal prosthesis, provided by a non-physician

Bill DME/MAC

✳ **L8048** Unspecified maxillofacial prosthesis, by report, provided by a non-physician

Bill DME/MAC

✳ **L8049** Repair or modification of maxillofacial prosthesis, labor component, 15 minute increments, provided by a non-physician

Bill DME/MAC

Trusses

⊚ **L8300** Truss, single with standard pad

Bill DME/MAC

IOM: 100-02, 15, 120; 100-03, 4, 280.11; 100-03, 4, 280.12; 100-04, 4, 240

⊚ **L8310** Truss, double with standard pads

Bill DME/MAC

IOM: 100-02, 15, 120; 100-03, 4, 280.11; 100-03, 4, 280.12; 100-04, 4, 240

⊚ **L8320** Truss, addition to standard pad, water pad

Bill DME/MAC

IOM: 100-02, 15, 120; 100-03, 4, 280.11; 100-03, 4, 280.12; 100-04, 4, 240

⊚ **L8330** Truss, addition to standard pad, scrotal pad

Bill DME/MAC

IOM: 100-02, 15, 120; 100-03, 4, 280.11; 100-03, 4, 280.12; 100-04, 4, 240

Prosthetic Socks

⊚ **L8400** Prosthetic sheath, below knee, each

Bill DME/MAC

IOM: 100-02, 15, 200

⊚ **L8410** Prosthetic sheath, above knee, each

Bill DME/MAC

IOM: 100-02, 15, 200

▶ **New** → **Revised** ✔ **Reinstated** ~~deleted~~ **Deleted**

⊚ **Special coverage instructions** ◆ **Not covered or valid by Medicare** ✳ **Carrier discretion**

⊚ **L8415** Prosthetic sheath, upper limb, each

Bill DME/MAC

IOM: 100-02, 15, 200

✳ **L8417** Prosthetic sheath/sock, including a gel cushion layer, below knee or above knee, each

Bill DME/MAC

⊚ **L8420** Prosthetic sock, multiple ply, below knee, each

Bill DME/MAC

IOM: 100-02, 15, 200

⊚ **L8430** Prosthetic sock, multiple ply, above knee, each

Bill DME/MAC

IOM: 100-02, 15, 200

⊚ **L8435** Prosthetic sock, multiple ply, upper limb, each

Bill DME/MAC

IOM: 100-02, 15, 200

⊚ **L8440** Prosthetic shrinker, below knee, each

Bill DME/MAC

IOM: 100-02, 15, 200

⊚ **L8460** Prosthetic shrinker, above knee, each

Bill DME/MAC

IOM: 100-02, 15, 200

⊚ **L8465** Prosthetic shrinker, upper limb, each

Bill DME/MAC

IOM: 100-02, 15, 200

⊚ **L8470** Prosthetic sock, single ply, fitting, below knee, each

Bill DME/MAC

IOM: 100-02, 15, 200

⊚ **L8480** Prosthetic sock, single ply, fitting, above knee, each

Bill DME/MAC

IOM: 100-02, 15, 200

⊚ **L8485** Prosthetic sock, single ply, fitting, upper limb, each

Bill DME/MAC

IOM: 100-02, 15, 200

✳ **L8499** Unlisted procedure for miscellaneous prosthetic services

Bill local carrier if repair of implanted prosthetic device. If other, bill DME/MAC

Prosthetic Implants

Larynx, Tracheoesophageal

⊚ **L8500** Artificial larynx, any type

Bill DME/MAC

IOM: 100-02, 15, 120; 100-03, 1, 50.2; 100-04, 4, 240

⊚ **L8501** Tracheostomy speaking valve

Bill DME/MAC

IOM: 100-03, 1, 50.4

✳ **L8505** Artificial larynx replacement battery/accessory, any type

Bill DME/MAC

✳ **L8507** Tracheo-esophageal voice prosthesis, patient inserted, any type, each

Bill DME/MAC

✳ **L8509** Tracheo-esophageal voice prosthesis, inserted by a licensed health care provider, any type

Bill DME/MAC

⊚ **L8510** Voice amplifier

Bill DME/MAC

IOM: 100-03, 1, 50.2

✳ **L8511** Insert for indwelling tracheoesophageal prosthesis, with or without valve, replacement only, each

Bill DME/MAC

✳ **L8512** Gelatin capsules or equivalent, for use with tracheoesophageal voice prosthesis, replacement only, per 10

Bill DME/MAC

✳ **L8513** Cleaning device used with tracheoesophageal voice prosthesis, pipet, brush, or equal, replacement only, each

Bill DME/MAC

✳ **L8514** Tracheoesophageal puncture dilator, replacement only, each

Bill DME/MAC

✳ **L8515** Gelatin capsule, application device for use with tracheoesophageal voice prosthesis, each

Bill DME/MAC

▶ **New** → **Revised** ✔ **Reinstated** ~~deleted~~ **Deleted**

⊚ **Special coverage instructions** ◆ **Not covered or valid by Medicare** ✳ **Carrier discretion**

Breast

⚙ **L8600**   Implantable breast prosthesis, silicone or equal

Bill local carrier

IOM: 100-02, 15, 120; 100-3, 2, 140.2

Urinary System

⚙ **L8603**   Injectable bulking agent, collagen implant, urinary tract, 2.5 ml syringe, includes shipping and necessary supplies

Bill local carrier

Bill on paper, acquisition cost invoice required

IOM: 100-03, 4, 280.1

＊ **L8604**   Injectable bulking agent, dextranomer/hyaluronic acid copolymer implant, urinary tract, 1 ml, includes shipping and necessary supplies

Bill local carrier

▶ ＊ **L8605**   Injectable bulking agent, dextranomer/hyaluronic acid copolymer implant, anal canal, 1 ml, includes shipping and necessary supplies

⚙ **L8606**   Injectable bulking agent, synthetic implant, urinary tract, 1 ml syringe, includes shipping and necessary supplies

Bill local carrier

Bill on paper, acquisition cost invoice required

IOM: 100-03, 4, 280.1

Head (Skull, Facial Bones, and Temporomandibular Joint)

＊ **L8609**   Artificial cornea

Bill local carrier

⚙ **L8610**   Ocular implant

Bill local carrier

IOM: 100-02, 15, 120

⚙ **L8612**   Aqueous shunt

Bill local carrier

IOM: 100-02, 15, 120

Cross Reference Q0074

⚙ **L8613**   Ossicula implant

Bill local carrier

IOM: 100-02, 15, 120

⚙ **L8614**   Cochlear device, includes all internal and external components

Bill local carrier

IOM: 100-02, 15, 120; 100-03, 1, 50.3

⚙ **L8615**   Headset/headpiece for use with cochlear implant device, replacement

Bill local carrier

IOM: 100-03, 1, 50.3

⚙ **L8616**   Microphone for use with cochlear implant device, replacement

Bill local carrier

IOM: 100-03, 1, 50.3

⚙ **L8617**   Transmitting coil for use with cochlear implant device, replacement

Bill local carrier

IOM: 100-03, 1, 50.3

⚙ **L8618**   Transmitter cable for use with cochlear implant device, replacement

Bill local carrier

IOM: 100-03, 1, 50.3

＊ **L8619**   Cochlear implant, external speech processor and controller, integrated system, replacement

Bill local carrier

IOM: 100-03, 1, 50.3

＊ **L8621**   Zinc air battery for use with cochlear implant device, replacement, each

Bill local carrier

＊ **L8622**   Alkaline battery for use with cochlear implant device, any size, replacement, each

Bill local carrier

＊ **L8623**   Lithium ion battery for use with cochlear implant device speech processor, other than ear level, replacement, each

Bill local carrier

＊ **L8624**   Lithium ion battery for use with cochlear implant device speech processor, ear level, replacement, each

Bill local carrier

⚙ **L8627**   Cochlear implant, external speech processor, component, replacement

Bill local carrier

IOM: 103-03, Part 1, 50.3

▶ New   → Revised   ✔ Reinstated   ~~deleted~~ Deleted

⚙ Special coverage instructions   ◆ Not covered or valid by Medicare   ＊ Carrier discretion

⊛ **L8628** Cochlear implant, external controller component, replacement

Bill local carrier

IOM: 103-03, Part 1, 50.3

⊛ **L8629** Transmitting coil and cable, integrated, for use with cochlear implant device, replacement

Bill local carrier

IOM: 103-03, Part 1, 50.3

Upper Extremity

⊛ **L8630** Metacarpophalangeal joint implant

Bill local carrier

IOM: 100-02, 15, 120

⊛ **L8631** Metacarpal phalangeal joint replacement, two or more pieces, metal (e.g., stainless steel or cobalt chrome), ceramic-like material (e.g., pyrocarbon), for surgical implantation (all sizes, includes entire system)

Bill local carrier

IOM: 100-02, 15, 120

Lower Extremity (Joint: Knee, Ankle, Toe)

⊛ **L8641** Metatarsal joint implant

Bill local carrier

IOM: 100-02, 15, 120

⊛ **L8642** Hallux implant

Bill local carrier

May be billed by ambulatory surgical center or surgeon

IOM: 100-02, 15, 120

Cross Reference CPT Q0073

Miscellaneous Muscular-Skeletal

⊛ **L8658** Interphalangeal joint spacer, silicone or equal, each

Bill local carrier

IOM: 100-02, 15, 120

⊛ **L8659** Interphalangeal finger joint replacement, 2 or more pieces, metal (e.g., stainless steel or cobalt chrome), ceramic-like material (e.g., pyrocarbon) for surgical implantation, any size

Bill local carrier

IOM: 100-02, 15, 120

Cardiovascular System

⊛ **L8670** Vascular graft material, synthetic, implant

Bill local carrier

IOM: 100-02, 15, 120

Neurostimulator

→ ◆ **L8680** Implantable neurostimulator electrode, each

Bill local carrier

Related CPT codes: 43647, 63650, 63655, 64553, 64555, 64560, 64561, 64565, 64573, 64575, 64577, 64580, 64581.

IOM: 100-03, 4, 280.4

⊛ **L8681** Patient programmer (external) for use with implantable programmable neurostimulator pulse generator, replacement only

Bill local carrier

IOM: 100-03, 4, 280.4

→ ◆ **L8682** Implantable neurostimulator radiofrequency receiver

Bill local carrier

IOM: 100-03, 4, 280.4

→ ◆ **L8683** Radiofrequency transmitter (external) for use with implantable neurostimulator radiofrequency receiver

Bill local carrier

IOM: 100-03, 4, 280.4

→ ◆ **L8684** Radiofrequency transmitter (external) for use with implantable sacral root neurostimulator receiver for bowel and bladder management, replacement

Bill local carrier

IOM: 100-03, 4, 280.4

→ ◆ **L8685** Implantable neurostimulator pulse generator, single array, rechargeable, includes extension

Bill local carrier

Related CPT codes: 61885, 64590, 63685.

IOM: 100-03, 4, 280.4

▶ **New** → **Revised** ✔ **Reinstated** ~~deleted~~ **Deleted**

⊛ **Special coverage instructions** ◆ **Not covered or valid by Medicare** ✳ **Carrier discretion**

→ ◆ **L8686** Implantable neurostimulator pulse generator, single array, non-rechargeable, includes extension

Bill local carrier

Related CPT codes: 61885, 64590, 63685.

IOM: 100-03, 4, 280.4

→ ◆ **L8687** Implantable neurostimulator pulse generator, dual array, rechargeable, includes extension

Bill local carrier

Related CPT codes: 64590, 63685, 61886.

IOM: 100-03, 4, 280.4

→ ◆ **L8688** Implantable neurostimulator pulse generator, dual array, non-rechargeable, includes extension

Bill local carrier

Related CPT codes: 61885, 64590, 63685.

IOM: 100-03, 4, 280.4

۞ **L8689** External recharging system for battery (internal) for use with implantable neurostimulator, replacement only

Bill local carrier

IOM: 100-03, 4, 280.4

✻ **L8690** Auditory osseointegrated device, includes all internal and external components

Bill local carrier

Related CPT codes: 69714, 69715, 69717, 69718.

✻ **L8691** Auditory osseointegrated device, external sound processor, replacement

Bill local carrier

◆ **L8692** Auditory osseointegrated device, external sound processor, used without osseointegration, body worn, includes headband or other means of external attachment

Bill local carrier

Medicare Statute 1862(a)(7)

✻ **L8693** Auditory osseointegrated device abutment, any length, replacement only

Bill local carrier

۞ **L8695** External recharging system for battery (external) for use with implantable neurostimulator, replacement only

Bill local carrier

IOM: 100-03, 4, 280.4

Genital

✻ **L8699** Prosthetic implant, not otherwise specified

Bill local carrier

✻ **L9900** Orthotic and prosthetic supply, accessory, and/or service component of another HCPCS "L" code

Bill local carrier if repair of implanted prosthetic device. If other, bill DME/MAC

▶ New   → Revised   ✔ Reinstated   ~~deleted~~ Deleted

۞ Special coverage instructions   ◆ Not covered or valid by Medicare   ✻ Carrier discretion

OTHER MEDICAL SERVICES (M0000-M0301)

M0064-M0301: Bill DME/MAC

⚙ **M0064** Brief office visit for the sole purpose of monitoring or changing drug prescriptions used in the treatment of mental psychoneurotic and personality disorders

Not to be reported separately from CPT codes 90785-90853

◆ **M0075** Cellular therapy

◆ **M0076** Prolotherapy

Prolotherapy stimulates production of new ligament tissue. Not covered by Medicare

◆ **M0100** Intragastric hypothermia using gastric freezing

◆ **M0300** IV chelation therapy (chemical endarterectomy)

Non-covered by Medicare

◆ **M0301** Fabric wrapping of abdominal aneurysm

Treatment for abdominal aneurysms that involves wrapping aneurysms with cellophane or fascia lata. Fabric wrapping of abdominal aneurysms is not a covered Medicare procedure.

LABORATORY SERVICES (P0000-P9999)

Chemistry and Toxicology Tests

P2028-P2038: Bill local carrier

⊗ **P2028** Cephalin floculation, blood

This code appears on a CMS list of codes that represent obsolete and unreliable tests and procedures. Verify before reporting.

IOM: 100-03, 4, 300.1

⊗ **P2029** Congo red, blood

This code appears on a CMS list of codes that represent obsolete and unreliable tests and procedures. Verify before reporting.

IOM: 100-03, 4, 300.1

◆ **P2031** Hair analysis (excluding arsenic)

IOM: 100-03, 4, 300.1

⊗ **P2033** Thymol turbidity, blood

This code appears on a CMS list of codes that represent obsolete and unreliable tests and procedures. Verify before reporting.

IOM: 100-03, 4, 300.1

⊗ **P2038** Mucoprotein, blood (seromucoid) (medical necessity procedure)

This code appears on a CMS list of codes that represent obsolete and unreliable tests and procedures. Verify before reporting.

IOM: 100-03, 4, 300.1

Pathology Screening Tests

P3000-P7001: Bill local carrier

⊗ **P3000** Screening Papanicolaou smear, cervical or vaginal, up to three smears, by technician under physician supervision

Co-insurance and deductible waived

Assign for Pap smear ordered for screening purposes only, conventional method, performed by technician

IOM: 100-03, 3, 190.2,

Laboratory Certification: Cytology

⊗ **P3001** Screening Papanicolaou smear, cervical or vaginal, up to three smears, requiring interpretation by physician

Co-insurance and deductible waived

Report professional component for Pap smears requiring physician interpretation. There are CPT codes assigned for diagnostic Paps, such as, 88141; HCPCS are for screening Paps

IOM: 100-03, 3, 190.2

Laboratory Certification: Cytology

Microbiology Tests

◆ **P7001** Culture, bacterial, urine; quantitative, sensitivity study

Cross Reference CPT

Laboratory Certification: Bacteriology

Miscellaneous Pathology

P9010-P9615: Bill local carrier

⊗ **P9010** Blood (whole), for transfusion, per unit

Blood furnished on an outpatient basis, subject to Medicare Part B blood deductible; applicable to first 3 pints of whole blood or equivalent units of packed red cells in calendar year

IOM: 100-01, 3, 20.5; 100-02, 1, 10

OPPS recognized blood/blood products

⊗ **P9011** Blood, split unit

Reports all splitting activities of any blood component

IOM: 100-01, 3, 20.5; 100-02, 1, 10

OPPS recognized blood/blood products

⊗ **P9012** Cryoprecipitate, each unit

IOM: 100-01, 3, 20.5; 100-02, 1, 10

OPPS recognized blood/blood products

⊗ **P9016** Red blood cells, leukocytes reduced, each unit

IOM: 100-01, 3, 20.5; 100-02, 1, 10

OPPS recognized blood/blood products

⊗ **P9017** Fresh frozen plasma (single donor), frozen within 8 hours of collection, each unit

IOM: 100-01, 3, 20.5; 100-02, 1, 10

OPPS recognized blood/blood products

⊗ **P9019** Platelets, each unit

IOM: 100-01, 3, 20.5; 100-02, 1, 10

OPPS recognized blood/blood products

▶ New → Revised ✔ Reinstated deleted Deleted

⊗ Special coverage instructions ◆ Not covered or valid by Medicare ✳ Carrier discretion

⚙ **P9020** Platelet rich plasma, each unit

IOM: 100-01, 3, 20.5; 100-02, 1, 10

OPPS recognized blood/blood products

⚙ **P9021** Red blood cells, each unit

IOM: 100-01, 3, 20.5; 100-02, 1, 10

OPPS recognized blood/blood products

⚙ **P9022** Red blood cells, washed, each unit

IOM: 100-01, 3, 20.5; 100-02, 1, 10

OPPS recognized blood/blood products

⚙ **P9023** Plasma, pooled multiple donor, solvent/detergent treated, frozen, each unit

IOM: 100-01, 3, 20.5; 100-02, 1, 10

OPPS recognized blood/blood products

⚙ **P9031** Platelets, leukocytes reduced, each unit

IOM: 100-01, 3, 20.5; 100-02, 1, 10

OPPS recognized blood/blood products

⚙ **P9032** Platelets, irradiated, each unit

IOM: 100-01, 3, 20.5; 100-02, 1, 10

OPPS recognized blood/blood products

⚙ **P9033** Platelets, leukocytes reduced, irradiated, each unit

IOM: 100-01, 3, 20.5; 100-02, 1, 10

OPPS recognized blood/blood products

⚙ **P9034** Platelets, pheresis, each unit

IOM: 100-01, 3, 20.5; 100-02, 1, 10

OPPS recognized blood/blood products

⚙ **P9035** Platelets, pheresis, leukocytes reduced, each unit

IOM: 100-01, 3, 20.5; 100-02, 1, 10

OPPS recognized blood/blood products

⚙ **P9036** Platelets, pheresis, irradiated, each unit

IOM: 100-01, 3, 20.5; 100-02, 1, 10

OPPS recognized blood/blood products

⚙ **P9037** Platelets, pheresis, leukocytes reduced, irradiated, each unit

IOM: 100-01, 3, 20.5; 100-02, 1, 10

OPPS recognized blood/blood products

⚙ **P9038** Red blood cells, irradiated, each unit

IOM: 100-01, 3, 20.5; 100-02, 1, 10

OPPS recognized blood/blood products

⚙ **P9039** Red blood cells, deglycerolized, each unit

IOM: 100-01, 3, 20.5; 100-02, 1, 10

OPPS recognized blood/blood products

⚙ **P9040** Red blood cells, leukocytes reduced, irradiated, each unit

IOM: 100-01, 3, 20.5; 100-02, 1, 10

OPPS recognized blood/blood products

✳ **P9041** Infusion, albumin (human), 5%, 50 ml

⚙ **P9043** Infusion, plasma protein fraction (human), 5%, 50 ml

IOM: 100-01, 3, 20.5; 100-02, 1, 10

OPPS recognized blood/blood products

⚙ **P9044** Plasma, cryoprecipitate reduced, each unit

IOM: 100-01, 3, 20.5; 100-02, 1, 10

OPPS recognized blood/blood products

✳ **P9045** Infusion, albumin (human), 5%, 250 ml

✳ **P9046** Infusion, albumin (human), 25%, 20 ml

✳ **P9047** Infusion, albumin (human), 25%, 50 ml

✳ **P9048** Infusion, plasma protein fraction (human), 5%, 250 ml

OPPS recognized blood/blood products

✳ **P9050** Granulocytes, pheresis, each unit

OPPS recognized blood/blood products

⚙ **P9051** Whole blood or red blood cells, leukocytes reduced, CMV-negative, each unit

Medicare Statute 1833(t)

OPPS recognized blood/blood products

⚙ **P9052** Platelets, HLA-matched leukocytes reduced, apheresis/pheresis, each unit

Medicare Statute 1833(t)

OPPS recognized blood/blood products

⚙ **P9053** Platelets, pheresis, leukocytes reduced, CMV-negative, irradiated, each unit

Freezing and thawing are reported separately, see Transmittal 1487 (Hospital outpatient)

Medicare Statute 1833(t)

OPPS recognized blood/blood products

⚙ **P9054** Whole blood or red blood cells, leukocytes reduced, frozen, deglycerol, washed, each unit

Medicare Statute 1833(t)

OPPS recognized blood/blood products

⚙ **P9055** Platelets, leukocytes reduced, CMV-negative, apheresis/pheresis, each unit

Medicare Statute 1833(t)

OPPS recognized blood/blood products

▶ **New** → **Revised** ✔ **Reinstated** ~~deleted~~ **Deleted**

⚙ **Special coverage instructions** ◆ **Not covered or valid by Medicare** ✳ **Carrier discretion**

⚙ **P9056** Whole blood, leukocytes reduced, irradiated, each unit

Medicare Statute 1833(t)

OPPS recognized blood/blood products

⚙ **P9057** Red blood cells, frozen/deglycerolized/ washed, leukocytes reduced, irradiated, each unit

Medicare Statute 1833(t)

OPPS recognized blood/blood products

⚙ **P9058** Red blood cells, leukocytes reduced, CMV-negative, irradiated, each unit

Medicare Statute 1833(t)

OPPS recognized blood/blood products

⚙ **P9059** Fresh frozen plasma between 8-24 hours of collection, each unit

Medicare Statute 1833(t)

OPPS recognized blood/blood products

⚙ **P9060** Fresh frozen plasma, donor retested, each unit

Medicare Statute 1833(t)

OPPS recognized blood/blood products

⚙ **P9603** Travel allowance one way in connection with medically necessary laboratory specimen collection drawn from home bound or nursing home bound patient; prorated miles actually traveled

Fee for clinical laboratory travel (P9603) is $0.96 per mile for CY2011

IOM: 100-04, 16, 60

⚙ **P9604** Travel allowance one way in connection with medically necessary laboratory specimen collection drawn from home bound or nursing home bound patient; prorated trip charge

For CY2010, the fee for clinical laboratory travel is $9.60 per flat rate trip for CY2011

IOM: 100-04, 16, 60

⚙ **P9612** Catheterization for collection of specimen, single patient, all places of service

NCCI edits indicate that when 51701 is comprehensive or is a Column 1 code, P9612 cannot be reported. When the catheter insertion is a component of another procedure, do not report straight catheterization separately.

IOM: 100-04, 16, 60

⚙ **P9615** Catheterization for collection of specimen(s) (multiple patients)

IOM: 100-04, 16, 60

▶ New   → Revised   ✔ Reinstated   ~~deleted~~ Deleted
⚙ Special coverage instructions   ◆ Not covered or valid by Medicare   ✳ Carrier discretion

TEMPORARY CODES ASSIGNED BY CMS (Q0000-Q9999)

Cardiokymography

⚙ **Q0035**   Cardiokymography

Bill local carrier

Report modifier 26 if professional component only

IOM: 100-03, 1, 20.24

Chemotherapy

Q0081-Q0085:   Bill local carrier

⚙ **Q0081**   Infusion therapy, using other than chemotherapeutic drugs, per visit

IV piggyback only assigned one time per patient encounter per day. Report for hydration or the intravenous administration of antibiotics, antiemetics, or analgesics. Bill on paper. Requires a report.

IOM: 100-03, 4, 280.14

✳ **Q0083**   Chemotherapy administration by other than infusion technique only (e.g., subcutaneous, intramuscular, push), per visit

⚙ **Q0084**   Chemotherapy administration by infusion technique only, per visit

IOM: 100-03, 4, 280.14

✳ **Q0085**   Chemotherapy administration by both infusion technique and other technique(s) (e.g., subcutaneous, intramuscular, push), per visit

Smear, Papanicolaou

⚙ **Q0091**   Screening Papanicolaou smear; obtaining, preparing and conveyance of cervical or vaginal smear to laboratory

Bill local carrier

Medicare does not cover comprehensive preventive medicine services; however, services described by G0101 and Q0091 (only for Medicare patients) are covered. Includes the services necessary to procure and transport the specimen to the laboratory.

IOM: 100-03, 3, 190.2

Equipment, X-Ray, Portable

⚙ **Q0092**   Set-up portable x-ray equipment

Bill local carrier

IOM: 100-04, 13, 90

Laboratory

Q0111-Q0115:   Bill local carrier

✳ **Q0111**   Wet mounts, including preparations of vaginal, cervical or skin specimens

Laboratory Certification: Bacteriology, Mycology, Parasitology

✳ **Q0112**   All potassium hydroxide (KOH) preparations

Laboratory Certification: Mycology

✳ **Q0113**   Pinworm examinations

Laboratory Certification: Parasitology

✳ **Q0114**   Fern test

Laboratory certification: Routine chemistry

✳ **Q0115**   Post-coital direct, qualitative examinations of vaginal or cervical mucous

Laboratory Certification: Hematology

Drugs

✳ **Q0138**   Injection, ferumoxytol, for treatment of iron deficiency anemia, 1 mg (non-ESRD use)

Feraheme is FDA approved for chronic kidney disease

NDC: Feraheme

▶ **New**   → **Revised**   ✔ **Reinstated**   ~~deleted~~ **Deleted**

⚙ **Special coverage instructions**   ◆ **Not covered or valid by Medicare**   ✳ **Carrier discretion**

✳ **Q0139**   Injection, ferumoxytol, for treatment of iron deficiency anemia, 1 mg (for ESRD on dialysis)

NDC: Feraheme

◆ **Q0144**   Azithromycin dihydrate, oral, capsules/powder, 1 gm

If incident to a physician's service, do not bill; otherwise, bill DME/MAC.

Other: Zithromax

✪ **Q0162**   Ondansetron 1 mg, oral, FDA-approved prescription anti-emetic, for use as a complete therapeutic substitute for an iv anti-emetic at the time of chemotherapy treatment, not to exceed a 48 hour dosage regimen

NDC: Zofran

Medicare Statute 4557

✪ **Q0163**   Diphenhydramine hydrochloride, 50 mg, oral, FDA approved prescription anti-emetic, for use as a complete therapeutic substitute for an IV anti-emetic at time of chemotherapy treatment not to exceed a 48 hour dosage regimen

Bill DME/MAC

Other: Alercap, Aler-Dryl, Allergy Children's, Allergy Relief Medicine, Allermax, Alertab, Anti-Hist, Antihistamine, Banophen, Complete Allergy Medication, Complete Allergy medicine, Diphedryl, Diphen, Diphenhist, Diphenyl, Dormin Sleep Aid, Geridryl, Good Sense Antihistamine Allergy Relief, Good Sense Nighttime Sleep Aid, Genahist, Hydramine, Medicine Shoppe Medi-Phedryl, Medicine Shoppe Nite Time Sleep, Mediphedryl, Night Time Sleep Aid, Nytol Quickcaps, Nytol Quickgels maximum strength, Q-Dryl, Quality Choice Sleep Aid, Quality Choice Rest Simply, Quenalin, Rite Aid Allergy, Serabrina La France, Siladryl Allergy, Silphen, Simply Sleep, Sleep Tabs, Sleep-ettes D, Sleepinal, Sominex, Twilite, Valu-Dryl Allergy

Medicare Statute 4557

✪ **Q0164**   Prochlorperazine maleate, 5 mg, oral, FDA approved prescription anti-emetic, for use as a complete therapeutic substitute for an IV anti-emetic at the time of chemotherapy treatment, not to exceed a 48 hour dosage regimen

Bill DME/MAC

Other: Compazine

Medicare Statute 4557

✪ **Q0165**   Prochlorperazine maleate, 10 mg, oral, FDA approved prescription anti-emetic, for use as a complete therapeutic substitute for an IV anti-emetic at the time of chemotherapy treatment, not to exceed a 48 hour dosage regimen

Bill DME/MAC

Other: Compazine

Medicare Statute 4557

✪ **Q0166**   Granisetron hydrochloride, 1 mg, oral, FDA approved prescription anti-emetic, for use as a complete therapeutic substitute for an IV anti-emetic at the time of chemotherapy treatment, not to exceed a 24 hour dosage regimen

Bill DME/MAC

Other: Kytril

Medicare Statute 4557

✪ **Q0167**   Dronabinol, 2.5 mg, oral, FDA approved prescription anti-emetic, for use as a complete therapeutic substitute for an IV anti-emetic at the time of chemotherapy treatment, not to exceed a 48 hour dosage regimen

Bill DME/MAC

NDC: Marinol

Medicare Statute 4557

✪ **Q0168**   Dronabinol, 5 mg, oral, FDA approved prescription anti-emetic, for use as a complete therapeutic substitute for an IV anti-emetic at the time of chemotherapy treatment, not to exceed a 48 hour dosage regimen

Bill DME/MAC

Other: Marinol

Medicare Statute 4557

✪ **Q0169**   Promethazine hydrochloride, 12.5 mg, oral, FDA approved prescription anti-emetic, for use as a complete therapeutic substitute for an IV anti-emetic at the time of chemotherapy treatment, not to exceed a 48 hour dosage regimen

Bill DME/MAC

Other: Phenergan

Medicare Statute 4557

▶ New   → Revised   ✔ Reinstated   ~~deleted~~ Deleted

✪ Special coverage instructions   ◆ Not covered or valid by Medicare   ✳ Carrier discretion

⊛ **Q0170** Promethazine hydrochloride, 25 mg, oral, FDA approved prescription anti-emetic, for use as a complete therapeutic substitute for an IV anti-emetic at the time of chemotherapy treatment, not to exceed a 48 hour dosage regimen

Bill DME/MAC

Other: Phenergan, Promacot

Medicare Statute 4557

⊛ **Q0171** Chlorpromazine hydrochloride, 10 mg, oral, FDA approved prescription anti-emetic, for use as a complete therapeutic substitute for an IV anti-emetic at the time of chemotherapy treatment, not to exceed a 48 hour dosage regimen

Bill DME/MAC

Medicare Statute 4557

⊛ **Q0172** Chlorpromazine hydrochloride, 25 mg, oral, FDA approved prescription anti-emetic, for use as a complete therapeutic substitute for an IV anti-emetic at the time of chemotherapy treatment, not to exceed a 48 hour dosage regimen

Bill DME/MAC

Medicare Statute 4557

⊛ **Q0173** Trimethobenzamide hydrochloride, 250 mg, oral, FDA approved prescription anti-emetic, for use as a complete therapeutic substitute for an IV anti-emetic at the time of chemotherapy treatment, not to exceed a 48 hour dosage regimen

Bill DME/MAC

Other: Ticon, Tigan

Medicare Statute 4557

⊛ **Q0174** Thiethylperazine maleate, 10 mg, oral, FDA approved prescription anti-emetic, for use as a complete therapeutic substitute for an IV anti-emetic at the time of chemotherapy treatment, not to exceed a 48 hour dosage regimen

Bill DME/MAC

Other: Torecan

Medicare Statute 4557

⊛ **Q0175** Perphenazine, 4 mg, oral, FDA approved prescription anti-emetic, for use as a complete therapeutic substitute for an IV anti-emetic at the time of chemotherapy treatment, not to exceed a 48 hour dosage regimen

Bill DME/MAC

Medicare Statute 4557

⊛ **Q0176** Perphenazine, 8 mg, oral, FDA approved prescription anti-emetic, for use as a complete therapeutic substitute for an IV anti-emetic at the time of chemotherapy treatment, not to exceed a 48 hour dosage regimen

Bill DME/MAC

Medicare Statute 4557

⊛ **Q0177** Hydroxyzine pamoate, 25 mg, oral, FDA approved prescription anti-emetic, for use as a complete therapeutic substitute for an IV anti-emetic at the time of chemotherapy treatment, not to exceed a 48 hour dosage regimen

Bill DME/MAC

Other: Vistaril

Medicare Statute 4557

⊛ **Q0178** Hydroxyzine pamoate, 50 mg, oral, FDA approved prescription anti-emetic, for use as a complete therapeutic substitute for an IV anti-emetic at the time of chemotherapy treatment, not to exceed a 48 hour dosage regimen

Bill DME/MAC

Other: Vistaril

Medicare Statute 4557

⊛ **Q0180** Dolasetron mesylate, 100 mg, oral, FDA approved prescription anti-emetic, for use as a complete therapeutic substitute for an IV anti-emetic at the time of chemotherapy treatment, not to exceed a 24 hour dosage regimen

Bill DME/MAC

NDC: Anzemet

Medicare Statute 4557

⊛ **Q0181** Unspecified oral dosage form, FDA approved prescription anti-emetic, for use as a complete therapeutic substitute for a IV anti-emetic at the time of chemotherapy treatment, not to exceed a 48 hour dosage regimen

Bill DME/MAC

Medicare Statute 4557

▶ **New**   → **Revised**   ✔ **Reinstated**   ~~deleted~~ **Deleted**

⊛ **Special coverage instructions**   ◆ **Not covered or valid by Medicare**   ✷ **Carrier discretion**

Miscellaneous Devices

→ ☼ **Q0478**   Power adapter for use with electric or electric/pneumatic ventricular assist device, vehicle type

CMS has determined the reasonable useful lifetime is one year. Add modifier -RA to claims to report when battery is replaced because it was lost, stolen, or irreparably damaged. (http://www.wpsmedicare.com/part_b/publications/communique/archived/_files/winter-2011-comm.pdf)

→ ☼ **Q0479**   Power module for use with electric or electric/pneumatic ventricular assist device, replacement only

CMS has determined the reasonable useful lifetime is one year. Add modifier -RA in cases where the battery is being replaced because it was lost, stolen, or irreparably damaged. (http://www.wpsmedicare.com/part_b/publications/communique/archived/_files/winter-2011-comm.pdf)

→ ☼ **Q0480**   Driver for use with pneumatic ventricular assist device, replacement only

Bill local carrier

→ ☼ **Q0481**   Microprocessor control unit for use with electric ventricular assist device, replacement only

Bill local carrier

→ ☼ **Q0482**   Microprocessor control unit for use with electric/pneumatic combination ventricular assist device, replacement only

Bill local carrier

→ ☼ **Q0483**   Monitor/display module for use with electric ventricular assist device, replacement only

Bill local carrier

→ ☼ **Q0484**   Monitor/display module for use with electric or electric/pneumatic ventricular assist device, replacement only

Bill local carrier

→ ☼ **Q0485**   Monitor control cable for use with electric ventricular assist device, replacement only

Bill local carrier

→ ☼ **Q0486**   Monitor control cable for use with electric/pneumatic ventricular assist device, replacement only

Bill local carrier

→ ☼ **Q0487**   Leads (pneumatic/electrical) for use with any type electric/pneumatic ventricular assist device, replacement only

Bill local carrier

→ ☼ **Q0488**   Power pack base for use with electric ventricular assist device, replacement only

Bill local carrier

→ ☼ **Q0489**   Power pack base for use with electric/pneumatic ventricular assist device, replacement only

Bill local carrier

→ ☼ **Q0490**   Emergency power source for use with electric ventricular assist device, replacement only

Bill local carrier

→ ☼ **Q0491**   Emergency power source for use with electric/pneumatic ventricular assist device, replacement only

Bill local carrier

→ ☼ **Q0492**   Emergency power supply cable for use with electric ventricular assist device, replacement only

Bill local carrier

→ ☼ **Q0493**   Emergency power supply cable for use with electric/pneumatic ventricular assist device, replacement only

Bill local carrier

→ ☼ **Q0494**   Emergency hand pump for use with electric or electric/pneumatic ventricular assist device, replacement only

Bill local carrier

→ ☼ **Q0495**   Battery/power pack charger for use with electric or electric/pneumatic ventricular assist device, replacement only

Bill local carrier

→ ✳ **Q0496**   Battery, other than lithium-ion, for use with electric or electric/pneumatic ventricular assist device, replacement only

Bill local carrier

Reasonable useful lifetime is 6 months (CR3931).

→ ☼ **Q0497**   Battery clips for use with electric or electric/pneumatic ventricular assist device, replacement only

Bill local carrier

▶ **New**   → **Revised**   ✔ **Reinstated**   ~~deleted~~ **Deleted**

☼ **Special coverage instructions**   ◆ **Not covered or valid by Medicare**   ✳ **Carrier discretion**

→ ✪ **Q0498** Holster for use with electric or electric/pneumatic ventricular assist device, replacement only

Bill local carrier

→ ✪ **Q0499** Belt/vest/bag for use to carry external peripheral components of any type ventricular assist device, replacement only

Bill local carrier

→ ✪ **Q0500** Filters for use with electric or electric/pneumatic ventricular assist device, replacement only

Bill local carrier

→ ✪ **Q0501** Shower cover for use with electric or electric/pneumatic ventricular assist device, replacement only

Bill local carrier

→ ✪ **Q0502** Mobility cart for pneumatic ventricular assist device, replacement only

Bill local carrier

→ ✪ **Q0503** Battery for pneumatic ventricular assist device, replacement only, each

Bill local carrier

Reasonable useful lifetime is 6 months (CR3931).

→ ✪ **Q0504** Power adapter for pneumatic ventricular assist device, replacement only, vehicle type

Bill local carrier

→ ✪ **Q0505** Miscellaneous supply or accessory for use with ventricular assist device

Bill local carrier

→ ✪ **Q0506** Battery, lithium-ion, for use with electric or electric/pneumatic, ventricular assist device, replacement only

Reasonable useful lifetime is 12 months. Add -RA for replacement if lost, stolen, or irreparable damage.

Fee, Pharmacy

Q0510-Q0515: Bill DME/MAC

✪ **Q0510** Pharmacy supply fee for initial immunosuppressive drug(s), first month following transplant

✪ **Q0511** Pharmacy supply fee for oral anti-cancer, oral anti-emetic or immunosuppressive drug(s); for the first prescription in a 30-day period

✪ **Q0512** Pharmacy supply fee for oral anti-cancer, oral anti-emetic or immunosuppressive drug(s); for a subsequent prescription in a 30-day period

✪ **Q0513** Pharmacy dispensing fee for inhalation drug(s); per 30 days

✪ **Q0514** Pharmacy dispensing fee for inhalation drug(s); per 90 days

✪ **Q0515** Injection, sermorelin acetate, 1 microgram

NDC: Geref Diagnostic

IOM: 100-02, 15, 50

Lens, Intraocular

Q1004-Q1005: Bill local carrier

✪ **Q1004** New technology intraocular lens category 4 as defined in Federal Register notice

✪ **Q1005** New technology intraocular lens category 5 as defined in Federal Register notice

Solutions and Drugs

✪ **Q2004** Irrigation solution for treatment of bladder calculi, for example renacidin, per 500 ml

Bill local carrier

IOM: 100-02, 15, 50

Medicare Statute 1861S2B

✳ **Q2009** Injection, fosphenytoin, 50 mg phenytoin equivalent

Bill local carrier

NDC: Cerebyx

IOM: 100-02, 15, 50

Medicare Statute 1861S2B

✪ **Q2017** Injection, teniposide, 50 mg

Bill local carrier

NDC: Vumon

IOM: 100-02, 15, 50

Medicare Statute 1861S2B

✪ **Q2026** Injection, radiesse, 0.1 ml

✪ **Q2027** Injection, sculptra, 0.1 ml

▶ New   → Revised   ✔ Reinstated   ~~deleted~~ Deleted

✪ Special coverage instructions   ◆ Not covered or valid by Medicare   ✳ Carrier discretion

▶ ✪ **Q2034**　Influenza virus vaccine, split virus, for intramuscular use (Agriflu) Sipuleucel-t, minimum of 50 million autologous CD54+ cells activated with PAP-GM-CSF, including leukapheresis and all other preparatory procedures, per infusion

IOM 100-02, 15, 50

✪ **Q2035**　Influenza virus vaccine, split virus, when administered to individuals 3 years of age and older, for intramuscular use (Afluria)

Preventive service; no deductible

IOM: 100-02, 15, 50

✪ **Q2036**　Influenza virus vaccine, split virus, when administered to individuals 3 years of age and older, for intramuscular use (Flulaval)

Preventive service; no deductible

IOM: 100-02, 15, 50

✪ **Q2037**　Influenza virus vaccine, split virus, when administered to individuals 3 years of age and older, for intramuscular use (Fluvirin)

Preventive service; no deductible

IOM: 100-02, 15, 50

✪ **Q2038**　Influenza virus vaccine, split virus, when administered to individuals 3 years of age or older, for intramuscular use (Fluzone)

Preventive service; no deductible

IOM: 100-02, 15, 50

✪ **Q2039**　Influenza virus vaccine, split virus, when administered to individuals 3 years of age and older, for intramuscular use (not otherwise specified)

Preventive service; no deductible

IOM: 100-02, 15, 50

✪ **Q2043**　Sipuleucel-T, minimum of 50 million autologous CD54+ cells activated with PAP-GM-CSF, including leukapheresis and all other preparatory procedures, per infusion

~~**Q2045**　Injection, human fibrinogen concentrate, 1 mg~~　✖

Cross Reference: J7178

~~**Q2046**　Injection, aflibercept, 1 mg~~　✖

Cross Reference: J7178

~~**Q2047**　Injection, peginesatide, 0. 1 mg (for ESRD on dialysis)~~　✖

Cross Reference: J0890

~~**Q2048**　Injection, doxorubicin hydrochloride, liposomal, doxil, 10 mg~~　✖

Cross Reference: J9002

▶ ✳ **Q2049**　Injection, doxorubicin hydrochloride, liposomal, imported lipodox, 10 mg

Brachytherapy Radioelements

✪ **Q3001**　Radioelements for brachytherapy, any type, each

IOM: 100-04, 12, 70; 100-04, 13, 20

Telehealth

✳ **Q3014**　Telehealth originating site facility fee

Bill local carrier

Effective January of each year, the fee for telehealth services is increased by the Medicare Economic Index (MEI). The telehealth originating facility site fee (HCPCS code Q3014) for 2011 was 80 percent of the lesser of the actual charge or $24.10.

Drugs

Q3025-Q3026:　Bill local carrier

✪ **Q3025**　Injection, interferon beta-1a, 11 mcg for intramuscular use

NDC: Avonex

IOM: 100-02, 15, 50

◆ **Q3026**　Injection, interferon beta-1a, 11 mcg for subcutaneous use

Other: Rebif

Test, Skin

✪ **Q3031**　Collagen skin test

Bill local carrier

IOM: 100-03, 4, 280.1

Supplies, Cast

Q4001-Q4051:　Bill local carrier

Payment on a reasonable charge basis is required for splints, casts by regulations contained in 42 CFR 405.501.

✳ **Q4001**　Casting supplies, body cast adult, with or without head, plaster

✳ **Q4002**　Cast supplies, body cast adult, with or without head, fiberglass

---

▶ New　→ Revised　✔ Reinstated　~~deleted~~ Deleted

✪ Special coverage instructions　◆ Not covered or valid by Medicare　✳ Carrier discretion

✳ **Q4003** Cast supplies, shoulder cast, adult (11 years +), plaster

✳ **Q4004** Cast supplies, shoulder cast, adult (11 years +), fiberglass

✳ **Q4005** Cast supplies, long arm cast, adult (11 years +), plaster

✳ **Q4006** Cast supplies, long arm cast, adult (11 years +), fiberglass

✳ **Q4007** Cast supplies, long arm cast, pediatric (0-10 years), plaster

✳ **Q4008** Cast supplies, long arm cast, pediatric (0-10 years), fiberglass

✳ **Q4009** Cast supplies, short arm cast, adult (11 years +), plaster

✳ **Q4010** Cast supplies, short arm cast, adult (11 years +), fiberglass

✳ **Q4011** Cast supplies, short arm cast, pediatric (0-10 years), plaster

✳ **Q4012** Cast supplies, short arm cast, pediatric (0-10 years), fiberglass

✳ **Q4013** Cast supplies, gauntlet cast (includes lower forearm and hand), adult (11 years +), plaster

✳ **Q4014** Cast supplies, gauntlet cast (includes lower forearm and hand), adult (11 years +), fiberglass

✳ **Q4015** Cast supplies, gauntlet cast (includes lower forearm and hand), pediatric (0-10 years), plaster

✳ **Q4016** Cast supplies, gauntlet cast (includes lower forearm and hand), pediatric (0-10 years), fiberglass

✳ **Q4017** Cast supplies, long arm splint, adult (11 years +), plaster

✳ **Q4018** Cast supplies, long arm splint, adult (11 years +), fiberglass

✳ **Q4019** Cast supplies, long arm splint, pediatric (0-10 years), plaster

✳ **Q4020** Cast supplies, long arm splint, pediatric (0-10 years), fiberglass

✳ **Q4021** Cast supplies, short arm splint, adult (11 years +), plaster

✳ **Q4022** Cast supplies, short arm splint, adult (11 years +), fiberglass

✳ **Q4023** Cast supplies, short arm splint, pediatric (0-10 years), plaster

✳ **Q4024** Cast supplies, short arm splint, pediatric (0-10 years), fiberglass

✳ **Q4025** Cast supplies, hip spica (one or both legs), adult (11 years +), plaster

✳ **Q4026** Cast supplies, hip spica (one or both legs), adult (11 years +), fiberglass

✳ **Q4027** Cast supplies, hip spica (one or both legs), pediatric (0-10 years), plaster

✳ **Q4028** Cast supplies, hip spica (one or both legs), pediatric (0-10 years), fiberglass

✳ **Q4029** Cast supplies, long leg cast, adult (11 years +), plaster

✳ **Q4030** Cast supplies, long leg cast, adult (11 years +), fiberglass

✳ **Q4031** Cast supplies, long leg cast, pediatric (0-10 years), plaster

✳ **Q4032** Cast supplies, long leg cast, pediatric (0-10 years), fiberglass

✳ **Q4033** Cast supplies, long leg cylinder cast, adult (11 years +), plaster

✳ **Q4034** Cast supplies, long leg cylinder cast, adult (11 years +), fiberglass

✳ **Q4035** Cast supplies, long leg cylinder cast, pediatric (0-10 years), plaster

✳ **Q4036** Cast supplies, long leg cylinder cast, pediatric (0-10 years), fiberglass

✳ **Q4037** Cast supplies, short leg cast, adult (11 years +), plaster

✳ **Q4038** Cast supplies, short leg cast, adult (11 years +), fiberglass

✳ **Q4039** Cast supplies, short leg cast, pediatric (0-10 years), plaster

✳ **Q4040** Cast supplies, short leg cast, pediatric (0-10 years), fiberglass

✳ **Q4041** Cast supplies, long leg splint, adult (11 years +), plaster

✳ **Q4042** Cast supplies, long leg splint, adult (11 years +), fiberglass

✳ **Q4043** Cast supplies, long leg splint, pediatric (0-10 years), plaster

✳ **Q4044** Cast supplies, long leg splint, pediatric (0-10 years), fiberglass

✳ **Q4045** Cast supplies, short leg splint, adult (11 years +), plaster

✳ **Q4046** Cast supplies, short leg splint, adult (11 years +), fiberglass

✳ **Q4047** Cast supplies, short leg splint, pediatric (0-10 years), plaster

✳ **Q4048** Cast supplies, short leg splint, pediatric (0-10 years), fiberglass

✳ **Q4049** Finger splint, static

✳ **Q4050** Cast supplies, for unlisted types and materials of casts

✳ **Q4051** Splint supplies, miscellaneous (includes thermoplastics, strapping, fasteners, padding and other supplies)

▶ New   → Revised   ✔ Reinstated   ~~deleted~~ Deleted

⊙ Special coverage instructions   ◆ Not covered or valid by Medicare   ✳ Carrier discretion

Drugs

＊ **Q4074** Iloprost, inhalation solution, FDA-approved final product, non-compounded, administered through DME, unit dose form, up to 20 micrograms

NDC: Ventavis

✪ **Q4081** Injection, epoetin alfa, 100 units (for ESRD on dialysis)

Bill DME/MAC for method II home dialysis. If other, bill DME/MAC.

NDC: Epogen, Procrit

＊ **Q4082** Drug or biological, not otherwise classified, Part B drug competitive acquisition program (CAP)

Bill local carrier

Skin Substitutes

＊ **Q4100** Skin substitute, not otherwise specified

Bill local carrier

Other: Orcel, Surgimend collagen matrix

＊ **Q4101** Apligraf, per square centimeter

Bill local carrier

＊ **Q4102** Oasis Wound Matrix, per square centimeter

Bill local carrier

＊ **Q4103** Oasis Burn Matrix, per square centimeter

Bill local carrier

＊ **Q4104** Integra Bilayer Matrix Wound Dressing (BMWD), per square centimeter

Bill local carrier

＊ **Q4105** Integra Dermal Regeneration Template (DRT), per square centimeter

Bill local carrier

＊ **Q4106** Dermagraft, per square centimeter

Bill local carrier

＊ **Q4107** Graftjacket, per square centimeter

Bill local carrier

NDC: Graftjacket Maxstrip, Graftjacket Small Ligament Repair Matrix, Graftjacket STD, Handjacket Scaffold Thin, Maxforce Thick, Ulcerjacket Scaffold, Ultra Maxforce

＊ **Q4108** Integra Matrix, per square centimeter

Bill local carrier

＊ **Q4110** Primatrix, per square centimeter

Bill local carrier

＊ **Q4111** GammaGraft, per square centimeter

Bill local carrier

＊ **Q4112** Cymetra, injectable, 1cc

＊ **Q4113** GraftJacket Xpress, injectable, 1cc

Bill local carrier

＊ **Q4114** Integra Flowable Wound Matrix, injectable, 1cc

Bill local carrier

＊ **Q4115** Alloskin, per square centimeter

Bill local carrier

＊ **Q4116** Alloderm, per square centimeter

Bill local carrier

＊ **Q4117** Hyalomatrix, per square centimeter

IOM: 100-02, 15, 50

＊ **Q4118** Matristem micromatrix, 1 mg

→ ＊ **Q4119** Matristem wound matrix, PSMX, RS, or PSM, per square centimeter

＊ **Q4120** Matristem burn matrix, per square centimeter

＊ **Q4121** Theraskin, per square centimeter

＊ **Q4122** Dermacell, per square centimeter

＊ **Q4123** AlloSkin RT, per square centimeter

＊ **Q4124** Oasis Ultra Tri-layer Wound Matrix, per square centimeter

＊ **Q4125** Arthroflex, per square centimeter

→ ＊ **Q4126** Memoderm, dermaspan, tranzgraft or integuply, per square centimeter

＊ **Q4127** Talymed, per square centimeter

→ ＊ **Q4128** FlexHD, Allopatch HD, or Matrix HD, per square centimeter

＊ **Q4129** Unite Biomatrix, per square centimeter

＊ **Q4130** Strattice TM, per square centimeter

▶ ＊ **Q4131** Epifix, per square centimeter

▶ ＊ **Q4132** Grafix core, per square centimeter

▶ ＊ **Q4133** Grafix prime, per square centimeter

▶ ＊ **Q4134** Hmatrix, per square centimeter

▶ ＊ **Q4135** Mediskin, per square centimeter

▶ ＊ **Q4136** Ez-derm, per square centimeter

▶ New　→ Revised　✔ Reinstated　~~deleted~~ Deleted
✪ Special coverage instructions　◆ Not covered or valid by Medicare　＊ Carrier discretion

Hospice Care

⊛ **Q5001** Hospice care provided in patient's home/residence

Bill local carrier

⊛ **Q5002** Hospice care provided in assisted living facility

Bill local carrier

⊛ **Q5003** Hospice care provided in nursing long term care facility (LTC) or non-skilled nursing facility (NF)

Bill local carrier

⊛ **Q5004** Hospice care provided in skilled nursing facility (SNF)

Bill local carrier

⊛ **Q5005** Hospice care provided in inpatient hospital

Bill local carrier

⊛ **Q5006** Hospice care provided in inpatient hospice facility

Bill local carrier

Hospice care provided in an inpatient hospice facility. These are residential facilities, which are places for patients to live while receiving routine home care or continuous home care. These hospice residential facilities are not certified by Medicare or Medicaid for provision of General Inpatient (GIP) or respite care, and regulations at 42 CFR 418.202(e) do not allow provision of GIP or respite care at hospice residential facilities. (http://www.palmettogba.com/Palmetto/Providers.Nsf/files/Hospice_Coalition_QAs_03-2011.pdf/$File/Hospice_Coalition_QAs_03-2011.pdf)

⊛ **Q5007** Hospice care provided in long term care facility

Bill local carrier

⊛ **Q5008** Hospice care provided in inpatient psychiatric facility

Bill local carrier

⊛ **Q5009** Hospice care provided in place not otherwise specified (NOS)

Bill local carrier

⊛ **Q5010** Hospice home care provided in a hospice facility

Contrast

⊛ **Q9951** Low osmolar contrast material, 400 or greater mg/ml iodine concentration, per ml

Bill local carrier

IOM: 100-04, 12, 70; 100-04, 13, 20; 100-04, 13, 90

⊛ **Q9953** Injection, iron-based magnetic resonance contrast agent, per ml

Bill local carrier

IOM: 100-04, 12, 70; 100-04, 13, 20; 100-04, 13, 90

⊛ **Q9954** Oral magnetic resonance contrast agent, per 100 ml

Bill local carrier

NDC: Gastromark

IOM: 100-04, 12, 70; 100-04, 13, 20; 100-04, 13, 90

✳ **Q9955** Injection, perflexane lipid microspheres, per ml

Bill local carrier

✳ **Q9956** Injection, octafluoropropane microspheres, per ml

Bill local carrier

NDC: Optison

✳ **Q9957** Injection, perflutren lipid microspheres, per ml

Bill local carrier

NDC: Definity

⊛ **Q9958** High osmolar contrast material, up to 149 mg/ml iodine concentration, per ml

Bill local carrier

NDC: Conray 30, Cysto-Conray II, Cystografin, Cystografin-Dilute, Reno-Dip

IOM: 100-04, 12, 70; 100-04, 13, 20; 100-04, 13, 90

⊛ **Q9959** High osmolar contrast material, 150-199 mg/ml iodine concentration, per ml

Bill local carrier

IOM: 100-04, 12, 70; 100-04, 13, 20; 100-04, 13, 90

▶ New → Revised ✔ Reinstated deleted Deleted
⊛ Special coverage instructions ◆ Not covered or valid by Medicare ✳ Carrier discretion

✪ **Q9960** High osmolar contrast material, 200-249 mg/ml iodine concentration, per ml

Bill local carrier

NDC: Conray 43

IOM: 100-04, 12, 70; 100-04, 13, 20; 100-04, 13, 90

✪ **Q9961** High osmolar contrast material, 250-299 mg/ml iodine concentration, per ml

Bill local carrier

NDC: Conray, Cholografin Meglumine

IOM: 100-04, 12, 70; 100-04, 13, 20; 100-04, 13, 90

✪ **Q9962** High osmolar contrast material, 300-349 mg/ml iodine concentration, per ml

Bill local carrier

IOM: 100-04, 12, 70; 100-04, 13, 20; 100-04, 13, 90

✪ **Q9963** High osmolar contrast material, 350-399 mg/ml iodine concentration, per ml

Bill local carrier

NDC: Gastrografin, Md-76R, Md Gastroview, Sinografin

IOM: 100-04, 12, 70; 100-04, 13, 20; 100-04, 13, 90

✪ **Q9964** High osmolar contrast material, 400 or greater mg/ml iodine concentration, per ml

Bill local carrier

IOM: 100-04, 12, 70; 100-04, 13, 20; 100-04, 13, 90

✪ **Q9965** Low osmolar contrast material, 100-199 mg/ml iodine concentration, per ml

Bill local carrier

NDC: Omnipaque, Ultravist

IOM: 100-04, 12, 70; 100-04, 13, 20; 100-04, 13, 90

✪ **Q9966** Low osmolar contrast material, 200-299 mg/ml iodine concentration, per ml

Bill local carrier

NDC: Isovue, Omnipaque, Optiray, Ultravist, Visipaque

IOM: 100-04, 12, 70; 100-04, 13, 20; 100-04, 13, 90

✪ **Q9967** Low osmolar contrast material, 300-399 mg/ml iodine concentration, per ml

Bill local carrier

NDC: Hexabrix 320, Isovue-300, Isovue-370, Omnipaque 300, Omnipaque 350, Optiray, Oxilan, Ultravist, Vispaque

IOM: 100-04, 12, 70; 100-04, 13, 20; 100-04, 13, 90

✳ **Q9968** Injection, non-radioactive, non-contrast, visualization adjunct (e.g., Methylene Blue, Isosulfan Blue), 1 mg

▶ ✳ **Q9969** Tc-99m from non-highly enriched uranium source, full cost recovery add-on, per study dose

---

▶ New → Revised ✔ Reinstated ~~deleted~~ Deleted

✪ Special coverage instructions ◆ Not covered or valid by Medicare ✳ Carrier discretion

DIAGNOSTIC RADIOLOGY SERVICES (R0000-R9999)

Transportation/Setup of Portable Equipment

R0070-R0076:   Bill local carrier

⊕ **R0070**   Transportation of portable x-ray equipment and personnel to home or nursing home, per trip to facility or location, one patient seen

CMS Transmittal B03-049; specific instructions to contractors on pricing

IOM: 100-04, 13, 90; 100-04, 13, 90.3

⊕ **R0075**   Transportation of portable x-ray equipment and personnel to home or nursing home, per trip to facility or location, more than one patient seenB

This code would not apply to the x-ray equipment if stored at the location where the x-ray was performed (e.g., a nursing home).

IOM: 100-04, 13, 90; 100-04, 13, 90.3

⊕ **R0076**   Transportation of portable ECG to facility or location, per patient

EKG procedure code 93000 or 93005 must be submitted on same claim as transportation code. Bundled status on physician fee schedule

IOM: 100-01, 5, 90.2; 100-02, 15, 80; 100-03, 1, 20.15; 100-04, 13, 90; 100-04, 16, 10; 100-04, 16, 110.4

▶ New   → Revised   ✔ Reinstated   ~~deleted~~ Deleted

⊕ Special coverage instructions   ◆ Not covered or valid by Medicare   ✳ Carrier discretion

TEMPORARY NATIONAL CODES ESTABLISHED BY PRIVATE PAYERS (S0000-S9999)

Medicare and other federal payers do not recognize "S" codes; however, S codes may be useful for claims to some private insurers.

- ◆ **S0012** Butorphanol tartrate, nasal spray, **25 mg**
- ◆ **S0014** Tacrine hydrochloride, **10 mg**
- ◆ **S0017** Injection, aminocaproic acid, **5 grams**
- ◆ **S0020** Injection, bupivacaine hydrochloride, **30 ml**
- ◆ **S0021** Injection, cefoperazone sodium, **1 gram**
- ◆ **S0023** Injection, cimetidine hydrochloride, **300 mg**
- ◆ **S0028** Injection, famotidine, **20 mg**
- ◆ **S0030** Injection, metronidazole, **500 mg**
- ◆ **S0032** Injection, nafcillin sodium, **2 grams**
- ◆ **S0034** Injection, ofloxacin, **400 mg**
- ◆ **S0039** Injection, sulfamethoxazole and tri-methoprim, **10 ml**
- ◆ **S0040** Injection, ticarcillin disodium and clavulanate potassium, **3.1 grams**
- ◆ **S0073** Injection, aztreonam, **500 mg**
- ◆ **S0074** Injection, cefotetan disodium, **500 mg**
- ◆ **S0077** Injection, clindamycin phosphate, **300 mg**
- ◆ **S0078** Injection, fosphenytoin sodium, **750 mg**
- ◆ **S0080** Injection, pentamidine isethionate, **300 mg**
- ◆ **S0081** Injection, piperacillin sodium, **500 mg**
- ◆ **S0088** Imatinib, **100 mg**
- ◆ **S0090** Sildenafil citrate, **25 mg**
- ◆ **S0091** Granisetron hydrochloride, **1 mg** (for circumstances falling under the Medicare Statute, use Q0166)
- ◆ **S0092** Injection, hydromorphone hydrochloride, **250 mg** (loading dose for infusion pump)
- ◆ **S0093** Injection, morphine sulfate, **500 mg** (loading dose for infusion pump)
- ◆ **S0104** Zidovudine, oral, **100 mg**
- ◆ **S0106** Bupropion HCl sustained release tablet, **150 mg,** per bottle of 60 tablets
- ◆ **S0108** Mercaptopurine, oral, **50 mg**
- ◆ **S0109** Methadone, oral, **5 mg**

- ◆ **S0117** Tretinoin, topical, **5 grams**
- ◆ **S0119** Ondansetron, oral, 4 mg (for circumstances falling under the medicare statute, use HCPCS Q code)
- ◆ **S0122** Injection, menotropins, **75 IU**
- ◆ **S0126** Injection, follitropin alfa, **75 IU**
- ◆ **S0128** Injection, follitropin beta, **75 IU**
- ◆ **S0132** Injection, ganirelix acetate, **250 mcg**
- ◆ **S0136** Clozapine, **25 mg**
- ◆ **S0137** Didanosine (DDI), **25 mg**
- ◆ **S0138** Finasteride, **5 mg**
- ◆ **S0139** Minoxidil, **10 mg**
- ◆ **S0140** Saquinavir, **200 mg**
- ◆ **S0142** Colistimethate sodium, inhalation solution administered through DME, concentrated form, **per mg**
- ◆ **S0145** Injection, pegylated interferon alfa-2a, **180 mcg per ml**
- ◆ **S0148** Injection, pegylated interferon ALFA-2b, **10 mcg**
- ◆ **S0155** Sterile dilutant for epoprostenol, **50 ml**
- ◆ **S0156** Exemestane, **25 mg**
- ◆ **S0157** Becaplermin gel 0.01%, **0.5 gm**
- ◆ **S0160** Dextroamphetamine sulfate, **5 mg**
- ◆ **S0164** Injection, pantoprazole sodium, **40 mg**
- ◆ **S0166** Injection, olanzapine, **2.5 mg**
- ◆ **S0169** Calcitrol, **0.25 microgram**
- ◆ **S0170** Anastrozole, oral, **1mg**
- ◆ **S0171** Injection, bumetanide, **0.5 mg**
- ◆ **S0172** Chlorambucil, oral, **2 mg**
- ◆ **S0174** Dolasetron mesylate, oral **50 mg** (for circumstances falling under the Medicare Statute, use Q0180)
- ◆ **S0175** Flutamide, oral, **125 mg**
- ◆ **S0176** Hydroxyurea, oral, **500 mg**
- ◆ **S0177** Levamisole hydrochloride, oral, **50 mg**
- ◆ **S0178** Lomustine, oral, **10 mg**
- ◆ **S0179** Megestrol acetate, oral, **20 mg**
- ◆ **S0182** Procarbazine hydrochloride, oral, **50 mg**
- ◆ **S0183** Prochlorperazine maleate, oral, **5 mg** (for circumstances falling under the Medicare Statute, use Q0164-Q0165)
- ◆ **S0187** Tamoxifen citrate, oral, **10 mg**
- ◆ **S0189** Testosterone pellet, **75 mg**
- ◆ **S0190** Mifepristone, oral, **200 mg**
- ◆ **S0191** Misoprostol, oral **200 mcg**

▶ New → Revised ✔ Reinstated ~~deleted~~ Deleted

◎ Special coverage instructions ◆ Not covered or valid by Medicare ✳ Carrier discretion

◆ **S0194**   Dialysis/stress vitamin supplement, oral, **100 capsules**

◆ **S0195**   Pneumococcal conjugate vaccine, polyvalent, intramuscular, for children from five years to nine years of age who have not previously received the vaccine

◆ **S0197**   Prenatal vitamins, 30-day supply

◆ **S0199**   Medically induced abortion by oral ingestion of medication including all associated services and supplies (e.g., patient counseling, office visits, confirmation of pregnancy by HCG, ultrasound to confirm duration of pregnancy, ultrasound to confirm completion of abortion) except drugs

◆ **S0201**   Partial hospitalization services, less than 24 hours, per diem

◆ **S0207**   Paramedic intercept, non-hospital-based ALS service (non-voluntary), non-transport

◆ **S0208**   Paramedic intercept, hospital-based ALS service (non-voluntary), non-transport

◆ **S0209**   Wheelchair van, mileage, per mile

◆ **S0215**   Non-emergency transportation; mileage per mile

◆ **S0220**   Medical conference by a physician with interdisciplinary team of health professionals or representatives of community agencies to coordinate activities of patient care (patient is present); approximately 30 minutes

◆ **S0221**   Medical conference by a physician with interdisciplinary team of health professionals or representatives of community agencies to coordinate activities of patient care (patient is present); approximately 60 minutes

◆ **S0250**   Comprehensive geriatric assessment and treatment planning performed by assessment team

◆ **S0255**   Hospice referral visit (advising patient and family of care options) performed by nurse, social worker, or other designated staff

◆ **S0257**   Counseling and discussion regarding advance directives or end of life care planning and decisions, with patient and/or surrogate (list separately in addition to code for appropriate evaluation and management service)

◆ **S0260**   History and physical (outpatient or office) related to surgical procedure (list separately in addition to code for appropriate evaluation and management service)

◆ **S0265**   Genetic counseling, under physician supervision, each 15 minutes

◆ **S0270**   Physician management of patient home care, standard monthly case rate (per 30 days)

◆ **S0271**   Physician management of patient home care, hospice monthly case rate (per 30 days)

◆ **S0272**   Physician management of patient home care, episodic care monthly case rate (per 30 days)

◆ **S0273**   Physician visit at member's home, outside of a capitation arrangement

◆ **S0274**   Nurse practitioner visit at member's home, outside of a capitation arrangement

◆ **S0280**   Medical home program, comprehensive care coordination and planning, initial plan

◆ **S0281**   Medical home program, comprehensive care coordination and planning, maintenance of plan

◆ **S0302**   Completed Early Periodic Screening Diagnosis and Treatment (EPSDT) service (list in addition to code for appropriate evaluation and management service)

◆ **S0310**   Hospitalist services (list separately in addition to code for appropriate evaluation and management service)

◆ **S0315**   Disease management program; initial assessment and initiation of the program

◆ **S0316**   Disease management program; follow-up/reassessment

◆ **S0317**   Disease management program; per diem

◆ **S0320**   Telephone calls by a registered nurse to a disease management program member for monitoring purposes; per month

◆ **S0340**   Lifestyle modification program for management of coronary artery disease, including all supportive services; first quarter/stage

◆ **S0341**   Lifestyle modification program for management of coronary artery disease, including all supportive services; second or third quarter/ stage

◆ **S0342**   Lifestyle modification program for management of coronary artery disease, including all supportive services; fourth quarter/stage

---

▶ New   → Revised   ✔ Reinstated   ~~deleted~~ Deleted

☺ Special coverage instructions   ◆ Not covered or valid by Medicare   ✳ Carrier discretion

▶ ✳ **S0353** Treatment planning and care coordination management for cancer, initial treatment

▶ ✳ **S0354** Treatment planning and care coordination management for cancer, established patient with a change of regimen

◆ **S0390** Routine foot care; removal and/or trimming of corns, calluses and/or nails and preventive maintenance in specific medical conditions (e.g. diabetes), per visit

◆ **S0395** Impression casting of a foot performed by a practitioner other than the manufacturer of the orthotic

◆ **S0400** Global fee for extracorporeal shock wave lithotripsy treatment of kidney stone(s)

◆ **S0500** Disposable contact lens, per lens

◆ **S0504** Single vision prescription lens (safety, athletic, or sunglass), per lens

◆ **S0506** Bifocal vision prescription lens (safety, athletic, or sunglass), per lens

◆ **S0508** Trifocal vision prescription lens (safety, athletic, or sunglass), per lens

◆ **S0510** Non-prescription lens (safety, athletic, or sunglass), per lens

◆ **S0512** Daily wear specialty contact lens, per lens

◆ **S0514** Color contact lens, per lens

◆ **S0515** Scleral lens, liquid bandage device, per lens

◆ **S0516** Safety eyeglass frames

◆ **S0518** Sunglasses frames

◆ **S0580** Polycarbonate lens (list this code in addition to the basic code for the lens)

◆ **S0581** Nonstandard lens (list this code in addition to the basic code for the lens)

◆ **S0590** Integral lens service, miscellaneous services reported separately

◆ **S0592** Comprehensive contact lens evaluation

◆ **S0595** Dispensing new spectacle lenses for patient supplied frame

▶ ⊙ **S0596** Phakic intraocular lens for correction of refractive error

◆ **S0601** Screening proctoscopy

◆ **S0610** Annual gynecological examination, new patient

◆ **S0612** Annual gynecological examination, established patient

◆ **S0613** Annual gynecological examination; clinical breast examination without pelvic evaluation

◆ **S0618** Audiometry for hearing aid evaluation to determine the level and degree of hearing loss

◆ **S0620** Routine ophthalmological examination including refraction; new patient

Many non-Medicare vision plans may require code for routine encounter, no complaints

◆ **S0621** Routine ophthalmological examination including refraction; established patient

Many non-Medicare vision plans may require code for routine encounter, no complaints

◆ **S0622** Physical exam for college, new or established patient (list separately) in addition to appropriate evaluation and management code

◆ **S0630** Removal of sutures; by a physician other than the physician who originally closed the wound

◆ **S0800** Laser in situ keratomileusis (LASIK)

◆ **S0810** Photorefractive keratectomy (PRK)

◆ **S0812** Phototherapeutic keratectomy (PTK)

◆ **S1001** Deluxe item, patient aware (list in addition to code for basic item)

◆ **S1002** Customized item (list in addition to code for basic item)

◆ **S1015** IV tubing extension set

◆ **S1016** Non-PVC (polyvinyl chloride) intravenous administration set, for use with drugs that are not stable in PVC e.g. paclitaxel

◆ **S1030** Continuous noninvasive glucose monitoring device, purchase (for physician interpretation of data, use CPT code)

◆ **S1031** Continuous noninvasive glucose monitoring device, rental, including sensor, sensor replacement, and download to monitor (for physician interpretation of data, use CPT code)

◆ **S1040** Cranial remolding orthosis, pediatric, rigid, with soft interface material, custom fabricated, includes fitting and adjustment(s)

▶ ◆ **S1090** Mometasone furoate sinus implant, 370 micrograms

◆ **S2053** Transplantation of small intestine and liver allografts

---

▶ **New**   → **Revised**   ✔ **Reinstated**   ~~deleted~~ **Deleted**

⊙ **Special coverage instructions**   ◆ **Not covered or valid by Medicare**   ✳ **Carrier discretion**

◆ **S2054** Transplantation of multivisceral organs

◆ **S2055** Harvesting of donor multivisceral organs, with preparation and maintenance of allografts; from cadaver donor

◆ **S2060** Lobar lung transplantation

◆ **S2061** Donor lobectomy (lung) for transplantation, living donor

◆ **S2065** Simultaneous pancreas kidney transplantation

◆ **S2066** Breast reconstruction with gluteal artery perforator (GAP) flap, including harvesting of the flap, microvascular transfer, closure of donor site and shaping the flap into a breast, unilateral

◆ **S2067** Breast reconstruction of a single breast with "stacked" deep inferior epigastric perforator (DIEP) flap(s) and/or gluteal artery perforator (GAP) flap(s), including harvesting of the flap(s), microvascular transfer, closure of donor site(s) and shaping the flap into a breast, unilateral

◆ **S2068** Breast reconstruction with deep inferior epigastric perforator (DIEP) flap, or superficial inferior epigastric artery (SIEA) flap, including harvesting of the flap, microvascular transfer, closure of donor site and shaping the flap into a breast, unilateral

◆ **S2070** Cystourethroscopy, with ureteroscopy and/or pyeloscopy; with endoscopic laser treatment of ureteral calculi (includes ureteral catheterization)

◆ **S2079** Laparoscopic esophagomyotomy (Heller type)

◆ **S2080** Laser-assisted uvulopalatoplasty (LAUP)

◆ **S2083** Adjustment of gastric band diameter via subcutaneous port by injection or aspiration of saline

◆ **S2095** Transcatheter occlusion or embolization for tumor destruction, percutaneous, any method, using yttrium-90 microspheres

◆ **S2102** Islet cell tissue transplant from pancreas; allogeneic

◆ **S2103** Adrenal tissue transplant to brain

◆ **S2107** Adoptive immunotherapy i.e. development of specific anti-tumor reactivity (e.g. tumor-infiltrating lymphocyte therapy) per course of treatment

◆ **S2112** Arthroscopy, knee, surgical for harvesting of cartilage (chondrocyte cells)

◆ **S2115** Osteotomy, periacetabular, with internal fixation

◆ **S2117** Arthroereisis, subtalar

◆ **S2118** Metal-on-metal total hip resurfacing, including acetabular and femoral components

◆ **S2120** Low density lipoprotein (LDL) apheresis using heparin-induced extracorporeal LDL precipitation

◆ **S2140** Cord blood harvesting for transplantation, allogeneic

◆ **S2142** Cord blood-derived stem cell transplantation, allogeneic

◆ **S2150** Bone marrow or blood-derived stem cells (peripheral or umbilical), allogeneic or autologous, harvesting, transplantation, and related complications; including: pheresis and cell preparation/storage; marrow ablative therapy; drugs, supplies, hospitalization with outpatient follow-up; medical/ surgical, diagnostic, emergency, and rehabilitative services; and the number of days of pre- and post-transplant care in the global definition

◆ **S2152** Solid organ(s), complete or segmental, single organ or combination of organs; deceased or living donor(s), procurement, transplantation, and related complications; including: drugs; supplies; hospitalization with outpatient follow-up; medical/surgical, diagnostic, emergency, and rehabilitative services, and the number of days of pre- and post-transplant care in the global definition

◆ **S2202** Echosclerotherapy

◆ **S2205** Minimally invasive direct coronary artery bypass surgery involving mini-thoracotomy or mini-sternotomy surgery, performed under direct vision; using arterial graft(s), single coronary arterial graft

◆ **S2206** Minimally invasive direct coronary artery bypass surgery involving mini-thoracotomy or mini-sternotomy surgery, performed under direct vision; using arterial graft(s), two coronary arterial grafts

◆ **S2207** Minimally invasive direct coronary artery bypass surgery involving mini-thoracotomy or mini-sternotomy surgery, performed under direct vision; using venous graft only, single coronary venous graft

---

▶ New → Revised ✔ Reinstated ~~deleted~~ Deleted

☺ Special coverage instructions ◆ Not covered or valid by Medicare ✳ Carrier discretion

◆ **S2208** Minimally invasive direct coronary artery bypass surgery involving mini-thoracotomy or mini-sternotomy surgery, performed under direct vision; using single arterial and venous graft(s), single venous graft

◆ **S2209** Minimally invasive direct coronary artery bypass surgery involving mini-thoracotomy or mini-sternotomy surgery, performed under direct vision; using two arterial grafts and single venous graft

◆ **S2225** Myringotomy, laser-assisted

◆ **S2230** Implantation of magnetic component of semi-implantable hearing device on ossicles in middle ear

◆ **S2235** Implantation of auditory brain stem implant

◆ **S2260** Induced abortion, 17 to 24 weeks

◆ **S2265** Induced abortion, 25 to 28 weeks

◆ **S2266** Induced abortion, 29 to 31 weeks

◆ **S2267** Induced abortion, 32 weeks or greater

◆ **S2300** Arthroscopy, shoulder, surgical; with thermally-induced capsulorrhaphy

◆ **S2325** Hip core decompression

◆ **S2340** Chemodenervation of abductor muscle(s) of vocal cord

◆ **S2341** Chemodenervation of adductor muscle(s) of vocal cord

◆ **S2342** Nasal endoscopy for post-operative debridement following functional endoscopic sinus surgery, nasal and/or sinus cavity(s), unilateral or bilateral

◆ **S2348** Decompression procedure, percutaneous, of nucleus pulpous of intervertebral disc, using radiofrequency energy, single or multiple levels, lumbar

◆ **S2350** Diskectomy, anterior, with decompression of spinal cord and/or nerve root(s), including osteophytectomy; lumbar, single interspace

◆ **S2351** Diskectomy, anterior, with decompression of spinal cord and/or nerve root(s) including osteophytectomy; lumbar, each additional interspace (list separately in addition to code for primary procedure)

◆ **S2360** Percutaneous vertebroplasty, one vertebral body, unilateral or bilateral injection; cervical

◆ **S2361** Each additional cervical vertebral body (list separately in addition to code for primary procedure)

◆ **S2400** Repair, congenital diaphragmatic hernia in the fetus using temporary tracheal occlusion, procedure performed in utero

◆ **S2401** Repair, urinary tract obstruction in the fetus, procedure performed in utero

◆ **S2402** Repair, congenital cystic adenomatoid malformation in the fetus, procedure performed in utero

◆ **S2403** Repair, extralobar pulmonary sequestration in the fetus, procedure performed in utero

◆ **S2404** Repair, myelomeningocele in the fetus, procedure performed in utero

◆ **S2405** Repair of sacrococcygeal teratoma in the fetus, procedure performed in utero

◆ **S2409** Repair, congenital malformation of fetus, procedure performed in utero, not otherwise classified

◆ **S2411** Fetoscopic laser therapy for treatment of twin-to-twin transfusion syndrome

◆ **S2900** Surgical techniques requiring use of robotic surgical system (list separately in addition to code for primary procedure)

◆ **S3000** Diabetic indicator; retinal eye exam, dilated, bilateral

◆ **S3005** Performance measurement, evaluation of patient self assessment, depression

◆ **S3600** STAT laboratory request (situations other than S3601)

◆ **S3601** Emergency STAT laboratory charge for patient who is homebound or residing in a nursing facility

◆ **S3620** Newborn metabolic screening panel, includes test kit, postage and the laboratory tests specified by the state for inclusion in this panel (e.g. galactose; hemoglobin, electrophoresis; hydroxyprogesterone, 17-D; phenylalanine (PKU); and thyroxine, total)

◆ **S3625** Maternal serum triple marker screen including alpha-fetoprotein (AFP), estriol, and human chorionic gonadotropin (HCG)

◆ **S3626** Maternal serum quadruple marker screen including alpha-fetoprotein (AFP), estriol, human chorionic gonadotropin (HCG) and inhibin a

◆ **S3630** Eosinophil count, blood, direct

▶ New → Revised ✔ Reinstated ~~deleted~~ Deleted
◎ Special coverage instructions ◆ Not covered or valid by Medicare ✳ Carrier discretion

◆ **S3645**   HIV-1 antibody testing of oral mucosal transudate

◆ **S3650**   Saliva test, hormone level; during menopause

◆ **S3652**   Saliva test, hormone level; to assess preterm labor risk

◆ **S3655**   Antisperm antibodies test (immunobead)

◆ **S3708**   Gastrointestinal fat absorption study

~~**S3711**   Circulating tumor cell test~~ ✖

~~**S3713**   KRAS mutation analysis testing~~ ✖

▶ ◆ **S3721**   Prostate cancer antigen 3 (PCA3) testing

◆ **S3722**   Dose optimization by area under the curve (AUC) analysis, for infusional 5-fluorouracil

◆ **S3800**   Genetic testing for amyotrophic lateral sclerosis (ALS)

~~**S3818**   Complete gene sequence analysis; BCRA1 gene~~ ✖

~~**S3819**   Complete gene sequence analysis; BCRA2 gene~~ ✖

~~**S3820**   Complete BCRA1 and BCRA2 gene sequence analysis for susceptibility to breast and ovarian cancer~~ ✖

~~**S3822**   Single mutation analysis (in individual with a known BCRA1 or BCRA2 mutation in the family) for susceptibility to breast and ovarian cancer~~ ✖

~~**S3823**   Three mutation brca1 and brca2 analysis for susceptibility to breast and ovarian cancer in Ashkenazi individuals~~ ✖

~~**S3828**   Complete gene sequence analysis; MLH1 gene~~ ✖

~~**S3829**   Complete gene sequence analysis; MSH2 gene~~ ✖

~~**S3830**   Complete MLH1 and MSH2 gene sequence analysis for hereditary nonpolyposis colorectal cancer (HNPCC) genetic testing~~ ✖

~~**S3831**   Single mutation analysis (in individual with a known MLH1 and MSH2 mutation in the family) for hereditary nonpolyposis colorectal cancer (HNPCC) genetic testing~~ ✖

◆ **S3833**   Complete APC gene sequence analysis for susceptibility to familial adenomatous polyposis (FAP) and attenuated FAP

◆ **S3834**   Single-mutation analysis (in individual with a known APC mutation in the family) for susceptibility to familial adenomatous polyposis (FAP) and attenuated FAP

~~**S3835**   Complete gene sequence analysis for cystic fibrosis genetic testing~~ ✖

~~**S3837**   Complete gene sequence analysis for hemochromatosis genetic testing~~ ✖

◆ **S3840**   DNA analysis for germline mutations of the RET proto-oncogene for susceptibility to multiple endocrine neoplasia type 2

◆ **S3841**   Genetic testing for retinoblastoma

◆ **S3842**   Genetic testing for von Hippel-Lindau disease

~~**S3843**   DNA analysis of the F5 gene for susceptibility to factor V Leiden thrombophilia~~ ✖

◆ **S3844**   DNA analysis of the connexin 26 gene (GJB2) for susceptibility to congenital, profound deafness

◆ **S3845**   Genetic testing for alpha-thalassemia

◆ **S3846**   Genetic testing for hemoglobin E beta-thalassemia

~~**S3847**   Genetic testing for Tay-sachs disease~~ ✖

~~**S3848**   Genetic testing for Gaucher disease~~ ✖

◆ **S3849**   Genetic testing for Niemann-Pick disease

◆ **S3850**   Genetic testing for sickle cell anemia

~~**S3851**   Genetic testing for Canavan disease~~ ✖

◆ **S3852**   DNA analysis for APOE epilson 4 allele for susceptibility to Alzheimer's disease

◆ **S3853**   Genetic testing for myotonic muscular dystrophy

◆ **S3854**   Gene expression profiling panel for use in the management of breast cancer treatment

◆ **S3855**   Genetic testing for detection of mutations in the presenilin - 1 gene

~~**S3860**   Genetic testing, comprehensive cardiac ion channel analysis, for variants in 5 major cardiac ion channel genes for individuals with high index of suspicion for familial long QT syndrome (LQTS) or related syndromes~~ ✖

◆ **S3861**   Genetic testing, sodium channel, voltage-gated, type V, alpha subunit (SCN5A) and variants for suspected Brugada syndrome

---

▶ **New**   → **Revised**   ✔ **Reinstated**   ~~deleted~~ **Deleted**

○ **Special coverage instructions**   ◆ **Not covered or valid by Medicare**   ✳ **Carrier discretion**

~~S3862~~ ~~Genetic testing, family-specific ion channel analysis, for blood relatives of individuals (index case) who have previously tested positive for a genetic variant of a cardiac ion channel syndrome using either one of the above test configurations or confirmed results from another laboratory~~ ✖

◆ **S3865** Comprehensive gene sequence analysis for hypertrophic cardiomyopathy

◆ **S3866** Genetic analysis for a specific gene mutation for hypertrophic cardiomyopathy (HCM) in an individual with a known HCM mutation in the family

◆ **S3870** Comparative genomic hybrization (CGH) microarray testing for developmental delay, autism spectrum disorder and/or mental retardation

◆ **S3890** DNA analysis, fecal, for colorectal cancer screening

◆ **S3900** Surface electromyography (EMG)

◆ **S3902** Ballistrocardiogram

◆ **S3904** Masters two step

Bill on paper. Requires a report.

◆ **S4005** Interim labor facility global (labor occurring but not resulting in delivery)

◆ **S4011** In vitro fertilization; including but not limited to identification and incubation of mature oocytes, fertilization with sperm, incubation of embryo(s), and subsequent visualization for determination of development

◆ **S4013** Complete cycle, gamete intrafallopian transfer (GIFT), case rate

◆ **S4014** Complete cycle, zygote intrafallopian transfer (ZIFT), case rate

◆ **S4015** Complete in vitro fertilization cycle, not otherwise specified, case rate

◆ **S4016** Frozen in vitro fertilization cycle, case rate

◆ **S4017** Incomplete cycle, treatment cancelled prior to stimulation, case rate

◆ **S4018** Frozen embryo transfer procedure cancelled before transfer, case rate

◆ **S4020** In vitro fertilization procedure cancelled before aspiration, case rate

◆ **S4021** In vitro fertilization procedure cancelled after aspiration, case rate

◆ **S4022** Assisted oocyte fertilization, case rate

◆ **S4023** Donor egg cycle, incomplete, case rate

◆ **S4025** Donor services for in vitro fertilization (sperm or embryo), case rate

◆ **S4026** Procurement of donor sperm from sperm bank

◆ **S4027** Storage of previously frozen embryos

◆ **S4028** Microsurgical epididymal sperm aspiration (MESA)

◆ **S4030** Sperm procurement and cryopreservation services; initial visit

◆ **S4031** Sperm procurement and cryopreservation services; subsequent visit

◆ **S4035** Stimulated intrauterine insemination (IUI), case rate

◆ **S4037** Cryopreserved embryo transfer, case rate

◆ **S4040** Monitoring and storage of cryopreserved embryos, per 30 days

◆ **S4042** Management of ovulation induction (interpretation of diagnostic tests and studies, non-face-to-face medical management of the patient), per cycle

◆ **S4981** Insertion of levonorgestrel-releasing intrauterine system

◆ **S4989** Contraceptive intrauterine device (e.g. Progestasert IUD), including implants and supplies

◆ **S4990** Nicotine patches, legend

◆ **S4991** Nicotine patches, non-legend

◆ **S4993** Contraceptive pills for birth control

Only billed by Family Planning Clinics

◆ **S4995** Smoking cessation gum

◆ **S5000** Prescription drug, generic

◆ **S5001** Prescription drug, brand name

◆ **S5010** 5% dextrose and 0.45% normal saline, **1000 ml**

◆ **S5011** 5% dextrose in lactated Ringer's, **1000 ml**

◆ **S5012** 5% dextrose with potassium chloride, **1000 ml**

◆ **S5013** 5% dextrose/0.45% normal saline with potassium chloride and magnesium sulfate, **1000 ml**

◆ **S5014** 5% dextrose/0.45% normal saline with potassium chloride and magnesium sulfate, **1500 ml**

◆ **S5035** Home infusion therapy, routine service of infusion device (e.g. pump maintenance)

◆ **S5036** Home infusion therapy, repair of infusion device (e.g. pump repair)

◆ **S5100** Day care services, adult; per 15 minutes

◆ **S5101** Day care services, adult; per half day

◆ **S5102** Day care services, adult; per diem

▶ New　　→ Revised　　✔ Reinstated　　~~deleted~~ Deleted

⊙ Special coverage instructions　　◆ Not covered or valid by Medicare　　✳ Carrier discretion

◆ **S5105**　Day care services, center-based; services not included in program fee, per diem

◆ **S5108**　Home care training to home care client, per 15 minutes

◆ **S5109**　Home care training to home care client, per session

◆ **S5110**　Home care training, family; per 15 minutes

◆ **S5111**　Home care training, family; per session

◆ **S5115**　Home care training, non-family; per 15 minutes

◆ **S5116**　Home care training, non-family; per session

◆ **S5120**　Chore services; per 15 minutes

◆ **S5121**　Chore services; per diem

◆ **S5125**　Attendant care services; per 15 minutes

◆ **S5126**　Attendant care services; per diem

◆ **S5130**　Homemaker service, NOS; per 15 minutes

◆ **S5131**　Homemaker service, NOS; per diem

◆ **S5135**　Companion care, adult (e.g. IADL/ADL); per 15 minutes

◆ **S5136**　Companion care, adult (e.g. IADL/ADL); per diem

◆ **S5140**　Foster care, adult; per diem

◆ **S5141**　Foster care, adult; per month

◆ **S5145**　Foster care, therapeutic, child; per diem

◆ **S5146**　Foster care, therapeutic, child; per month

◆ **S5150**　Unskilled respite care, not hospice; per 15 minutes

◆ **S5151**　Unskilled respite care, not hospice; per diem

◆ **S5160**　Emergency response system; installation and testing

◆ **S5161**　Emergency response system; service fee, per month (excludes installation and testing)

◆ **S5162**　Emergency response system; purchase only

◆ **S5165**　Home modifications; per service

◆ **S5170**　Home delivered meals, including preparation; per meal

◆ **S5175**　Laundry service, external, professional; per order

◆ **S5180**　Home health respiratory therapy, initial evaluation

◆ **S5181**　Home health respiratory therapy, NOS, per diem

◆ **S5185**　Medication reminder service, non-face-to-face; per month

◆ **S5190**　Wellness assessment, performed by non-physician

◆ **S5199**　Personal care item, NOS, each

◆ **S5497**　Home infusion therapy, catheter care/maintenance, not otherwise classified; includes administrative services, professional pharmacy services, care coordination, and all necessary supplies and equipment (drugs and nursing visits coded separately), per diem

◆ **S5498**　Home infusion therapy, catheter care/maintenance, simple (single lumen), includes administrative services, professional pharmacy services, care coordination and all necessary supplies and equipment, (drugs and nursing visits coded separately), per diem

◆ **S5501**　Home infusion therapy, catheter care/maintenance, complex (more than one lumen), includes administrative services, professional pharmacy services, care coordination, and all necessary supplies and equipment (drugs and nursing visits coded separately), per diem

◆ **S5502**　Home infusion therapy, catheter care/maintenance, implanted access device, includes administrative services, professional pharmacy services, care coordination, and all necessary supplies and equipment, (drugs and nursing visits coded separately), per diem (use this code for interim maintenance of vascular access not currently in use)

◆ **S5517**　Home infusion therapy, all supplies necessary for restoration of catheter patency or declotting

◆ **S5518**　Home infusion therapy, all supplies necessary for catheter repair

◆ **S5520**　Home infusion therapy, all supplies (including catheter) necessary for a peripherally inserted central venous catheter (PICC) line insertion

　　　　　Bill on paper. Requires a report.

◆ **S5521**　Home infusion therapy, all supplies (including catheter) necessary for a midline catheter insertion

◆ **S5522**　Home infusion therapy, insertion of peripherally inserted central venous catheter (PICC), nursing services only (no supplies or catheter included)

◆ **S5523**　Home infusion therapy, insertion of midline central venous catheter, nursing services only (no supplies or catheter included)

▶ New　→ Revised　✔ Reinstated　deleted Deleted
○ Special coverage instructions　◆ Not covered or valid by Medicare　✳ Carrier discretion

◆ **S5550** Insulin, rapid onset, **5 units**

◆ **S5551** Insulin, most rapid onset (Lispro or Aspart); **5 units**

◆ **S5552** Insulin, intermediate acting (NPH or Lente); **5 units**

◆ **S5553** Insulin, long acting; **5 units**

◆ **S5560** Insulin delivery device, reusable pen; **1.5 ml** size

◆ **S5561** Insulin delivery device, reusable pen; **3 ml** size

◆ **S5565** Insulin cartridge for use in insulin delivery device other than pump; **150 units**

◆ **S5566** Insulin cartridge for use in insulin delivery device other than pump; **300 units**

◆ **S5570** Insulin delivery device, disposable pen (including insulin); **1.5 ml** size

◆ **S5571** Insulin delivery device, disposable pen (including insulin); **3 ml** size

◆ **S8030** Scleral application of tantalum ring(s) for localization of lesions for proton beam therapy

◆ **S8035** Magnetic source imaging

◆ **S8037** Magnetic resonance cholangiopancreatography (MRCP)

◆ **S8040** Topographic brain mapping

◆ **S8042** Magnetic resonance imaging (MRI), low-field

~~S8049~~ ~~Intraoperative radiation therapy (single administration)~~ ✱

◆ **S8055** Ultrasound guidance for multifetal pregnancy reduction(s), technical component (only to be used when the physician doing the reduction procedure does not perform the ultrasound, guidance is included in the CPT code for multifetal pregnancy reduction - 59866)

◆ **S8080** Scintimammography (radioimmunoscintigraphy of the breast), unilateral, including supply of radiopharmaceutical

◆ **S8085** Fluorine-18 fluorodeoxyglucose (F-18 FDG) imaging using dual-head coincidence detection system (non-dedicated PET scan)

◆ **S8092** Electron beam computed tomography (also known as ultrafast CT, cine CT)

◆ **S8096** Portable peak flow meter

◆ **S8097** Asthma kit (including but not limited to portable peak expiratory flow meter, instructional video, brochure, and/or spacer)

◆ **S8100** Holding chamber or spacer for use with an inhaler or nebulizer; without mask

◆ **S8101** Holding chamber or spacer for use with an inhaler or nebulizer; with mask

◆ **S8110** Peak expiratory flow rate (physician services)

◆ **S8120** Oxygen contents, gaseous, 1 unit equals 1 cubic foot

◆ **S8121** Oxygen contents, liquid, 1 unit equals 1 pound

◆ **S8130** Interferential current stimulator, 2 channel

◆ **S8131** Interferential current stimulator, 4 channel

◆ **S8185** Flutter device

◆ **S8186** Swivel adaptor

◆ **S8189** Tracheostomy supply, not otherwise classified

◆ **S8210** Mucus trap

◆ **S8262** Mandibular orthopedic repositioning device, each

◆ **S8265** Haberman feeder for cleft lip/palate

◆ **S8270** Enuresis alarm, using auditory buzzer and/or vibration device

◆ **S8301** Infection control supplies, not otherwise specified

◆ **S8415** Supplies for home delivery of infant

◆ **S8420** Gradient pressure aid (sleeve and glove combination), custom made

◆ **S8421** Gradient pressure aid (sleeve and glove combination), ready made

◆ **S8422** Gradient pressure aid (sleeve), custom made, medium weight

◆ **S8423** Gradient pressure aid (sleeve), custom made, heavy weight

◆ **S8424** Gradient pressure aid (sleeve), ready made

◆ **S8425** Gradient pressure aid (glove), custom made, medium weight

◆ **S8426** Gradient pressure aid (glove), custom made, heavy weight

◆ **S8427** Gradient pressure aid (glove), ready made

◆ **S8428** Gradient pressure aid (gauntlet), ready made

◆ **S8429** Gradient pressure exterior wrap

◆ **S8430** Padding for compression bandage, roll

◆ **S8431** Compression bandage, roll

◆ **S8450** Splint, prefabricated, digit (specify digit by use of modifier)

◆ **S8451** Splint, prefabricated, wrist or ankle

▶ **New** → **Revised** ✔ **Reinstated** ~~deleted~~ **Deleted**

☺ **Special coverage instructions** ◆ **Not covered or valid by Medicare** ✱ **Carrier discretion**

◆ **S8452** Splint, prefabricated, elbow

◆ **S8460** Camisole, post-mastectomy

◆ **S8490** Insulin syringes (100 syringes, any size)

▶◆ **S8930** Electrical stimulation of auricular acupuncture points; each 15 minutes of personal one-on-one contact with the patient

◆ **S8940** Equestrian/Hippotherapy, per session

◆ **S8948** Application of a modality (requiring constant provider attendance) to one or more areas; low-level laser; each 15 minutes

◆ **S8950** Complex lymphedema therapy, each 15 minutes

◆ **S8990** Physical or manipulative therapy performed for maintenance rather than restoration

◆ **S8999** Resuscitation bag (for use by patient on artificial respiration during power failure or other catastrophic event)

◆ **S9001** Home uterine monitor with or without associated nursing services

◆ **S9007** Ultrafiltration monitor

◆ **S9015** Automated EEG monitoring

◆ **S9024** Paranasal sinus ultrasound

◆ **S9025** Omnicardiogram/cardiointegram

◆ **S9034** Extracorporeal shockwave lithotripsy for gall stones (if performed with ERCP, use 43265)

◆ **S9055** Procuren or other growth factor preparation to promote wound healing

◆ **S9056** Coma stimulation per diem

◆ **S9061** Home administration of aerosolized drug therapy (e.g., pentamidine); administrative services, professional pharmacy services, care coordination, all necessary supplies and equipment (drugs and nursing visits coded separately), per diem

◆ **S9083** Global fee urgent care centers

◆ **S9088** Services provided in an urgent care center (list in addition to code for service)

◆ **S9090** Vertebral axial decompression, per session

◆ **S9097** Home visit for wound care

◆ **S9098** Home visit, phototherapy services (e.g. Bili-Lite), including equipment rental, nursing services, blood draw, supplies, and other services, per diem

~~S9109~~ ~~Congestive heart failure~~ ✖
~~telemonitoring, equipment rental,~~
~~including telescale, computer system~~
~~and software, telephone connections,~~
~~and maintenance, per month~~

▶◆ **S9110** Telemonitoring of patient in their home, including all necessary equipment; computer system, connections, and software; maintenance; patient education and support; per month

◆ **S9117** Back school, per visit

◆ **S9122** Home health aide or certified nurse assistant, providing care in the home; per hour

◆ **S9123** Nursing care, in the home; by registered nurse, per hour (use for general nursing care only, not to be used when CPT codes 99500-99602 can be used)

◆ **S9124** Nursing care, in the home; by licensed practical nurse, per hour

◆ **S9125** Respite care, in the home, per diem

◆ **S9126** Hospice care, in the home, per diem

◆ **S9127** Social work visit, in the home, per diem

◆ **S9128** Speech therapy, in the home, per diem

◆ **S9129** Occupational therapy, in the home, per diem

◆ **S9131** Physical therapy; in the home, per diem

◆ **S9140** Diabetic management program, follow-up visit to non-MD provider

◆ **S9141** Diabetic management program, follow-up visit to MD provider

◆ **S9145** Insulin pump initiation, instruction in initial use of pump (pump not included)

◆ **S9150** Evaluation by ocularist

◆ **S9152** Speech therapy, re-evaluation

◆ **S9208** Home management of preterm labor, including administrative services, professional pharmacy services, care coordination, and all necessary supplies or equipment (drugs and nursing visits coded separately), per diem (do not use this code with any home infusion per diem code)

◆ **S9209** Home management of preterm premature rupture of membranes (PPROM), including administrative services, professional pharmacy services, care coordination, and all necessary supplies or equipment (drugs and nursing visits coded separately), per diem (do not use this code with any home infusion per diem code)

◆ **S9211** Home management of gestational hypertension, includes administrative services, professional pharmacy services, care coordination, and all necessary supplies and equipment (drugs and nursing visits coded separately); per diem (do not use this code with any home infusion per diem code)

| ▶ New | → Revised | ✔ Reinstated | ~~deleted~~ Deleted |

☺ Special coverage instructions ◆ Not covered or valid by Medicare ✳ Carrier discretion

◆ **S9212** Home management of postpartum hypertension, includes administrative services, professional pharmacy services, care coordination, and all necessary supplies and equipment (drugs and nursing visits coded separately), per diem (do not use this code with any home infusion per diem code)

◆ **S9213** Home management of preeclampsia, includes administrative services, professional pharmacy services, care coordination, and all necessary supplies and equipment (drugs and nursing services coded separately); per diem (do not use this code with any home infusion per diem code)

◆ **S9214** Home management of gestational diabetes, includes administrative services, professional pharmacy services, care coordination, and all necessary supplies and equipment (drugs and nursing visits coded separately); per diem (do not use this code with any home infusion per diem code)

◆ **S9325** Home infusion therapy, pain management infusion; administrative services, professional pharmacy services, care coordination, and all necessary supplies and equipment, (drugs and nursing visits coded separately), per diem (do not use this code with S9326, S9327 or S9328)

◆ **S9326** Home infusion therapy, continuous (twenty-four hours or more) pain management infusion; administrative services, professional pharmacy services, care coordination, and all necessary supplies and equipment (drugs and nursing visits coded separately), per diem

◆ **S9327** Home infusion therapy, intermittent (less than twenty-four hours) pain management infusion; administrative services, professional pharmacy services, care coordination, and all necessary supplies and equipment (drugs and nursing visits coded separately), per diem

◆ **S9328** Home infusion therapy, implanted pump pain management infusion; administrative services, professional pharmacy services, care coordination, and all necessary supplies and equipment (drugs and nursing visits coded separately), per diem

◆ **S9329** Home infusion therapy, chemotherapy infusion; administrative services, professional pharmacy services, care coordination, and all necessary supplies and equipment (drugs and nursing visits coded separately), per diem (do not use this code with S9330 or S9331)

◆ **S9330** Home infusion therapy, continuous (twenty-four hours or more) chemotherapy infusion; administrative services, professional pharmacy services, care coordination, and all necessary supplies and equipment (drugs and nursing visits coded separately), per diem

◆ **S9331** Home infusion therapy, intermittent (less than twenty-four hours) chemotherapy infusion; administrative services, professional pharmacy services, care coordination, and all necessary supplies and equipment (drugs and nursing visits coded separately), per diem

◆ **S9335** Home therapy, hemodialysis; administrative services, professional pharmacy services, care coordination, and all necessary supplies and equipment (drugs and nursing services coded separately), per diem

◆ **S9336** Home infusion therapy, continuous anticoagulant infusion therapy (e.g. heparin), administrative services, professional pharmacy services, care coordination, and all necessary supplies and equipment (drugs and nursing visits coded separately), per diem

◆ **S9338** Home infusion therapy, immunotherapy, administrative services, professional pharmacy services, care coordination, and all necessary supplies and equipment (drug and nursing visits coded separately), per diem

◆ **S9339** Home therapy; peritoneal dialysis, administrative services, professional pharmacy services, care coordination and all necessary supplies and equipment (drugs and nursing visits coded separately), per diem

◆ **S9340** Home therapy; enteral nutrition; administrative services, professional pharmacy services, care coordination, and all necessary supplies and equipment (enteral formula and nursing visits coded separately), per diem

---

▶ New → Revised ✔ Reinstated ~~deleted~~ Deleted

☉ Special coverage instructions ◆ Not covered or valid by Medicare ✳ Carrier discretion

◆ **S9341** Home therapy; enteral nutrition via gravity; administrative services, professional pharmacy services, care coordination, and all necessary supplies and equipment (enteral formula and nursing visits coded separately), per diem

◆ **S9342** Home therapy; enteral nutrition via pump; administrative services, professional pharmacy services, care coordination, and all necessary supplies and equipment (enteral formula and nursing visits coded separately), per diem

◆ **S9343** Home therapy; enteral nutrition via bolus; administrative services, professional pharmacy services, care coordination, and all necessary supplies and equipment (enteral formula and nursing visits coded separately), per diem

◆ **S9345** Home infusion therapy, anti-hemophilic agent infusion therapy (e.g. Factor VIII); administrative services, professional pharmacy services, care coordination, and all necessary supplies and equipment (drugs and nursing visits coded separately), per diem

◆ **S9346** Home infusion therapy, alpha-1-proteinase inhibitor (e.g., Prolastin); administrative services, professional pharmacy services, care coordination, and all necessary supplies and equipment (drugs and nursing visits coded separately), per diem

◆ **S9347** Home infusion therapy, uninterrupted, long-term, controlled rate intravenous or subcutaneous infusion therapy (e.g. Epoprostenol); administrative services, professional pharmacy services, care coordination, and all necessary supplies and equipment (drugs and nursing visits coded separately), per diem

◆ **S9348** Home infusion therapy, sympathomimetic/inotropic agent infusion therapy (e.g., Dobutamine); administrative services, professional pharmacy services, care coordination, all necessary supplies and equipment (drugs and nursing visits coded separately), per diem

◆ **S9349** Home infusion therapy, tocolytic infusion therapy; administrative services, professional pharmacy services, care coordination, and all necessary supplies and equipment (drugs and nursing visits coded separately), per diem

◆ **S9351** Home infusion therapy, continuous or intermittent anti-emetic infusion therapy; administrative services, professional pharmacy services, care coordination, and all necessary supplies and equipment (drugs and visits coded separately), per diem

◆ **S9353** Home infusion therapy, continuous insulin infusion therapy; administrative services, professional pharmacy services, care coordination, and all necessary supplies and equipment (drugs and nursing visits coded separately), per diem

◆ **S9355** Home infusion therapy, chelation therapy; administrative services, professional pharmacy services, care coordination, and all necessary supplies and equipment (drugs and nursing visits coded separately), per diem

◆ **S9357** Home infusion therapy, enzyme replacement intravenous therapy; (e.g. Imiglucerase); administrative services, professional pharmacy services, care coordination, and all necessary supplies and equipment (drugs and nursing visits coded separately), per diem

◆ **S9359** Home infusion therapy, anti-tumor necrosis factor intravenous therapy; (e.g. Infliximab); administrative services, professional pharmacy services, care coordination, and all necessary supplies and equipment (drugs and nursing visits coded separately), per diem

◆ **S9361** Home infusion therapy, diuretic intravenous therapy; administrative services, professional pharmacy services, care coordination, and all necessary supplies and equipment (drugs and nursing visits coded separately), per diem

◆ **S9363** Home infusion therapy, anti-spasmotic therapy; administrative services, professional pharmacy services, care coordination, and all necessary supplies and equipment (drugs and nursing visits coded separately), per diem

◆ **S9364** Home infusion therapy, total parenteral nutrition (TPN); administrative services, professional pharmacy services, care coordination, and all necessary supplies and equipment including standard TPN formula (lipids, specialty amino acid formulas, drugs other than in standard formula, and nursing visits coded separately) per diem (do not use with home infusion codes S9365-S9368 using daily volume scales)

▶ New → Revised ✔ Reinstated ~~deleted~~ Deleted

☺ Special coverage instructions ◆ Not covered or valid by Medicare ✳ Carrier discretion

◆ **S9365** Home infusion therapy, total parenteral nutrition (TPN); one liter per day, administrative services, professional pharmacy services, care coordination, and all necessary supplies and equipment including standard TPN formula (lipids, specialty amino acid formulas, drugs other than in standard formula and nursing visits coded separately), per diem

◆ **S9366** Home infusion therapy, total parenteral nutrition (TPN); more than one liter but no more than two liters per day, administrative services, professional pharmacy services, care coordination, and all necessary supplies and equipment including standard TPN formula; (lipids, specialty amino acid formulas, drugs other than in standard formula and nursing visits coded separately), per diem

◆ **S9367** Home infusion therapy, total parenteral nutrition (TPN); more than two liters but no more than three liters per day, administrative services, professional pharmacy services, care coordination, and all necessary supplies and equipment including standard TPN formula; (lipids, specialty amino acid formulas, drugs other than in standard formula and nursing visits coded separately), per diem

◆ **S9368** Home infusion therapy, total parenteral nutrition (TPN); more than three liters per day, administrative services, professional pharmacy services, care coordination, and all necessary supplies and equipment (including standard TPN formula; lipids, specialty amino acid formulas, drugs other than in standard formula and nursing visits coded separately), per diem

◆ **S9370** Home therapy, intermittent anti-emetic injection therapy; administrative services, professional pharmacy services, care coordination, and all necessary supplies and equipment (drugs and nursing visits coded separately), per diem

◆ **S9372** Home therapy; intermittent anticoagulant injection therapy (e.g., heparin); administrative services, professional pharmacy services, care coordination, and all necessary supplies and equipment (drugs and nursing visits coded separately), per diem (do not use this code for flushing of infusion devices with heparin to maintain patency)

◆ **S9373** Home infusion therapy, hydration therapy; administrative services, professional pharmacy services, care coordination, and all necessary supplies and equipment (drugs and nursing visits coded separately), per diem (do not use with hydration therapy codes S9374-S9377 using daily volume scales)

◆ **S9374** Home infusion therapy, hydration therapy; one liter per day, administrative services, professional pharmacy services, care coordination, and all necessary supplies and equipment (drugs and nursing visits coded separately), per diem

◆ **S9375** Home infusion therapy, hydration therapy; more than one liter but no more than two liters per day, administrative services, professional pharmacy services, care coordination, and all necessary supplies and equipment (drugs and nursing visits coded separately), per diem

◆ **S9376** Home infusion therapy, hydration therapy; more than two liters but no more than three liters per day, administrative services, professional pharmacy services, care coordination, and all necessary supplies and equipment (drugs and nursing visits coded separately), per diem

◆ **S9377** Home infusion therapy, hydration therapy; more than three liters per day, administrative services, professional pharmacy services, care coordination, and all necessary supplies (drugs and nursing visits coded separately), per diem

◆ **S9379** Home infusion therapy, infusion therapy, not otherwise classified; administrative services, professional pharmacy services, care coordination, and all necessary supplies and equipment (drugs and nursing visits coded separately), per diem

◆ **S9381** Delivery or service to high risk areas requiring escort or extra protection, per visit

◆ **S9401** Anticoagulation clinic, inclusive of all services except laboratory tests, per session

◆ **S9430** Pharmacy compounding and dispensing services

◆ **S9433** Medical food nutritionally complete, administered orally, providing 100% of nutritional intake

▶ New → Revised ✔ Reinstated ~~deleted~~ Deleted

☺ Special coverage instructions ◆ Not covered or valid by Medicare ✳ Carrier discretion

◆ **S9434** Modified solid food supplements for inborn errors of metabolism

◆ **S9435** Medical foods for inborn errors of metabolism

◆ **S9436** Childbirth preparation/Lamaze classes, non-physician provider, per session

◆ **S9437** Childbirth refresher classes, non-physician provider, per session

◆ **S9438** Cesarean birth classes, non-physician provider, per session

◆ **S9439** VBAC (vaginal birth after cesarean) classes, non-physician provider, per session

◆ **S9441** Asthma education, non-physician provider, per session

◆ **S9442** Birthing classes, non-physician provider, per session

◆ **S9443** Lactation classes, non-physician provider, per session

◆ **S9444** Parenting classes, non-physician provider, per session

◆ **S9445** Patient education, not otherwise classified, non-physician provider, individual, per session

◆ **S9446** Patient education, not otherwise classified, non-physician provider, group, per session

◆ **S9447** Infant safety (including CPR) classes, non-physician provider, per session

◆ **S9449** Weight management classes, non-physician provider, per session

◆ **S9451** Exercise classes, non-physician provider, per session

◆ **S9452** Nutrition classes, non-physician provider, per session

◆ **S9453** Smoking cessation classes, non-physician provider, per session

◆ **S9454** Stress management classes, non-physician provider, per session

◆ **S9455** Diabetic management program, group session

◆ **S9460** Diabetic management program, nurse visit

◆ **S9465** Diabetic management program, dietitian visit

◆ **S9470** Nutritional counseling, dietitian visit

◆ **S9472** Cardiac rehabilitation program, non-physician provider, per diem

◆ **S9473** Pulmonary rehabilitation program, non-physician provider, per diem

◆ **S9474** Enterostomal therapy by a registered nurse certified in enterostomal therapy, per diem

◆ **S9475** Ambulatory setting substance abuse treatment or detoxification services, per diem

◆ **S9476** Vestibular rehabilitation program, non-physician provider, per diem

◆ **S9480** Intensive outpatient psychiatric services, per diem

◆ **S9482** Family stabilization services, per 15 minutes

◆ **S9484** Crisis intervention mental health services, per hour

◆ **S9485** Crisis intervention mental health services, per diem

◆ **S9490** Home infusion therapy, corticosteroid infusion; administrative services, professional pharmacy services, care coordination, and all necessary supplies and equipment (drugs and nursing visits coded separately), per diem

◆ **S9494** Home infusion therapy, antibiotic, antiviral, or antifungal therapy; administrative services, professional pharmacy services, care coordination, and all necessary supplies and equipment (drugs and nursing visits coded separately) per diem, (do not use this code with home infusion codes for hourly dosing schedules S9497-S9504)

◆ **S9497** Home infusion therapy, antibiotic, antiviral, or antifungal therapy; once every 3 hours; administrative services, professional pharmacy services, care coordination, and all necessary supplies and equipment (drugs and nursing visits coded separately), per diem

◆ **S9500** Home infusion therapy, antibiotic, antiviral, or antifungal therapy; once every 24 hours; administrative services, professional pharmacy services, care coordination, and all necessary supplies and equipment (drugs and nursing visits coded separately), per diem

◆ **S9501** Home infusion therapy, antibiotic, antiviral, or antifungal therapy; once every 12 hours; administrative services, professional pharmacy services, care coordination, and all necessary supplies and equipment (drugs and nursing visits coded separately), per diem

◆ **S9502** Home infusion therapy, antibiotic, antiviral, or antifungal therapy; once every 8 hours, administrative services, professional pharmacy services, care coordination, and all necessary supplies and equipment (drugs and nursing visits coded separately), per diem

---

▶ New   → Revised   ✔ Reinstated   ~~deleted~~ Deleted

☯ Special coverage instructions   ◆ Not covered or valid by Medicare   ✳ Carrier discretion

◆ **S9503** Home infusion therapy, antibiotic, antiviral, or antifungal; once every 6 hours; administrative services, professional pharmacy services, care coordination, and all necessary supplies and equipment (drugs and nursing visits coded separately), per diem

◆ **S9504** Home infusion therapy, antibiotic, antiviral, or antifungal; once every 4 hours; administrative services, professional pharmacy services, care coordination, and all necessary supplies and equipment (drugs and nursing visits coded separately), per diem

◆ **S9529** Routine venipuncture for collection of specimen(s), single home bound, nursing home, or skilled nursing facility patient

◆ **S9537** Home therapy; hematopoietic hormone injection therapy (e.g. erythropoietin, G-CSF, GM-CSF); administrative services, professional pharmacy services, care coordination, and all necessary supplies and equipment (drugs and nursing visits coded separately), per diem

◆ **S9538** Home transfusion of blood product(s); administrative services, professional pharmacy services, care coordination, and all necessary supplies and equipment (blood products, drugs, and nursing visits coded separately), per diem

◆ **S9542** Home injectable therapy; not otherwise classified, including administrative services, professional pharmacy services, care coordination, and all necessary supplies and equipment (drugs and nursing visits coded separately), per diem

◆ **S9558** Home injectable therapy; growth hormone, including administrative services, professional pharmacy services, care coordination, and all necessary supplies and equipment (drugs and nursing visits coded separately), per diem

◆ **S9559** Home injectable therapy; interferon, including administrative services, professional pharmacy services, care coordination, and all necessary supplies and equipment (drugs and nursing visits coded separately), per diem

◆ **S9560** Home injectable therapy; hormonal therapy (e.g., Leuprolide, Goserelin), including administrative services, professional pharmacy services, care coordination, and all necessary supplies and equipment (drugs and nursing visits coded separately), per diem

◆ **S9562** Home injectable therapy, palivizumab, including administrative services, professional pharmacy services, care coordination, and all necessary supplies and equipment (drugs and nursing visits coded separately), per diem

◆ **S9590** Home therapy, irrigation therapy (e.g. sterile irrigation of an organ or anatomical cavity); including administrative services, professional pharmacy services, care coordination, and all necessary supplies and equipment (drugs and nursing visits coded separately), per diem

◆ **S9810** Home therapy; professional pharmacy services for provision of infusion, specialty drug administration, and/or disease state management, not otherwise classified, per hour (do not use this code with any per diem code)

◆ **S9900** Services by journal-listed Christian Science Practitioner for the purpose of healing, per diem

◆ **S9970** Health club membership, annual

◆ **S9975** Transplant related lodging, meals and transportation, per diem

◆ **S9976** Lodging, per diem, not otherwise classified

◆ **S9977** Meals, per diem, not otherwise specified

◆ **S9981** Medical records copying fee, administrative

◆ **S9982** Medical records copying fee, per page

◆ **S9986** Not medically necessary service (patient is aware that service not medically necessary)

◆ **S9988** Services provided as part of a Phase I clinical trial

◆ **S9989** Services provided outside of the United States of America (list in addition to code(s) for services(s))

◆ **S9990** Services provided as part of a Phase II clinical trial

◆ **S9991** Services provided as part of a Phase III clinical trial

◆ **S9992** Transportation costs to and from trial location and local transportation costs (e.g., fares for taxicab or bus) for clinical trial participant and one caregiver/companion

◆ **S9994** Lodging costs (e.g., hotel charges) for clinical trial participant and one caregiver/companion

◆ **S9996** Meals for clinical trial participant and one caregiver/companion

◆ **S9999** Sales tax

▶ New   → Revised   ✔ Reinstated   ~~deleted~~ Deleted

✺ Special coverage instructions   ◆ Not covered or valid by Medicare   ✱ Carrier discretion

TEMPORARY NATIONAL CODES ESTABLISHED BY MEDICAID (T1000-T9999)

Not Valid For Medicare

◆ **T1000** Private duty/independent nursing service(s) - licensed, up to 15 minutes

◆ **T1001** Nursing assessment/evaluation

◆ **T1002** RN services, up to 15 minutes

◆ **T1003** LPN/LVN services, up to 15 minutes

◆ **T1004** Services of a qualified nursing aide, up to 15 minutes

◆ **T1005** Respite care services, up to 15 minutes

◆ **T1006** Alcohol and/or substance abuse services, family/couple counseling

◆ **T1007** Alcohol and/or substance abuse services, treatment plan development and/or modification

◆ **T1009** Child sitting services for children of the individual receiving alcohol and/or substance abuse services

◆ **T1010** Meals for individuals receiving alcohol and/or substance abuse services (when meals not included in the program)

◆ **T1012** Alcohol and/or substance abuse services, skills development

◆ **T1013** Sign language or oral interpretive services, per 15 minutes

◆ **T1014** Telehealth transmission, per minute, professional services bill separately

◆ **T1015** Clinic visit/encounter, all-inclusive

◆ **T1016** Case Management, each 15 minutes

◆ **T1017** Targeted Case Management, each 15 minutes

◆ **T1018** School-based individualized education program (IEP) services, bundled

◆ **T1019** Personal care services, per 15 minutes, not for an inpatient or resident of a hospital, nursing facility, ICF/MR or IMD, part of the individualized plan of treatment (code may not be used to identify services provided by home health aide or certified nurse assistant)

◆ **T1020** Personal care services, per diem, not for an inpatient or resident of a hospital, nursing facility, ICF/MR or IMD, part of the individualized plan of treatment (code may not be used to identify services provided by home health aide or certified nurse assistant)

◆ **T1021** Home health aide or certified nurse assistant, per visit

◆ **T1022** Contracted home health agency services, all services provided under contract, per day

◆ **T1023** Screening to determine the appropriateness of consideration of an individual for participation in a specified program, project or treatment protocol, per encounter

◆ **T1024** Evaluation and treatment by an integrated, specialty team contracted to provide coordinated care to multiple or severely handicapped children, per encounter

◆ **T1025** Intensive, extended multidisciplinary services provided in a clinic setting to children with complex medical, physical, mental and psychosocial impairments, per diem

◆ **T1026** Intensive, extended multidisciplinary services provided in a clinic setting to children with complex medical, physical, medical and psychosocial impairments, per hour

◆ **T1027** Family training and counseling for child development, per 15 minutes

◆ **T1028** Assessment of home, physical and family environment, to determine suitability to meet patient's medical needs

◆ **T1029** Comprehensive environmental lead investigation, not including laboratory analysis, per dwelling

◆ **T1030** Nursing care, in the home, by registered nurse, per diem

◆ **T1031** Nursing care, in the home, by licensed practical nurse, per diem

◆ **T1502** Administration of oral, intramuscular and/or subcutaneous medication by health care agency/professional, per visit

◆ **T1503** Administration of medication, other than oral and/or injectable, by a health care agency/professional, per visit

◆ **T1505** Electronic medication compliance management device, includes all components and accessories, not otherwise classified

◆ **T1999** Miscellaneous therapeutic items and supplies, retail purchases, not otherwise classified; identify product in "remarks"

◆ **T2001** Non-emergency transportation; patient attendant/escort

---

▶ New   → Revised   ✔ Reinstated   deleted Deleted

☉ Special coverage instructions   ◆ Not covered or valid by Medicare   ✳ Carrier discretion

◆ **T2002** Non-emergency transportation; per diem

◆ **T2003** Non-emergency transportation; encounter/trip

◆ **T2004** Non-emergency transport; commercial carrier, multi-pass

◆ **T2005** Non-emergency transportation: stretcher van

◆ **T2007** Transportation waiting time, air ambulance and non-emergency vehicle, one-half (1/2) hour increments

◆ **T2010** Preadmission screening and resident review (PASRR) level I identification screening, per screen

◆ **T2011** Preadmission screening and resident review (PASRR) level II evaluation, per evaluation

◆ **T2012** Habilitation, educational, waiver; per diem

◆ **T2013** Habilitation, educational, waiver; per hour

◆ **T2014** Habilitation, prevocational, waiver; per diem

◆ **T2015** Habilitation, prevocational, waiver; per hour

◆ **T2016** Habilitation, residential, waiver; per diem

◆ **T2017** Habilitation, residential, waiver; 15 minutes

◆ **T2018** Habilitation, supported employment, waiver; per diem

◆ **T2019** Habilitation, supported employment, waiver; per 15 minutes

◆ **T2020** Day habilitation, waiver; per diem

◆ **T2021** Day habilitation, waiver; per 15 minutes

◆ **T2022** Case management, per month

◆ **T2023** Targeted case management; per month

◆ **T2024** Service assessment/plan of care development, waiver

◆ **T2025** Waiver services; not otherwise specified (NOS)

◆ **T2026** Specialized childcare, waiver; per diem

◆ **T2027** Specialized childcare, waiver; per 15 minutes

◆ **T2028** Specialized supply, not otherwise specified, waiver

◆ **T2029** Specialized medical equipment, not otherwise specified, waiver

◆ **T2030** Assisted living, waiver; per month

◆ **T2031** Assisted living; waiver, per diem

◆ **T2032** Residential care, not otherwise specified (NOS), waiver; per month

◆ **T2033** Residential care, not otherwise specified (NOS), waiver; per diem

◆ **T2034** Crisis intervention, waiver; per diem

◆ **T2035** Utility services to support medical equipment and assistive technology/devices, waiver

◆ **T2036** Therapeutic camping, overnight, waiver; each session

◆ **T2037** Therapeutic camping, day, waiver; each session

◆ **T2038** Community transition, waiver; per service

◆ **T2039** Vehicle modifications, waiver; per service

◆ **T2040** Financial management, self-directed, waiver; per 15 minutes

◆ **T2041** Supports brokerage, self-directed, waiver; per 15 minutes

◆ **T2042** Hospice routine home care; per diem

◆ **T2043** Hospice continuous home care; per hour

◆ **T2044** Hospice inpatient respite care; per diem

◆ **T2045** Hospice general inpatient care; per diem

◆ **T2046** Hospice long term care, room and board only; per diem

◆ **T2048** Behavioral health; long-term care residential (non-acute care in a residential treatment program where stay is typically longer than 30 days), with room and board, per diem

◆ **T2049** Non-emergency transportation; stretcher van, mileage; per mile

◆ **T2101** Human breast milk processing, storage and distribution only

◆ **T4521** Adult sized disposable incontinence product, brief/diaper, small, each
  IOM: 100-03, 4, 280.1

◆ **T4522** Adult sized disposable incontinence product, brief/diaper, medium, each
  IOM: 100-03, 4, 280.1

◆ **T4523** Adult sized disposable incontinence product, brief/diaper, large, each
  IOM: 100-03, 4, 280.1

◆ **T4524** Adult sized disposable incontinence product, brief/diaper, extra large, each
  IOM: 100-03, 4, 280.1

▶ **New**   → **Revised**   ✔ **Reinstated**   ~~deleted~~ **Deleted**

☺ **Special coverage instructions**   ◆ **Not covered or valid by Medicare**   ✳ **Carrier discretion**

◆ **T4525** Adult sized disposable incontinence product, protective underwear/pull-on, small size, each

IOM: 100-03, 4, 280.1

◆ **T4526** Adult sized disposable incontinence product, protective underwear/pull-on, medium size, each

IOM: 100-03, 4, 280.1

◆ **T4527** Adult sized disposable incontinence product, protective underwear/pull-on, large size, each

IOM: 100-03, 4, 280.1

◆ **T4528** Adult sized disposable incontinence product, protective underwear/pull-on, extra large size, each

IOM: 100-03, 4, 280.1

◆ **T4529** Pediatric sized disposable incontinence product, brief/diaper, small/medium size, each

IOM: 100-03, 4, 280.1

◆ **T4530** Pediatric sized disposable incontinence product, brief/diaper, large size, each

IOM: 100-03, 4, 280.1

◆ **T4531** Pediatric sized disposable incontinence product, protective underwear/pull-on, small/medium size, each

IOM: 100-03, 4, 280.1

◆ **T4532** Pediatric sized disposable incontinence product, protective underwear/pull-on, large size, each

IOM: 100-03, 4, 280.1

◆ **T4533** Youth sized disposable incontinence product, brief/diaper, each

IOM: 100-03, 4, 280.1

◆ **T4534** Youth sized disposable incontinence product, protective underwear/pull-on, each

IOM: 100-03, 4, 280.1

◆ **T4535** Disposable liner/shield/guard/pad/undergarment, for incontinence, each

IOM: 100-03, 4, 280.1

◆ **T4536** Incontinence product, protective underwear/pull-on, reusable, any size, each

IOM: 100-03, 4, 280.1

◆ **T4537** Incontinence product, protective underpad, reusable, bed size, each

IOM: 100-03, 4, 280.1

◆ **T4538** Diaper service, reusable diaper, each diaper

IOM: 100-03, 4, 280.1

◆ **T4539** Incontinence product, diaper/brief, reusable, any size, each

IOM: 100-03, 4, 280.1

◆ **T4540** Incontinence product, protective underpad, reusable, chair size, each

IOM: 100-03, 4, 280.1

◆ **T4541** Incontinence product, disposable underpad, large, each

◆ **T4542** Incontinence product, disposable underpad, small size, each

◆ **T4543** Disposable incontinence product, brief/diaper, bariatric, each

IOM: 100-03, 4, 280.1

◆ **T5001** Positioning seat for persons with special orthopedic needs, supply, not otherwise specified

◆ **T5999** Supply, not otherwise specified

▶ New	→ Revised	✔ Reinstated	~~deleted~~ Deleted
☺ Special coverage instructions	◆ Not covered or valid by Medicare	✳ Carrier discretion	

VISION SERVICES (V0000-V2999)

Frames

V2020-V2025: Bill DME/MAC

⊙ **V2020** Frames, purchases

Includes cost of frame/replacement and dispensing fee. One unit of service represents one pair of eyeglass frames.

IOM: 100-02, 15, 120

◆ **V2025** Deluxe frame

Not a benefit. Billing deluxe frames— submit V2020 on one line; V2025 on second line

IOM: 100-04, 1, 30.3.5

Spectacle Lenses

NOTE: If a CPT procedure code for supply of spectacles or a permanent prosthesis is reported, recode with the specific lens type listed below. For aphakic temporary spectacle correction, see CPT.

Single Vision, Glass or Plastic

✳ **V2100** Sphere, single vision, plano to plus or minus 4.00, per lens

Bill DME/MAC

✳ **V2101** Sphere, single vision, plus or minus 4.12 to plus or minus 7.00d, per lens

Bill DME/MAC

✳ **V2102** Sphere, single vision, plus or minus 7.12 to plus or minus 20.00d, per lens

Bill DME/MAC

✳ **V2103** Spherocylinder, single vision, plano to plus or minus 4.00d sphere, .12 to 2.00d cylinder, per lens

Bill DME/MAC

✳ **V2104** Spherocylinder, single vision, plano to plus or minus 4.00d sphere, 2.12 to 4.00d cylinder, per lens

Bill DME/MAC

✳ **V2105** Spherocylinder, single vision, plano to plus or minus 4.00d sphere, 4.25 to 6.00d cylinder, per lens

Bill DME/MAC

✳ **V2106** Spherocylinder, single vision, plano to plus or minus 4.00d sphere, over 6.00d cylinder, per lens

Bill DME/MAC

✳ **V2107** Spherocylinder, single vision, plus or minus 4.25 to plus or minus 7.00 sphere, .12 to 2.00d cylinder, per lens

Bill DME/MAC

✳ **V2108** Spherocylinder, single vision, plus or minus 4.25d to plus or minus 7.00d sphere, 2.12 to 4.00d cylinder, per lens

Bill DME/MAC

✳ **V2109** Spherocylinder, single vision, plus or minus 4.25 to plus or minus 7.00d sphere, 4.25 to 6.00d cylinder, per lens

Bill DME/MAC

✳ **V2110** Sperocylinder, single vision, plus or minus 4.25 to 7.00d sphere, over 6.00d cylinder, per lens

Bill DME/MAC

✳ **V2111** Spherocylinder, single vision, plus or minus 7.25 to plus or minus 12.00d sphere, .25 to 2.25d cylinder, per lens

Bill DME/MAC

✳ **V2112** Spherocylinder, single vision, plus or minus 7.25 to plus or minus 12.00d sphere, 2.25d to 4.00d cylinder, per lens

Bill DME/MAC

✳ **V2113** Spherocylinder, single vision, plus or minus 7.25 to plus or minus 12.00d sphere, 4.25 to 6.00d cylinder, per lens

Bill DME/MAC

✳ **V2114** Spherocylinder, single vision, sphere over plus or minus 12.00d, per lens

Bill DME/MAC

✳ **V2115** Lenticular, (myodisc), per lens, single vision

Bill DME/MAC

✳ **V2118** Aniseikonic lens, single vision

Bill DME/MAC

⊙ **V2121** Lenticular lens, per lens, single

Bill DME/MAC

IOM: 100-02, 15, 120; 100-04, 3, 10.4

✳ **V2199** Not otherwise classified, single vision lens

Bill DME/MAC

Bill on paper. Requires report of type of single vision lens and optical lab invoice.

Bifocal, Glass or Plastic

✳ **V2200** Sphere, bifocal, plano to plus or minus 4.00d, per lens

Bill DME/MAC

▶ New   → Revised   ✔ Reinstated   ~~deleted~~ Deleted
⊙ Special coverage instructions   ◆ Not covered or valid by Medicare   ✳ Carrier discretion

* **V2201** Sphere, bifocal, plus or minus 4.12 to plus or minus 7.00d, per lens

Bill DME/MAC

* **V2202** Sphere, bifocal, plus or minus 7.12 to plus or minus 20.00d, per lens

Bill DME/MAC

* **V2203** Spherocylinder, bifocal, plano to plus or minus 4.00d sphere, .12 to 2.00d cylinder, per lens

Bill DME/MAC

* **V2204** Spherocylinder, bifocal, plano to plus or minus 4.00d sphere, 2.12 to 4.00d cylinder, per lens

Bill DME/MAC

* **V2205** Spherocylinder, bifocal, plano to plus or minus 4.00d sphere, 4.25 to 6.00d cylinder, per lens

Bill DME/MAC

* **V2206** Spherocylinder, bifocal, plano to plus or minus 4.00d sphere, over 6.00d cylinder, per lens

Bill DME/MAC

* **V2207** Spherocylinder, bifocal, plus or minus 4.25 to plus or minus 7.00d sphere, .12 to 2.00d cylinder, per lens

Bill DME/MAC

* **V2208** Spherocylinder, bifocal, plus or minus 4.25 to plus or minus 7.00d sphere, 2.12 to 4.00d cylinder, per lens

Bill DME/MAC

* **V2209** Spherocylinder, bifocal, plus or minus 4.25 to plus or minus 7.00d sphere, 4.25 to 6.00d cylinder, per lens

Bill DME/MAC

* **V2210** Spherocylinder, bifocal, plus or minus 4.25 to plus or minus 7.00d sphere, over 6.00d cylinder, per lens

Bill DME/MAC

* **V2211** Spherocylinder, bifocal, plus or minus 7.25 to plus or minus 12.00d sphere, .25 to 2.25d cylinder, per lens

Bill DME/MAC

* **V2212** Spherocylinder, bifocal, plus or minus 7.25 to plus or minus 12.00d sphere, 2.25 to 4.00d cylinder, per lens

Bill DME/MAC

* **V2213** Spherocylinder, bifocal, plus or minus 7.25 to plus or minus 12.00d sphere, 4.25 to 6.00d cylinder, per lens

Bill DME/MAC

* **V2214** Spherocylinder, bifocal, sphere over plus or minus 12.00d, per lens

Bill DME/MAC

* **V2215** Lenticular (myodisc), per lens, bifocal

Bill DME/MAC

* **V2218** Aniseikonic, per lens, bifocal

Bill DME/MAC

* **V2219** Bifocal seg width over 28mm

Bill DME/MAC

* **V2220** Bifocal add over 3.25d

Bill DME/MAC

☺ **V2221** Lenticular lens, per lens, bifocal

Bill DME/MAC

IOM: 100-02, 15, 120; 100-04, 3, 10.4

* **V2299** Specialty bifocal (by report)

Bill DME/MAC

Bill on paper. Requires report of type of specialty bifocal lens and optical lab invoice.

Trifocal, Glass or Plastic

* **V2300** Sphere, trifocal, plano to plus or minus 4.00d, per lens

Bill DME/MAC

* **V2301** Sphere, trifocal, plus or minus 4.12 to plus or minus 7.00d per lens

Bill DME/MAC

* **V2302** Sphere, trifocal, plus or minus 7.12 to plus or minus 20.00, per lens

Bill DME/MAC

* **V2303** Spherocylinder, trifocal, plano to plus or minus 4.00d sphere, .12 to 2.00d cylinder, per lens

Bill DME/MAC

* **V2304** Spherocylinder, trifocal, plano to plus or minus 4.00d sphere, 2.25-4.00d cylinder, per lens

Bill DME/MAC

* **V2305** Spherocylinder, trifocal, plano to plus or minus 4.00d sphere, 4.25 to 6.00 cylinder, per lens

Bill DME/MAC

* **V2306** Spherocylinder, trifocal, plano to plus or minus 4.00d sphere, over 6.00d cylinder, per lens

Bill DME/MAC

▶ New   → Revised   ✔ Reinstated   ~~deleted~~ Deleted
☺ Special coverage instructions   ◆ Not covered or valid by Medicare   * Carrier discretion

* **V2307** Spherocylinder, trifocal, plus or minus 4.25 to plus or minus 7.00d sphere, .12 to 2.00d cylinder, per lens

Bill DME/MAC

* **V2308** Spherocylinder, trifocal, plus or minus 4.25 to plus or minus 7.00d sphere, 2.12 to 4.00d cylinder, per lens

Bill DME/MAC

* **V2309** Spherocylinder, trifocal, plus or minus 4.25 to plus or minus 7.00d sphere, 4.25 to 6.00d cylinder, per lens

Bill DME/MAC

* **V2310** Spherocylinder, trifocal, plus or minus 4.25 to plus or minus 7.00d sphere, over 6.00d cylinder, per lens

Bill DME/MAC

* **V2311** Spherocylinder, trifocal, plus or minus 7.25 to plus or minus 12.00d sphere, .25 to 2.25d cylinder, per lens

Bill DME/MAC

* **V2312** Spherocylinder, trifocal, plus or minus 7.25 to plus or minus 12.00d sphere, 2.25 to 4.00d cylinder, per lens

Bill DME/MAC

* **V2313** Spherocylinder, trifocal, plus or minus 7.25 to plus or minus 12.00d sphere, 4.25 to 6.00d cylinder, per lens

Bill DME/MAC

* **V2314** Spherocylinder, trifocal, sphere over plus or minus 12.00d, per lens

Bill DME/MAC

* **V2315** Lenticular, (myodisc), per lens, trifocal

Bill DME/MAC

* **V2318** Aniseikonic lens, trifocal

Bill DME/MAC

* **V2319** Trifocal seg width over 28 mm

Bill DME/MAC

* **V2320** Trifocal add over 3.25d

Bill DME/MAC

☉ **V2321** Lenticular lens, per lens, trifocal

Bill DME/MAC

IOM: 100-02, 15, 120; 100-04, 3, 10.4

* **V2399** Specialty trifocal (by report)

Bill DME/MAC

Bill on paper. Requires report of type of trifocal lens and optical lab invoice.

Variable Asphericity

* **V2410** Variable asphericity lens, single vision, full field, glass or plastic, per lens

Bill DME/MAC

* **V2430** Variable asphericity lens, bifocal, full field, glass or plastic, per lens

Bill DME/MAC

* **V2499** Variable sphericity lens, other type

Bill DME/MAC

Bill on paper. Requires report of other type of lens and optical lab invoice.

Contact Lenses

If a CPT procedure code for supply of contact lens is reported, recode with specific lens type listed below (per lens).

* **V2500** Contact lens, PMMA, spherical, per lens

Bill DME/MAC

Requires prior authorization for patients under age 21.

* **V2501** Contact lens, PMMA, toric or prism ballast, per lens

Bill DME/MAC

Requires prior authorization for clients under age 21.

* **V2502** Contact lens PMMA, bifocal, per lens

Bill DME/MAC

Requires prior authorization for clients under age 21. Bill on paper. Requires optical lab invoice.

* **V2503** Contact lens PMMA, color vision deficiency, per lens

Bill DME/MAC

Requires prior authorization for clients under age 21. Bill on paper. Requires optical lab invoice.

* **V2510** Contact lens, gas permeable, spherical, per lens

Bill DME/MAC

Requires prior authorization for clients under age 21.

* **V2511** Contact lens, gas permeable, toric, prism ballast, per lens

Bill DME/MAC

Requires prior authorization for clients under age 21.

▶ New → Revised ✔ Reinstated ~~deleted~~ Deleted
☉ Special coverage instructions ◆ Not covered or valid by Medicare * Carrier discretion

✳ **V2512**   Contact lens, gas permeable, bifocal, per lens

Bill DME/MAC

Requires prior authorization for clients under age 21.

✳ **V2513**   Contact lens, gas permeable, extended wear, per lens

Bill DME/MAC

Requires prior authorization for clients under age 21.

⊙ **V2520**   Contact lens, hydrophilic, spherical, per lens

If "incident to" a physician service, do not bill; otherwise, bill DME/MAC

Requires prior authorization for clients under age 21.

IOM: 100-03, 1, 80.1; 100-03, 1, 80.4

⊙ **V2521**   Contact lens, hydrophilic, toric, or prism ballast, per lens

If "incident to" a physician's service, do not bill; otherwise, bill DME/MAC.

Requires prior authorization for clients under age 21.

IOM: 100-03, 1, 80.1; 100-03, 1, 80.4

⊙ **V2522**   Contact lens, hydrophilic, bifocal, per lens

If "incident to" a physician's service, do not bill; otherwise, bill DME/MAC.

Requires prior authorization for clients under age 21.

IOM: 100-03, 1, 80.1; 100-03, 1, 80.4

⊙ **V2523**   Contact lens, hydrophilic, extended wear, per lens

If "incident to" a physician's service, do not bill; otherwise, bill DME/MAC.

Requires prior authorization for clients under age 21.

IOM: 100-03, 1, 80.1; 100-03, 1, 80.4

✳ **V2530**   Contact lens, scleral, gas impermeable, per lens (for contact lens modification, see 92325)

Bill DME/MAC

Requires prior authorization for clients under age 21.

⊙ **V2531**   Contact lens, scleral, gas permeable, per lens (for contact lens modification, see 92325)

Bill DME/MAC

Requires prior authorization for clients under age 21. Bill on paper. Requires optical lab invoice.

IOM: 100-03, 1, 80.5

✳ **V2599**   Contact lens, other type

If "incident to" a physician's service, do not bill; otherwise, bill DME/MAC.

Requires prior authorization for clients under age 21. Bill on paper. Requires report of other type of contact lens and optical invoice.

Low Vision Aids

If a CPT procedure code for supply of low vision aid is reported, recode with specific systems listed below.

✳ **V2600**   Hand held low vision aids and other nonspectacle mounted aids

Bill DME/MAC

Requires prior authorization.

✳ **V2610**   Single lens spectacle mounted low vision aids

Bill DME/MAC

Requires prior authorization.

✳ **V2615**   Telescopic and other compound lens system, including distance vision telescopic, near vision telescopes and compound microscopic lens system

Bill DME/MAC

Requires prior authorization. Bill on paper. Requires optical lab invoice.

Prosthetic Eye

⊙ **V2623**   Prosthetic eye, plastic, custom

Bill DME/MAC

DME regional carrier. Requires prior authorization. Bill on paper. Requires optical lab invoice.

✳ **V2624**   Polishing/resurfacing of ocular prosthesis

Bill DME/MAC

Requires prior authorization. Bill on paper. Requires optical lab invoice.

▶ **New**   → **Revised**   ✔ **Reinstated**   ~~deleted~~ **Deleted**
⊙ **Special coverage instructions**   ◆ **Not covered or valid by Medicare**   ✳ **Carrier discretion**

✳ **V2625** Enlargement of ocular prosthesis

Bill DME/MAC

Requires prior authorization. Bill on paper. Requires optical lab invoice.

✳ **V2626** Reduction of ocular prosthesis

Bill DME/MAC

Requires prior authorization. Bill on paper. Requires optical lab invoice.

✿ **V2627** Scleral cover shell

Bill DME/MAC

DME regional carrier

Requires prior authorization. Bill on paper. Requires optical lab invoice.

IOM: 100-03, 4, 280.2

✳ **V2628** Fabrication and fitting of ocular conformer

Bill DME/MAC

Requires prior authorization. Bill on paper. Requires optical lab invoice.

✳ **V2629** Prosthetic eye, other type

Bill DME/MAC

Requires prior authorization. Bill on paper. Requires optical lab invoice.

Intraocular Lenses

✿ **V2630** Anterior chamber intraocular lens

Bill local carrier

IOM: 100-02, 15, 120

✿ **V2631** Iris supported intraocular lens

Bill local carrier

IOM: 100-02, 15, 120

✿ **V2632** Posterior chamber intraocular lens

Bill local carrier

IOM: 100-02, 15, 120

Miscellaneous

✳ **V2700** Balance lens, per lens

Bill DME/MAC

◆ **V2702** Deluxe lens feature

Bill DME/MAC

IOM: 100-02, 15, 120; 100-04, 3, 10.4

✳ **V2710** Slab off prism, glass or plastic, per lens

Bill DME/MAC

✳ **V2715** Prism, per lens

Bill DME/MAC

✳ **V2718** Press-on lens, Fresnel prism, per lens

Bill DME/MAC

✳ **V2730** Special base curve, glass or plastic, per lens

Bill DME/MAC

✿ **V2744** Tint, photochromatic, per lens

Bill DME/MAC

Requires prior authorization.

IOM: 100-02, 15, 120; 100-04, 3, 10.4

✿ **V2745** Addition to lens, tint, any color, solid, gradient or equal, excludes photochroatic, any lens material, per lens

Bill DME/MAC

Includes photochromatic lenses (V2744) used as sunglasses, which are prescribed in addition to regular prosthetic lenses for aphakic patient will be denied as not medically necessary.

IOM: 100-02, 15, 120; 100-04, 3, 10.4

✿ **V2750** Anti-reflective coating, per lens

Bill DME/MAC

Requires prior authorization.

IOM: 100-02, 15, 120; 100-04, 3, 10.4

✿ **V2755** U-V lens, per lens

Bill DME/MAC

IOM: 100-02, 15, 120; 100-04, 3, 10.4

✳ **V2756** Eye glass case

Bill DME/MAC

✳ **V2760** Scratch resistant coating, per lens

Bill DME/MAC

✿ **V2761** Mirror coating, any type, solid, gradient or equal, any lens material, per lens

Bill DME/MAC

IOM: 100-02, 15, 120; 100-04, 3, 10.4

✿ **V2762** Polarization, any lens material, per lens

Bill DME/MAC

IOM: 100-02, 15, 120; 100-04, 3, 10.4

✳ **V2770** Occluder lens, per lens

Bill DME/MAC

Requires prior authorization.

✳ **V2780** Oversize lens, per lens

Bill DME/MAC

Requires prior authorization.

✳ **V2781** Progressive lens, per lens

Bill DME/MAC

Requires prior authorization.

▶ New   → Revised   ✔ Reinstated   ~~deleted~~ Deleted

✿ Special coverage instructions   ◆ Not covered or valid by Medicare   ✳ Carrier discretion

⊘ **V2782** Lens, index 1.54 to 1.65 plastic or 1.60 to 1.79 glass, excludes polycarbonate, per lens

Bill DME/MAC

Do not bill in addition to V2784

IOM: 100-02, 15, 120; 100-04, 3, 10.4

⊘ **V2783** Lens, index greater than or equal to 1.66 plastic or greater than or equal to 1.80 glass, excludes polycarbonate, per lens

Bill DME/MAC

Do not bill in addition to V2784

IOM: 100-02, 15, 120; 100-04, 3, 10.4

⊘ **V2784** Lens, polycarbonate or equal, any index, per lens

Bill DME/MAC

Covered only for patients with functional vision in one eye—in this situation, an impact-resistant material is covered for both lenses if eyeglasses are covered. Claims with V2784 that do not meet this coverage criterion will be denied as not medically necessary.

IOM: 100-02, 15, 120; 100-04, 3, 10.4

✳ **V2785** Processing, preserving and transporting corneal tissue

Bill local carrier

Bill on paper. Must attach eye bank invoice to claim.

⊘ **V2786** Specialty occupational multifocal lens, per lens

Bill DME/MAC

IOM: 100-02, 15, 120; 100-04, 3, 10.4

◆ **V2787** Astigmatism correcting function of intraocular lens

Bill local carrier

Medicare Statute 1862(a)(7)

◆ **V2788** Presbyopia correcting function of intraocular lens

Bill local carrier

Medicare Statute 1862a7

✳ **V2790** Amniotic membrane for surgical reconstruction, per procedure

Bill local carrier

✳ **V2797** Vision supply, accessory and/or service component of another HCPCS vision code

Bill DME/MAC

✳ **V2799** Vision service, miscellaneous

Bill DME/MAC

Bill on paper. Requires report of miscellaneous service and optical lab invoice.

HEARING SERVICES (V5000-V5999)

NOTE: These codes are for non-physician services.

V5008-V5299: Bill local carrier

◆ **V5008** Hearing screening

IOM: 100-02, 16, 90

◆ **V5010** Assessment for hearing aid

Medicare Statute 1862a7

◆ **V5011** Fitting/orientation/checking of hearing aid

Medicare Statute 1862a7

◆ **V5014** Repair/modification of a hearing aid

Medicare Statute 1862a7

◆ **V5020** Conformity evaluation

Medicare Statute 1862a7

◆ **V5030** Hearing aid, monaural, body worn, air conduction

Medicare Statute 1862a7

◆ **V5040** Hearing aid, monaural, body worn, bone conduction

Medicare Statute 1862a7

◆ **V5050** Hearing aid, monaural, in the ear

Medicare Statute 1862a7

◆ **V5060** Hearing aid, monaural, behind the ear

Medicare Statute 1862a7

◆ **V5070** Glasses, air conduction

Medicare Statute 1862a7

◆ **V5080** Glasses, bone conduction

Medicare Statute 1862a7

◆ **V5090** Dispensing fee, unspecified hearing aid

Medicare Statute 1862a7

◆ **V5095** Semi-implantable middle ear hearing prosthesis

Medicare Statute 1862a7

◆ **V5100** Hearing aid, bilateral, body worn

Medicare Statute 1862a7

◆ **V5110** Dispensing fee, bilateral

Medicare Statute 1862a7

◆ **V5120** Binaural, body

Medicare Statute 1862a7

▶ **New** → **Revised** ✔ **Reinstated** ~~deleted~~ **Deleted**

⊘ **Special coverage instructions** ◆ **Not covered or valid by Medicare** ✳ **Carrier discretion**

◆ **V5130** Binaural, in the ear
Medicare Statute 1862a7

◆ **V5140** Binaural, behind the ear
Medicare Statute 1862a7

◆ **V5150** Binaural, glasses
Medicare Statute 1862a7

◆ **V5160** Dispensing fee, binaural
Medicare Statute 1862a7

◆ **V5170** Hearing aid, CROS, in the ear
Medicare Statute 1862a7

◆ **V5180** Hearing aid, CROS, behind the ear
Medicare Statute 1862a7

◆ **V5190** Hearing aid, CROS, glasses
Medicare Statute 1862a7

◆ **V5200** Dispensing fee, CROS
Medicare Statute 1862a7

◆ **V5210** Hearing aid, BICROS, in the ear
Medicare Statute 1862a7

◆ **V5220** Hearing aid, BICROS, behind the ear
Medicare Statute 1862a7

◆ **V5230** Hearing aid, BICROS, glasses
Medicare Statute 1862a7

◆ **V5240** Dispensing fee, BICROS
Medicare Statute 1862a7

◆ **V5241** Dispensing fee, monaural hearing aid, any type
Medicare Statute 1862a7

◆ **V5242** Hearing aid, analog, monaural, CIC (completely in the ear canal)
Medicare Statute 1862a7

◆ **V5243** Hearing aid, analog, monaural, ITC (in the canal)
Medicare Statute 1862a9

◆ **V5244** Hearing aid, digitally programmable analog, monaural, CIC
Medicare Statute 1862a7

◆ **V5245** Hearing aid, digitally programmable, analog, monaural, ITC
Medicare Statute 1862a7

◆ **V5246** Hearing aid, digitally programmable analog, monaural, ITE (in the ear)
Medicare Statute 1862a7

◆ **V5247** Hearing aid, digitally programmable analog, monaural, BTE (behind the ear)
Medicare Statute 1862a7

◆ **V5248** Hearing aid, analog, binaural, CIC
Medicare Statute 1862a7

◆ **V5249** Hearing aid, analog, binaural, ITC
Medicare Statute 1862a7

◆ **V5250** Hearing aid, digitally programmable analog, binaural, CIC
Medicare Statute 1862a7

◆ **V5251** Hearing aid, digitally programmable analog, binaural, ITC
Medicare Statute 1862a7

◆ **V5252** Hearing aid, digitally programmable, binaural, ITE
Medicare Statute 1862a7

◆ **V5253** Hearing aid, digitally programmable, binaural, BTE
Medicare Statute 1862a7

◆ **V5254** Hearing aid, digital, monaural, CIC
Medicare Statute 1862a7

◆ **V5255** Hearing aid, digital, monaural, ITC
Medicare Statute 1862a7

◆ **V5256** Hearing aid, digital, monaural, ITE
Medicare Statute 1862a7

◆ **V5257** Hearing aid, digital, monaural, BTE
Medicare Statute 1862a7

◆ **V5258** Hearing aid, digital, binaural, CIC
Medicare Statute 1862a7

◆ **V5259** Hearing aid, digital, binaural, ITC
Medicare Statute 1862a7

◆ **V5260** Hearing aid, digital, binaural, ITE
Medicare Statute 1862a7

◆ **V5261** Hearing aid, digital, binaural, BTE
Medicare Statute 1862a7

◆ **V5262** Hearing aid, disposable, any type, monaural
Medicare Statute 1862a7

◆ **V5263** Hearing aid, disposable, any type, binaural
Medicare Statute 1862a7

◆ **V5264** Ear mold/insert, not disposable, any type
Medicare Statute 1862a7

◆ **V5265** Ear mold/insert, disposable, any type
Medicare Statute 1862a7

◆ **V5266** Battery for use in hearing device
Medicare Statute 1862a7

▶ New   → Revised   ✔ Reinstated   ~~deleted~~ Deleted
☉ Special coverage instructions   ◆ Not covered or valid by Medicare   ✳ Carrier discretion

→ ◆ **V5267** Hearing aid or assistive listening device/supplies/accessories, not otherwise specified

Medicare Statute 1862a7

◆ **V5268** Assistive listening device, telephone amplifier, any type

Medicare Statute 1862a7

◆ **V5269** Assistive listening device, alerting, any type

Medicare Statute 1862a7

◆ **V5270** Assistive listening device, television amplifier, any type

Medicare Statute 1862a7

◆ **V5271** Assistive listening device, television caption decoder

Medicare Statute 1862a7

◆ **V5272** Assistive listening device, TDD

Medicare Statute 1862a7

◆ **V5273** Assistive listening device, for use with cochlear implant

Medicare Statute 1862a7

◆ **V5274** Assistive listening device, not otherwise specified

Medicare Statute 1862a7

◆ **V5275** Ear impression, each

Medicare Statute 1862a7

▶ ◆ **V5281** Assistive listening device, personal FM/DM system, monaural, (1 receiver, transmitter, microphone), any type

Medicare Statute 1862a7

▶ ◆ **V5282** Assistive listening device, personal FM/DM system, binaural, (2 receivers, transmitter, microphone), any type

Medicare Statute 1862a7

▶ ◆ **V5283** Assistive listening device, personal FM/DM neck, loop induction receiver

Medicare Statute 1862a7

▶ ◆ **V5284** Assistive listening device, personal FM/DM, ear level receiver

Medicare Statute 1862a7

▶ ◆ **V5285** Assistive listening device, personal FM/DM, direct audio input receiver

Medicare Statute 1862a7

▶ ◆ **V5286** Assistive listening device, personal blue tooth FM/DM receiver

Medicare Statute 1862a7

▶ ◆ **V5287** Assistive listening device, personal FM/DM receiver, not otherwise specified

Medicare Statute 1862a7

▶ ◆ **V5288** Assistive listening device, personal FM/DM transmitter assistive listening device

Medicare Statute 1862a7

▶ ◆ **V5289** Assistive listening device, personal FM/DM adapter/boot coupling device for receiver, any type

Medicare Statute 1862a7

▶ ◆ **V5290** Assistive listening device, transmitter microphone, any type

Medicare Statute 1862a7

◆ **V5298** Hearing aid, not otherwise classified

Medicare Statute 1862a7

⊘ **V5299** Hearing service, miscellaneousᴮ

IOM: 100-02, 16, 90

Speech-Language Pathology Services

NOTE: These codes are for non-physician services.

◆ **V5336** Repair/modification of augmentative communicative system or device (excludes adaptive hearing aid)

Bill DME/MAC

Medicare Statute 1862a7

◆ **V5362** Speech screening

Bill local carrier

Medicare Statute 1862a7

◆ **V5363** Language screening

Bill local carrier

Medicare Statute 1862a7

◆ **V5364** Dysphagia screening

Bill local carrier

Medicare Statute 1862a7

▶ **New**   → **Revised**   ✔ **Reinstated**   deleted **Deleted**

⊘ **Special coverage instructions**   ◆ **Not covered or valid by Medicare**   ✳ **Carrier discretion**

Trust Elsevier.
We've got you covered.

When it comes to preparing for ICD-10,

we've got you covered.

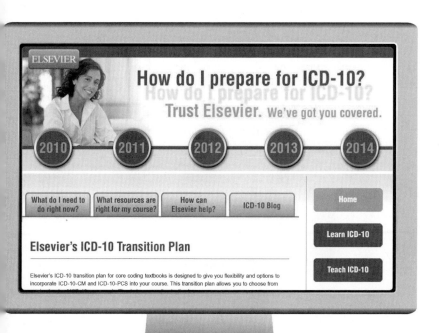

- Learn how to transition from ICD-9-CM to ICD-10-CM/PCS.

- Develop your plan to teach ICD-10-CM/PCS to students.

- Articles, updates, and webinars provide guidance for integrating ICD-10 into your program.

Count on the leader in coding education for everything you need to train your staff, teach your students, and transition your program.

Learn more at www.icd10educators.com!

A